Applied Neurotoxicology

Editors

MICHAEL R. DOBBS
MAM IBRAHEEM

NEUROLOGIC CLINICS

www.neurologic.theclinics.com

Consulting Editor
RANDOLPH W. EVANS

November 2020 • Volume 38 • Number 4

ELSEVIER

1600 John F. Kennedy Boulevard • Suite 1800 • Philadelphia, Pennsylvania, 19103-2899

http://www.theclinics.com

NEUROLOGIC CLINICS Volume 38, Number 4
November 2020 ISSN 0733-8619, ISBN-13: 978-0-323-71291-0

Editor: Stacy Eastman
Developmental Editor: Donald Mumford

Neurologic Clinics (ISSN 0733-8619) is published quarterly by Elsevier Inc., 360 Park Avenue South, New York, NY 10010–1710. Months of issue are February, May, August, and November. Periodicals postage paid at New York, NY, and additional mailing offices. Subscription prices are $326.00 per year for US individuals, $696.00 per year for US institutions, $100.00 per year for US students, $408.00 per year for Canadian individuals, $843.00 per year for Canadian institutions, $427.00 per year for international individuals, $843.00 per year for international institutions, $210.00 for foreign students/residents, and $100.00 for Canadian students/residents. To receive student/resident rate, orders must be accompanied by name of affiliated institution, date of term, and the *signature* of program/residency coordinator on institution letterhead. Orders will be billed at individual rate until proof of status is received. Foreign air speed delivery is included in all *Clinics* subscription prices. All prices are subject to change without notice. **POSTMASTER:** Send address changes to *Neurologic Clinics*, Elsevier Health Sciences Division, Subscription Customer Service, 3251 Riverport Lane, Maryland Heights, MO 63043. **Customer Service: Telephone: 1-800-654-2452 (U.S. and Canada); 314-447-8871 (outside U.S. and Canada). Fax: 314-447-8029. E-mail: journalscustomerservice-usa@elsevier.com (for print support); journalsonlinesupport-usa@elsevier.com (for online support).**

Reprints. For copies of 100 or more of articles in this publication, please contact the Commercial Reprints Department, Elsevier Inc., 360 Park Avenue South, New York, New York, 10010-1710; Tel.: +1-212-633-3874; Fax: +1-212-633-3820, and E-mail: reprints@elsevier.com.

Neurologic Clinics is also published in Spanish by Nueva Editorial Interamericana S.A., Mexico City, Mexico.

Neurologic Clinics is covered in *Current Contents/Clinical Medicine, MEDLINE/PubMed (Index Medicus), EMBASE/Excerpta Medica, and PsycINFO, and ISI/BIOMED.*

Contributors

CONSULTING EDITOR

RANDOLPH W. EVANS, MD
Clinical Professor, Department of Neurology, Baylor College of Medicine, Houston, Texas

EDITORS

MICHAEL R. DOBBS, MD, MHCM
Vice Dean of Clinical Affairs, Professor and Chair of Neurology, Department of Neurology, UT Health RGV Chief Medical Officer, University of Texas, Rio Grande Valley School of Medicine, Edinburg, Texas

MAM IBRAHEEM, MD, MPH, CPH, ABPN Diplomate
Assistant Professor of Neurology, University of Kentucky College of Medicine, Department of Neurology, Assistant Professor of Epidemiology, University of Kentucky College of Public Health, Department of Epidemiology, Alternate Neurology Service Chief, United States Department of Veterans Affairs, Lexington VA Medical Center-Troy Bowling Campus, Lexington, Kentucky

AUTHORS

MADELINE C. AULISIO, MPH
Department of Health Management and Policy, University of Kentucky College of Public Health, Lexington, Kentucky

JED A. BARASH, MD, MHS
Medical Director, Soldiers' Home, Chelsea, Massachusetts

CASSANDRA BEZI, MPH
Division of Infectious Diseases, Department of Pediatrics, Cincinnati Children's Hospital Medical Center, Cincinnati, Ohio

JOSEPH D. BURNS, MD
Associate Professor of Neurology and Neurosurgery, Department of Neurology, Tufts University School of Medicine, Staff Neurologist, Lahey Hospital and Medical Center, Burlington, Massachusetts

ALICE CAI, MD
Neurology Resident, Department of Neurology, University of Pennsylvania, Philadelphia, Pennsylvania

XUEMEI CAI, MD
Assistant Professor, Departments of Neurology and Neurosurgery, Tufts Medical Center, Boston, Massachusetts

RACHEL A. CAPLAN, MD
Resident Physician, Department of Neurology, Massachusetts General Hospital, Brigham and Women's Hospital, Harvard Medical School, Boston, Massachusetts

KIM M. CECIL, PhD
Department of Radiology, University of Cincinnati College of Medicine, Imaging Research Center, Cincinnati Children's Hospital Medical Center, Department of Environmental Health, University of Cincinnati College of Medicine, Cincinnati, Ohio

CHRISTOPHER L. COE, MD
Assistant Professor of Clinical Medicine, Division of Internal Medicine and Public Health, Department of Medicine, Vanderbilt University Medical Center, Nashville, Tennessee

MICHAEL R. DOBBS, MD, MHCM
Vice Dean of Clinical Affairs, Professor and Chair of Neurology, Department of Neurology, UT Health RGV Chief Medical Officer, University of Texas, Rio Grande Valley School of Medicine, Edinburg, Texas

KATELYN DOLBEC, MD
Department of Neurology, Beth Israel Deaconess Medical Center, Boston, Massachusetts

DAVID EDMONDSON, PhD
Department of Radiology, University of Cincinnati College of Medicine, Imaging Research Center, Cincinnati Children's Hospital Medical Center, Cincinnati, Ohio

COREY R. FEHNEL, MD, MPH
Associate Director, Neuroscience Intensive Care Unit, Beth Israel Deaconess Medical Center, Assistant Professor of Neurology, Harvard Medical School, Assistant Scientist, Hinda and Arthur Marcus Institute for Aging Research, Boston, Massachusetts

AMANDA C. GLUECK, PhD
Assistant Professor, Department of Neurology, University of Kentucky College of Medicine, Lexington, Kentucky

NAWAZ HACK, MD, LCDR, MC, USN
Neurology Department, Department of Defense, Walter Reed National Military Medical Center, Bethesda, Maryland; Assistant Professor, Department of Neurology, Armed Forces University of the Health Sciences

DONG Y. HAN, PsyD, CELM, FANA
Chief, UK Neuropsychology Service – Clinical Section, Professor, Departments of Neurology, Neurosurgery, and Physical Medicine and Rehabilitation, Kentucky Neuroscience Institute, UK Spinal Cord & Brain Injury Research Center, UK Epilepsy Center | Epilepsy & Brain Metabolism Alliance, University of Kentucky College of Medicine, Lexington, Kentucky

ERIN N. HAYNES, DrPH, MS
Department of Epidemiology, College of Public Health, University of Kentucky, Lexington, Kentucky

AMY HESSLER, DO, FAAN
Associate Professor, Director of Women's Neurology, Neurology, University of Kentucky, Lexington, Kentucky

SARA HOCKER, MD, FAAN
Professor of Neurology, Chair, Division of Neurocritical Care and Hospital Neurology, Department of Neurology, Mayo Clinic College of Medicine, Rochester, Minnesota

SARAH N. HORST, MD, MPH
Associate Professor of Medicine, Division of Gastroenterology, Hepatology and Nutrition, Vanderbilt University Medical Center, Nashville, Tennessee

MAM IBRAHEEM, MD, MPH, CPH, ABPN Diplomate
Assistant Professor of Neurology, University of Kentucky College of Medicine, Department of Neurology, Assistant Professor of Epidemiology, University of Kentucky College of Public Health, Department of Epidemiology, Alternate Neurology Service Chief, United States Department of Veterans Affairs, Lexington VA Medical Center-Troy Bowling Campus, Lexington, Kentucky

MANHAL J. IZZY, MD
Assistant Professor of Medicine, Division of Gastroenterology, Hepatology and Nutrition, Vanderbilt University Medical Center, Transplant Hepatology, Nashville, Tennessee

JACQUELINE JANECEK, MD
Neurology Resident, Department of Neurology and Rehabilitation Medicine, University of Cincinnati, Cincinnati, Ohio

SAAD S. KENDERIAN, MD
T Cell Engineering, Division of Hematology, Departments of Molecular Medicine and Immunology, Mayo Clinic, Rochester, Minnesota

MONICA KRAUSE, MD
Neurology Resident, Department of Neurology, Mayo Clinic College of Medicine, Rochester, Minnesota

HANI KUSHLAF, MD
Associate Professor of Neurology and Pathology, Departments of Neurology and Rehabilitation Medicine, and Pathology and Laboratory Medicine, University of Cincinnati, Cincinnati, Ohio

DAVID P. LERNER, MD
Assistant Professor, Department of Neurology, Tufts University School of Medicine, Staff Neurologist, Lahey Hospital and Medical Center, Burlington, Massachusetts

KAITLIN V. MARTIN, PhD, MPH
Department of Epidemiology, College of Public Health, University of Kentucky, Lexington, Kentucky

DANI McBRIDE, BS
Department of Environmental Health, University of Cincinnati College of Medicine, Cincinnati, Ohio

STEVEN McKNIGHT, MD, CPT, MC, USA
Neurology Department, Department of Defense, Walter Reed National Military Medical Center, Bethesda, Maryland

SANDRO PASAGIC, BSN
Department of Neurology, University of Kentucky College of Medicine, Lexington, Kentucky

HALEY N. PHILLIPS, MD
Resident Physician, Department of Neurology, Indiana University, Indiana University Neuroscience Center, Indianapolis, Indiana

MICHAEL W. RUFF, MD
T Cell Engineering, Department of Neurology, Mayo Clinic, Rochester, Minnesota

JAMES J. SEJVAR, MD
Division of High-Consequence Pathogens and Pathology, National Center for Emerging and Zoonotic Infectious Diseases, Centers for Disease Control and Prevention, Atlanta, Georgia

ELIZABETH L. SIEGLER, PhD
T Cell Engineering, Division of Hematology, Mayo Clinic, Rochester, Minnesota

ALEKSEY TADEVOSYAN, MD
Staff Neurologist, Department of Neurology, Lahey Hospital and Medical Center, Burlington, Massachusetts

MICHEL TOLEDANO, MD
Assistant Professor, Department of Neurology, Mayo Clinic, Rochester, Minnesota

LAURA TORMOEHLEN, MD, FACMT, FAAN
Associate Professor of Clinical Neurology and Emergency Medicine-Toxicology, Departments of Neurology and Emergency Medicine, Indiana University, Indiana University Neuroscience Center, Indianapolis, Indiana

MIRIAM LEAHSHEA VANCE
Department of Epidemiology, College of Public Health, University of Kentucky, Lexington, Kentucky

JONAH P. ZUFLACHT, MD
Resident Physician, Department of Neurology, Beth Israel Deaconess Medical Center, Boston Children's Hospital, Harvard Medical School, Boston, Massachusetts

Contents

Clinical neurotoxicology is an unrecognized neurologic subspecialty. Few neurology residency programs offer an organized education or training in the field. Nevertheless, neurotoxic exposures and subsequent injuries are common. This article provides a basic approach to clinical assessment and causal inference. It addresses the knowledge gap for clinical practice and provides a thematic structure to use interdisciplinary resources.

Peripheral neuropathies secondary to neurotoxicants are frequently considered but can be difficult to diagnose. Accurate diagnosis is important to avoid unnecessary testing, prevent further exposure, and initiate treatment when available. This article reviews key features of some of the more common or representative toxic neuropathies, including those caused by occupational and environmental exposure, medications, and chemotherapeutic agents.

Channelopathies, neuromuscular junction disorders, and myopathies represent multiple mechanisms by which toxins can affect the peripheral nervous system. These toxins include ciguatoxin, tetrodotoxin, botulinum toxin, metabolic poisons, venomous snake bites, and several medications. These toxins are important to be aware of because they can lead to serious symptoms, disability, or even death, and many can be treated if recognized ear.

Acute delirium is a transient state of cerebral dysfunction reflecting an underlying medical decompensation. Toxicity from medications and other substances are a common cause of delirium. History and laboratory testing may be limited by alteration and lack of specific tests for certain compounds. Classes of compounds produce a constellation of symptoms and examination findings recognized as a toxidrome. Cessation of the offending agent, supportive care, and specific antidotal therapy are key to treatment. This article reviews the presentations of the anticholinergic toxidrome, sympathomimetic toxidrome, hallucinogenic toxidrome, γ-aminobutyric acid withdrawal, and Wernicke encephalopathy, as well as their mechanisms and basic management.

Subacute toxic encephalopathies are challenging to identify due to their often insidious tempo of evolution, nonspecific manifestations, relative infrequency as individual entities, and frequent lack of specific diagnostic testing. Yet they are crucial to recognize—in aggregate, subacute toxic encephalopathies are a common problem that can lead to severe, irreversible harm if not diagnosed and treated efficiently. This article reviews the clinically relevant aspects of some of the more important subacute toxic encephalopathy syndromes caused by inorganic toxins, carbon monoxide, antibiotics, antineoplastic agents, and psychiatric medications.

Many medications and toxins may induce central nervous system (CNS) depression. Even when the intention is to induce CNS depression, other nervous system adverse effects may occur, such as with anesthetics. Pain medications produce characteristic CNS toxicities. Sedative hypnotics may induce altered mentation among systemic toxicities. Stimulants may mimic coma when discontinued abruptly. Acute and chronic carbon monoxide poisoning can lead to altered mental status and prolonged cognitive difficulties. Some medications and environmental toxins can mimic brain death. High clinical suspicion and early recognition of these effects is vital to treatment, most of which is supportive.

The cerebellum plays an important role in motor and nonmotor systems, with damage resulting in clinical manifestations presenting as weakness, ataxia, dysarthria, and nystagmus. There are numerous environmental and industrial agents as well as medications that, through either accidental or intentional use, can result in a range of neurologic presentations. The variability in the presentation is important to recognize promptly so that early cessation in exposure, use, or abuse can be initiated to reduce the severity of symptoms. Recognition of an agent causing the particular pathology is important so that the route of exposure, and subsequent treatment options can be identified.

Toxins identified as causing parkinsonism and being related to overall idiopathic Parkinson disease risk range from heavy metals to pesticides to contaminants in synthetic heroin. Several described in this article exhibit significant oxidative stress on neurons of the central nervous system and have a particular predilection toward damage of dopaminergic neurons. Although many of these toxins have well-established connections with Parkinson disease risk, a few continue to be studied with data still being produced. The parkinsonisms caused by these agents have variable responses to dopaminergic therapies. This article discusses manganese, mercury, MPTP, organochlorines, organophosphates, paraquat, rotenone, and Agent Orange.

New toxins are emerging all the time. In this article, the authors review common toxins that cause seizure, their mechanisms, associated toxidromes, and treatments. Stimulants, cholinergic agents, gamma-aminobutyric acid antagonists, glutamate agonists, histamine and adenosine antagonists, and withdrawal states are highlighted. Understanding current mechanisms for common toxin-induced seizures can promote understanding for future toxins and predicting if seizure may occur as a result of toxicity.

Nerve agents and neurobiological weapons are among the most devastating and lethal of weapons. Acetylcholinesterase inhibitors act by increasing the amount of acetylcholine in the neuromuscular junction, resulting in flaccid paralysis. Tabun, VX, soman, and sarin are the major agents in this category. Exposure to nerve agents can be inhalational or through dermal contact. Neurotoxins may have peripheral and central effects on the nervous system. Atropine is an effective antidote to nerve agents. Neurobiological weapons entail using whole organisms or organism-synthesized toxins as agents. Some organisms that can be used as biological weapons include smallpox virus.

Management of the pregnant patient with neurologic disease is challenging. Ideally, preconception planning can optimize the woman's neurologic condition before pregnancy. More than half of pregnancies are unplanned which makes careful consideration of medications vitally important. This article focuses on potential toxic risk to the fetus of medications deemed necessary to manage several common maternal neurologic issues: multiple sclerosis, epilepsy, and headache during pregnancy and postpartum. It is important for the practitioner to have an understanding beyond the category system to understand the potential toxic risks to the infant.

contains relatively few studies of such chemoreceptive dysfunction in the context of toxic exposure, this review explores the strength of such published associations. Several studies collectively demonstrated moderately strong evidence for an association between manganese dust exposure and olfactory deficits. Evidence of associations between individual chemicals, therapeutics, and composites, such as World Trade Center debris, and olfactory and gustatory deficits remains limited or mixed. Further need for controlled studies for clinical management, exposure limits, and policy development is identified.

Substance use disorders—and their associated neurologic complications—are frequently encountered by neurologists as well as emergency room physicians, internists, psychiatrists, and medical intensivists. Prominent neurologic sequelae of drug abuse, such as seizure and stroke, are common and often result in patients receiving medical attention. However, less overt neurologic manifestations, such as dysautonomia and perceptual disturbances, may be initially misattributed to primary medical or psychiatric illness, respectively. This article focuses on the epidemiology, pharmacology, and complications associated with commonly used recreational drugs, including opioids, alcohol, marijuana, cocaine, and hallucinogens.

NEUROLOGIC CLINICS

THE CLINICS ARE AVAILABLE ONLINE!
Access your subscription at:
www.theclinics.com

Preface

Next Steps for Clinical Neurotoxicology

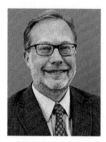   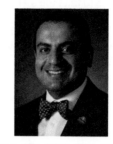

Michael R. Dobbs, MD, MHCM   Mam Ibraheem, MD, MPH, CPH, ABPN Diplomate
Editors

Clinical neurotoxicology is a heavy weight on those few who practice it. There are probably more than 1000 substantially neurotoxic substances, with exposure annually worldwide in the tens to hundreds of millions of people. Lead toxicity alone is reported as responsible for more than 1 million deaths yearly and devastates entire populations in cognitive development. Neurotoxic exposures may span all levels of society and the lifespan, although the developing nervous system has special risks. There are many examples of inequity in exposure risk, such as the lead exposure catastrophe of Flint, Michigan. There are meanwhile very few neurologists who are equipped to deal with neurotoxic problems.

Currently, diagnosis and management of neurotoxic problems are highly fragmented between public health, emergency medicine, occupational medicine, preventive medicine, and neurology. There are many excellent practitioners, but no one is really taking responsibility for the discipline.

Clinician neurotoxicology has a huge amount of material to learn, and there are serious gaps in neurology training. We are not aware of a single comprehensive neurotoxicology curriculum in a neurology residency, let alone a clinical neurotoxicology fellowship.

We need more neurologists trained in neurotoxicology. Emergency neurotoxic syndromes can be mislabeled, and a trained consulting neurologist can help to find the correct diagnosis. It is difficult for ambulatory patients to find clinical neurotoxicology expertise, and they will travel far. One of us ran a niche practice in ambulatory neurotoxicology for several years, and patients routinely came from distant states for consultation. We are aware of a very few isolated similar consultative clinics in Clinical Neurotoxicology in the United States.

Both editors of this issue of *Neurologic Clinics* have an interest in and passion for clinical neurotoxicology. Both of us also are pulled in many other directions and have precious little time to devote to advancement of our field. At this point, we would very much like to see more individual academic neurologists who develop and share a passion for neurotoxicology.

This issue of *Neurologic Clinics* follows on the heels of other neurotoxicology-themed issues, such as Toxic and Environmental Neurology (2005) and Frontiers in Clinical Neurotoxicology (2011). An issue that applies lessons in clinical neurotoxicology was a logical next step.

Furthermore, it is time to take the steps toward formalizing a curriculum in neurotoxicology for neurology residency training and to begin to offer advanced fellowship training in the discipline. We hope that this issue, Applied Neurotoxicology, will serve as at least a small step in that direction. We are grateful to the authors of this issue for their excellent contributions.

Michael R. Dobbs, MD, MHCM
University of Texas
Rio Grande Valley School of Medicine
1201 West University Drive
Edinburg, TX 78501, USA

Mam Ibraheem, MD, MPH, CPH, ABPN Diplomate
Department of Neurology
University of Kentucky
United States Department of Veterans Affairs
Lexington VA Medical Center–
Troy Bowling Campus
740 South Limestone
KY Clinic, J401
Lexington, KY 40536, USA

E-mail addresses:
Michael.dobbs@utrgv.edu (M.R. Dobbs)
Mam.Ibraheem@uky.edu (M. Ibraheem)

Neurotoxicology
Clinical Approach and Causal Inference

Mam Ibraheem, MD, MPH, CPH, ABPN Diplomate[a,b,*],
Dong Y. Han, PsyD, CELM[a,c,d], Michael R. Dobbs, MD, MHCM[e]

KEYWORDS

- Toxicology • Evidence-based toxicology • Epidemiology • Causality • Neurology

KEY POINTS

- Neurotoxic syndromes are recognizable, especially with comprehensive history and examination.
- Occupational and social histories are critical in neurotoxicology.
- Neurotoxins can affect all areas of the nervous system.
- Establishing causation is critical to the diagnosis and the treatment of neurotoxic syndromes.
- Causation methods include multiple approaches such as Epid-Tox framework and evidence-based toxicology.

INTRODUCTION

Neurotoxins are compounds that are toxic, or potentially toxic, to the nervous system. Capable of mimicking neurologic syndromes, neurotoxins can be classified into 3 main categories: (1) drugs (prescription, over the counter, and illicit), (2) chemicals (industrial, household, and abused agents), (3) environmental (biologic agents and naturally occurring chemicals). Neurotoxic presentations may be divided into 3 categories: acute, chronic, and sequelae of resolved exposures. The nervous system has unique physiologic characteristics, and thus is especially susceptible to toxic injury. Those characteristics are described in **Box 1**.[1]

Establishing causation is paramount to the correct diagnosis and the treatment of any patient suspected of neurotoxic poisoning. A knowledge base of common

M. Ibraheem and D.Y. Han are cofirst authors.
[a] Department of Neurology, University of Kentucky, 740 South Limestone, KY Clinic, J401, Lexington, KY 40536, USA; [b] US Department of Veterans Affairs, Lexington VA Medical Center, Troy Bowling Campus, 1101 Veterans Drive, Room A303a, Mail Code: 127-CD, Lexington, KY 40502, USA; [c] Department of Neurosurgery, University of Kentucky College of Medicine, Lexington, KY, USA; [d] Department of Physical Medicine and Rehabilitation, University of Kentucky College of Medicine, Lexington, KY, USA; [e] Department of Neurology, University of Texas Rio Grande Valley School of Medicine, 2102 Treasure Hills, Harlingen, TX 78550, USA
* Corresponding author.
E-mail address: Mam.Ibraheem@uky.edu

Box 1
Factors rendering the nervous system susceptible to toxic injuries

1. Neurons and their processes have a high surface area, increasing their exposure risk.

2. High lipid content of neuronal structures results in accumulation and retention of lipophilic substances.

3. Neurons have high metabolic demands and are strongly affected by energy or nutrient depletion.

4. High blood flow in the central nervous system increases effective exposure to circulating toxins.

5. Chemical toxins can interfere with normal neurotransmission by mimicking structures of endogenous molecules.

6. Following toxic injury, recovery of normal, complex interneuronal and intraneuronal connections is typically imperfect.

7. Neurons typically are postmitotic and do not divide.

Adapted from Firestone JA, Longstreth WT. Central Nervous System Diseases, In: Rosenstock L, et al., eds. Textbook of Clinical Occupational and Environmental Medicine. 2nd ed. London: Elsevier Saunders; 2004; with permission.

---

neurotoxins and associated syndromes is important. Coupled with a solid foundation in neurologic principles, this prepares practitioners to adequately recognize most cases of neurotoxicity. From there, initial assessment can be started, and a specialized provider can be consulted, if needed.

This article is not intended to be a comprehensive approach to neurotoxicology. Instead, it provides a basic framework to guide clinicians in their approach to patients with possible neurotoxic illnesses and to assess causality.

GENERAL PRINCIPLES

The clinical approach includes taking a relevant history, performing a focused examination, and formulating an assessment plan to guide further diagnostic and management plans.

It is often challenging to obtain an accurate and complete history in clinical neurotoxicology. However, it is sometimes very simple: the patient has a documented exposure to a known toxin, and either has not developed symptoms or has classic clinical symptoms of intoxication. At the other end of the spectrum are patients who cannot provide a history, such as comatose patients and those who have no idea that they have been exposed to something toxic. Most patients are somewhere in between.

Marshall and colleagues[2] developed the CH2OPD2 mnemonic (community, home, hobbies, occupation, personal habits, diet and drugs) as a tool to identify a patient's history of exposures to potentially toxic environmental contaminants. This tool is useful when screening for potential neurotoxic exposures.

Sometimes practitioners minimize the social history in their approach to a patient, limiting it to a few focused questions or even skipping it entirely. Clinicians cannot afford to minimize the social history in the case of possible neurotoxic exposure, because often therein lie clues to the diagnosis.

Occupational history is vital, because many toxic exposures occur in the workplace. At-risk jobs include farmers or farm workers (pesticides), painters (solvents or lead), deep miners (raw ore such as manganese), welders (manganese, arsenic), carpenters (lead), and warehousemen (carbon monoxide).[3–6]

Assessing home environment is important. Houses built in prior eras may contain paint with toxic levels of lead, or have been framed with arsenic-treated wood. If patients depend on well water, they risk exposure to minerals that seep in from groundwater. High inorganic arsenic levels have been found in wells around the world. Reverse osmosis filters can reduce arsenic concentrations from private water sources. However, such filters do not guarantee safe drinking water and, despite regulatory standards, some people continue to be exposed to very high arsenic concentrations. This possibility is particularly concerning in developing countries.[7–12]

Outside interests and hobbies can be sources of exposure. Recreational welders may become exposed to manganese, antique firearms aficionados may encounter toxic amounts of lead while crafting bullets, and builders of model vehicles can be exposed to toluene or other solvents. There have also been many casual gardeners who have become intoxicated from neurotoxic pesticides. Other people in the homes of these hobbyists may also be at risk of toxicity from these substances.

Travel history can be revealing. Travelers may venture into dangerous environments or try local cuisine or traditions to which they are unaccustomed. Travelers' naive physiologies may not be tolerant of exposure to toxins with which locals have come to coexist.

When aware of the nature of the toxic substance, be sure to ask about the source of the putative exposure, the amount of toxic substance, the length of exposure time, the environmental conditions, and the route of contact. Be aware that the patient may have been exposed to other toxic compounds that complicate the issue at hand. Patients exposed to organic toxins in industry, for example, are rarely exposed to just a single potentially toxic chemical substance. In complicated cases, it may be necessary to obtain records of compounds used at the patient's place of exposure.

Differentiating neurotoxic disorders from those of other causes might be the most challenging aspect of clinical neurotoxicology. Because toxins can affect all areas of the nervous system, there is a toxic mimic for nearly every neurologic syndrome.

In examining patients, prepared practitioners are aware of potential nonneurologic findings. Specific clues may be found in other body systems. Pay particular attention to the skin, hair, and nails.

The examination may contain several clues pointing toward a toxic cause. Many signs are general rather than neurologic, and clinicians cannot afford to rush through the general physical examination. Examples of helpful general examination signs include blue gums in lead intoxication, Mees lines (white transverse markings on the fingernails) with arsenic, alopecia with thallium, and acrodynia with mercury poisoning. Patients with arsenic and lead poisoned may both show serious abdominal colic, often acutely[13].

In the absence of a known exposure, there are few specific neurologic signs that point to toxic causes. However, notable neurologic clues may manifest in some toxic disorders. For example, bilateral trigeminal (and occasionally other cranial nerve) palsies may be seen in trichloroethylene encephalopathy.[14] There is also conflicting evidence on trichloroethylene as a cause of trigeminal neuropathy.[15] With lead encephalopathy, patients may concurrently show classic radial or peroneal nerve palsy. In arsenic, coexisting encephalopathy and peripheral polyneuropathy may occur. The neuropathy of arsenic exposure can mimic Guillain-Barré syndrome.[16,17]

FOCAL VERSUS DIFFUSE DEFICITS

Sympathomimetic drugs such as cocaine or amphetamines cause focal deficits from brain ischemia. Diffuse neurologic deficits, such as encephalopathy or polyneuropathy, are seen with many neurotoxins. Example toxins causing diffuse injury include organic solvents, lead, arsenic, and botulinum toxin. Some toxins may show focal neurologic deficits superimposed on a generalized encephalopathy. For example, manganese and carbon monoxide may cause focal parkinsonism from basal ganglia damage while showing general cerebral or psychiatric symptoms.

ACUTE EXPOSURES

Patients with acute, high-dose exposure to a neurotoxin often show substantial symptoms. However, sometimes the patients realize that they have been exposed and seek treatment before symptoms arise. In acute cases, it is highly desirable to remove the toxin from the patient's body before full absorption occurs. Timely administration of appropriate antidotes or antitoxins is prudent if they exist and are available.

Patients who realize they have had a major toxic exposure and can receive effective treatment before symptomatic damage ensues are fortunate. However, in many patients, this is not the case. Symptoms and signs may be the initial clue that someone has been exposed. Practitioners need to be able to recognize and differentiate common acute neurotoxic syndromes in order to save the exposed individual's nervous system from further damage.

This article centers on the basic toxidromes of acute encephalopathy, acute neuropathy, and neuromuscular junction dysfunction, and briefly discusses other syndromes.

TOXIC ENCEPHALOPATHY

Acute toxic encephalopathies show symptoms and signs that include mild confusion, attention deficits, seizures, and coma. Central nervous system (CNS) capillary damage, hypoxia, and cerebral edema play major roles.[18] Sometimes neurologic symptoms resolve with removal from exposure. However, a single short exposure to some toxins can cause permanent deficits or death.

Most classes of neurotoxins can show encephalopathic effects. Classic acute examples include carbon monoxide intoxication, neuromanganism, lead encephalopathy, mixed solvent encephalopathy, Korsakoff alcoholic encephalopathy (technically a nutritional problem rather than an intoxication), neurotoxic mushroom poisoning, and acute ethylene glycol poisoning. Organophosphate-intoxicated patients may show seizures, encephalopathy, poor vision from pupillary miosis, and effects in other systems.

Toxic encephalopathy beyond the acute phase may accompany lingering impairments in cognition, including attention, executive functioning, and memory (especially short-term memory).[19,20] Common neuropsychiatric sequelae also include increased anxiety, depression, irritability, impulsiveness, and psychosis.[20–26]

TOXIC NEUROPATHY

Acute toxic neuropathies can be focal or diffuse. Focal motor neuropathy is commonly seen in adult lead overexposure. This palsy is classically of the radial nerve and causes wrist drop, although other motor nerves can be affected. Buckthorn berry (coyotillo) intoxication shows the classic acute peripheral polyneuropathy, and is clinically indistinguishable from the acute inflammatory demyelinating polyradiculoneuropathy (AIDP).[27] Diphtheria toxin and tick paralysis toxin are other toxins that can mimic AIDP[28,29].

TOXIC NEUROMUSCULAR JUNCTION DYSFUNCTION

Botulinum toxin and organophosphates are among the toxic agents that act at the neuromuscular junction. Cranial nerve palsies superimposed on diffuse muscular weakness are commonly seen. Respiratory muscle weakness can be so severe as to cause respiratory failure.[30]

Organophosphate insecticides and military-grade nerve agents have the same basic mechanism of action. Organophosphates reversibly inhibit acetylcholinesterase, resulting in excess acetylcholine at the receptor and a syndrome of cholinergic overload. Fulminant cases show muscular twitching, followed by weakness, followed by paralysis and respiratory failure. In general, military-grade nerve agents are more rapidly cleared from the body and respond more quickly to antidotes than organophosphate insecticides. Antidotal treatment of organophosphates includes reversal agents such as pralidoxime, antiseizure agents such as diazepam, and atropine. Pyridostigmine can inhibit nerve agents if given before exposure, and is approved by the US Food and Drug Administration for pretreatment of exposure to soman.[31]

Botulinum toxin is found in nature in several forms. Typically, the toxin is found in poorly canned foods where the bacterium *Clostridium botulinum* has released exotoxin. On ingestion, botulinum toxin is absorbed and disseminates to cause a rapidly progressive descending presynaptic neuromuscular paralysis. Other than descending paralysis, hallmarks that differentiate botulism from AIDP include preserved reflexes and fixed dilated pupils. There is antitoxin available for treatment of botulism, which may shorten the duration of the illness.[30,32,33]

MISCELLANEOUS ACUTE NEUROTOXICITY

Nitrous oxide affects the posterior columns of the spinal cord preferentially, leading to deficits in position and vibratory sensation. Patients with nitrous oxide poisoning could show substantial myelopathic dysfunction in severe cases.[34]

Animal toxins include marine snake venoms, cone snail toxins, the blue-ringed octopus, neurotoxic terrestrial snake venoms (the cobras and other elapids), some scorpions, and certain spider venoms (eg, the black widow in North America). The patients are often aware that they have been exposed. Fulminant symptoms and death can ensue from some biological toxins. Antivenoms are available for many regionally. Clinicians should be aware of common toxic animals in their regions.

CHRONIC EXPOSURES

Chronic sequelae of neurotoxins may be caused by chronic nervous system injury from a single large exposure, or by slow accumulation of neurotoxins causing persistent effects. A toxin that may be fatal or highly damaging in a large, acute dose may go undetected for a long time, only manifesting in subtle symptoms after substantial damage has ensued. Lead, arsenic, organophosphate pesticides, organic solvents, and low-level carbon monoxide are all examples of toxins that may kill in large doses but cause milder symptoms with low exposures over time.

Sometimes it is difficult to ascertain whether a chronic, peripheral polyneuropathy is from a toxic agent or from some other cause. This difficulty is particularly compounded in patients who have underlying illnesses that are prone to neuropathy (eg, diabetes mellitus or acquired immunodeficiency syndrome) and are on multiple medications that can cause neuropathy as well. Chronic toxic neuropathies can present as axonopathies, myelinopathies, or mixed pictures depending on the individual toxic agent.

CONFIRMATORY TESTS

There are many testing resources available, the utility of which may vary from situation to situation. Blood and urine tests are accurate and standardized for many toxins, such as some heavy metals, alcohols, and drugs of abuse. For many, it becomes a challenging question of when to use blood testing versus urine testing. Hair or fingernail testing is useful to document exposure for some toxins, such as arsenic. There are also useful ancillary tests that help to guide diagnosis and treatment in some exposures.

Lead poisoning is a good example. A whole-blood lead level confirms the diagnosis. A blood level greater than 10 μg/dL is cause for concern, but, like many neurotoxins, the levels for toxicity are not known and may vary. In adults, 20 μg/dL is the threshold for neurotoxicity, and encephalopathy is usually not seen until levels of 100 μg/dL are reached.[35] Children should not exceed 5 μg/dL, according to the US Centers for Disease Control and Prevention. The hemogram may show a microcytic hypochromic anemia. Chemistry profiles may reveal uric acid derangements or other abnormalities. Radiographs of the abdomen may show lead foreign bodies. Radiographs of long bones may show characteristic findings of lead poisoning. A computed tomography (CT) scan or MRI of the brain may be useful to look for cerebral edema in cases of acute intoxication with encephalopathy. During treatment of lead poisoning with chelation therapy, urine levels are used to monitor excretion followed by repeat blood levels to assess for recurrence.[35,36]

LABORATORY TESTING

Laboratory testing for most neurotoxins is not a perfect science. However, a simple whole-blood or serum level is not always reflective of the amount of toxin in someone's body. Some toxins, particularly certain metals in the chronic state, can accumulate in body structures such as bone or nervous tissue, leading to a falsely low serum or urine level. Many organic toxins have no reliable confirmatory tests.

BLOOD AND SERUM

Blood testing is probably useful in intoxications caused by thallium, ethanol, methanol, and ethylene glycol. Whole-blood level testing is useful for cyanide, manganese, mercury, and lead. Arsenic may be underestimated in blood or serum testing, and these should be used only for acute exposure. Typically, inorganic arsenic is more likely to cause toxic exposure, and so speciation of arsenic levels is advised. Increased carboxyhemoglobin level indicates exposure to carbon monoxide, with a level greater than 10% likely being toxic.

There are surrogate blood tests available for organophosphate insecticide intoxication (red blood cell cholinesterase and serum pseudocholinesterase), but these tests are not commonly available quickly in an emergency setting. Testing for red blood cell cholinesterase or serum pseudocholinesterase is therefore not very useful for acute organophosphate poisonings, but is worthwhile to document and follow in cases of chronic exposure.

Because blood and serum testing for many toxins is not well standardized, it is prudent to become familiar with the ranges and limits for abnormal values in the patient population. Local clinical laboratory supervisors and poison control centers may be able to help.

URINE

In general, a 24-hour urine collection is preferred to a random sample. Some toxins are released in a diurnal pattern, and collection over 24 hours maximizes the likelihood of a positive study. Urine testing is the preferred test for arsenic intoxication. Urine drug screens may be useful for establishing recent ingestion of illicit substances.[37]

HAIR

Several laboratories offer hair analysis for traces of minerals and other toxins. It is used by health care providers and promoted by laboratories as a clinical tool to identify toxic exposures. The validity of these tests is questionable, and reproducibility of similar values among laboratories has been questioned by multiple scientific studies. Analysis of elements that bind to hair can be used to approximate when an exposure occurred. If a clinician uses hair analysis as a clinical assessment tool, caution is advised. Using hair analysis as a screening test is not routinely recommended.

NEUROPHYSIOLOGY

Only in rare instances does a neurophysiology study such as electroencephalography (EEG) or electromyography (EMG) definitively diagnose a neurointoxication. Their sensitivity far outweighs specificity in neurologic toxic exposures. For example, many intoxications show diffuse, generalized slowing suggestive of encephalopathy on the EEG. This finding does not suggest a particular toxic exposure; it merely provides objective evidence of encephalopathy in the intoxicated patient. It is also vital to remember that the absence of any abnormality on appropriately ordered neurophysiologic tests argues against an organic, toxic cause for the patient's symptoms. The utility of neurophysiologic testing in the practice of clinical neurotoxicology is largely that of an ancillary role, albeit an important one.

IMAGING

Normal CT or MRI scanning of the CNS does not rule out a toxic CNS disorder. In contrast, certain neurotoxic syndromes are recognized in large part from characteristic findings on neuroimaging. As an example, manganese can deposit in the basal ganglia, showing as hyperintense regions on T1-weighted imaging.

CONFIRMING AND RECONSIDERING NEUROTOXIC DISEASE

After reasonable diagnostic procedures are completed, the clinician must establish a probability that the patient's disorder is caused by exposure to a neurotoxin. Then the clinician should treat as indicated. Often, it is difficult to establish neurotoxicity with certainty because of a lack of biomarkers for most toxins. However, when reasonably established, it is obligatory to inform the appropriate authorities of the nature and source of exposure so that others can be protected. If additional signs or symptoms develop over time that point to another cause, then clinicians should be ready to backtrack and consider other possible causes for the patient's problem.

MEDICAL-LEGAL ISSUES

In many cases of neurotoxic exposures, the patients think they have been unjustly harmed and there are questions of fault. Patients who claim that they have been injured by toxic exposures may believe they have a right to collect damages. Litigation may ensue. These legal points could obscure the picture.

ISSUES OF IMPAIRMENT AND DISABILITY

Impairment and disability are different terms. People may be impaired functionally, but not disabled from doing their jobs. Disability is job dependent, and what may be disabling to one person in one job may not be to another. If a clinical neurologist loses a right index finger to an accident, the neurologist could still probably swing a reflex hammer well enough to do the job. However, a surgeon who loses an index finger might be disabled from performing surgery. The impairments (the loss of a finger) would be equal, but the disabilities would be different.

Neurotoxins may cause impairments or disabilities to differing degrees depending on the toxin, exposure route, dose, treatment, and individual susceptibility. Most toxic exposures are dynamic processes. Impaired or disabled neurotoxic patients may be back to normal at some time in the future. Then again, they may have permanent impairment and disability.

There is also often apprehension on returning to a place of exposure for fear that exposure may occur again. If exposure occurred at the workplace, this phobia could truly be disabling. In these cases, it is not only important to treat the patient's fears through appropriate medication and counseling but also to ensure that the risks of future exposures are reduced to the fullest possible extent by the patient's place of work.

CAUSATION METHODOLOGIES

Establishing causation is paramount to the correct diagnosis and the treatment of any patient suspected of neurotoxic poisoning. The disciplines of toxicology and epidemiology ask the question: can a substance cause a particular effect in humans? Recently 2 approaches to establishing causation in neurotoxicology were proposed. Adami and colleagues[38] proposed Epid-Tox causation framework incorporating data obtained in toxicologic and epidemiologic studies. The framework adopted some of the widely accepted causation criteria originally published and discussed by Sir Austin Bradford Hill (discussed later). The framework implied that data obtained in toxicologic and epidemiologic studies do not always lead to straightforward interpretation, and often different observers differ in their conclusions. This possibility is the problem inherent in the use of both weight of evidence and authoritative analyses.[39]

In contrast, a second approach adopted by the Institute of Medicine (IOM) uses methods of mapping the widely accepted logic underlying evidence-based medicine in toxicology to provide a consistent, objective, and rule-based methodology for evaluating human and animal toxicology data to determine whether a chemical creates a human health risk.[40]

Evidence-based toxicology (EBT) is driven by a methodology where the quality of evidence for each study is derived from logical ranking and rating of system that allows the evidence to lead to a causation conclusion in a more rigorous and transparent analysis.

The IOM panel pointed out the uncertainties associated with animal-to-human extrapolations that are inherent to toxicology test data and reiterated differences in physiology, the magnitude of dose tested, biology, and genetics as reasons why animal species do not always accurately predict the human hazard. Thus, the IOM effectively disagreed with the Epid-Tox approach, which assumes that animal data alone can be sufficiently conclusive when human data are either absent or too limited to reach a causal conclusion.

SIR AUSTIN BRADFORD HILL: CAUSATION CRITERIA

Exposure: did an exposure occur? Requires quantifying the level of a toxin in biological specimens (blood, urine, hair) or in the environment (air, water). In some cases, historical features alone may be adequate.[41]

Temporality: did symptoms begin concurrent with or after the exposure? A few toxins have long latent periods before symptoms develop but most cause symptoms shortly after the exposure.

Dose/response: do persons receiving higher doses and/or longer exposures have more severe symptoms?

Similarity to reported cases: are the symptoms similar to those previously reported?

Improvement as exposure is eliminated: do symptoms improve when the exposure is eliminated or reduced? Most toxin-induced symptoms improve after cessation of exposure, although a period of worsening symptoms, or even permanent symptoms, can occur after exposure to a few toxins.

Existence of animal model: do animal studies establish biological feasibility? Animal studies can be helpful to predict toxicity in the absence of human studies; some toxins do not have animal models and some toxins have different effects in different animals.

Other causes eliminated: are nontoxicologic causes excluded?

CASE 1

A 9-year-old right-handed boy presents with history of chronic lead exposure with recently identified blood lead concentration of 48 μg/dL. Environmental exposure turned out to be the causal factor, and the child was removed from the exposure environment. After toxicity had been medically managed, the patient was assessed for chronic cognitive deficit after exposure. Full-scale intelligence quotient (IQ) score of 83 revealed a low average IQ, but functional performance deficits were exacerbated by slowed processing speed, executive deficits, and impaired verbal memory. Most notable impairment was in visuospatial skills, which were also affected by poor motor control compared with peers. Comment: lead exposure is common and can lead to systemic toxicity, which includes neurocognitive developmental deficits. Assessment for cognition and psychological functioning in lead exposure should be added to routine diagnostics and treatment planning.

CASE 2

A 44-year-old right-handed man presents with a history of toxic exposure to thiourea (organosulfur compound with the formula $SC(NH_2)_2$) 3 years before presentation. The patient denies gross neurologic symptoms but reports vertigo and left-sided headaches with minimal relief from topiramate 100 mg twice a day. Accordingly, the patient was sent to us for posttoxicity headache assessment. Then the patient also reports mild memory and phonemic verbal fluency deficits, along with moderate executive dysfunction, suggesting post–toxic exposure neurocognitive sequelae. Affect was notable for depression without suicidality. Of note, there was pending litigation involving toxic exposure, and formal neuropsychological testing revealed suboptimal effort on test performances. Comment: this example highlights the importance of thorough evaluation in patients with toxic exposure, pending litigation or not, because clinical features can also be confounded by suboptimally reliable patient symptom report. Some of these situations can benefit from formal testing in neuropsychology that includes measures of malingering, especially when secondary gain as a confounding factor to the clinical picture is identified.

SUMMARY

The clinical history is vital in neurotoxicology, including the occupational history. Neurologic examination findings are often nonspecific, although nonneurologic signs may be present in select intoxications. Confirmatory testing is important, but the reference laboratories may not have standardized values for all substances. At times it may be advisable to involve an occupational, environmental, or toxicology medicine specialist to help review the data and determine relevance.[37]

Neurotoxins affect all areas of the nervous system. Cognitive effects are common. Damage may accumulate over time. Eliminating or reducing exposure is the primary principle, with treatment as indicated, in order to minimize permanent damage.

Establishing causation is critical to the correct diagnosis and the treatment of any patient suspected of neurotoxic poisoning. EBT can provide a consistent, objective, and rule-based methodology for evaluating human and animal toxicology data to determine whether a chemical creates a human health risk. Some of the critical steps involved in determining whether a neurotoxin is the causative agent are those established by Sir Austin Bradford Hill in differentiating association from causation in epidemiologic studies.

Neurotoxicology remains an underserved and under-recognized area of neurology. A few neurologists have developed interest or advanced training in toxicology over the past several years. A standardized training curriculum related to clinical neurotoxicology has yet to be developed. Likewise, care standards and clinical evidence remain scarce. An opportunity exists for pedagogy in neurology to further proliferate this area.

DISCLOSURE

The authors have no commercial or financial conflicts of interest to disclose.

REFERENCES

1. Firestone JA, Longstreth WT. Central nervous system diseases. In: Rosenstock L, editor. Textbook of Clinical occupational and environmental medicine. 2nd edition. London: Elsevier Saunders; 2004. p. 50–75.
2. Marshall L, Weir E, Abelsohn A, et al. Identifying and managing adverse environmental health effects: 1. Taking an exposure history. CMAJ 2002;166(8):1049–55.
3. National Institute for Occupational Safety and Health. National Occupational hazard Survey, 1972–74. DHEW Publication No. (NIOSH) 78-114. Cincinnati (OH): NIOSH; 1977.
4. Sriram K, Lin GX, Jefferson AM, et al. Modifying welding process parameters can reduce the neurotoxic potential of manganese-containing welding fumes. Toxicology 2015;328:168–78.
5. Sińczuk-walczak H, Janasik BM, Trzcinka-ochocka M, et al. Neurological and neurophysiological examinations of workers exposed to arsenic levels exceeding hygiene standards. Int J Occup Med Environ Health 2014;27(6):1013–25.
6. Myers J, London L, Lucchini RG. Neurotoxicology and development: human, environmental and social impacts. Neurotoxicology 2014;45:217–9.
7. George CM, Smith AH, Kalman DA, et al. Reverse osmosis filter use and high arsenic levels in private well water. Arch Environ Occup Health 2006;61(4):171–5.
8. Ishi K, Tamaoka A. [Ten-years records of organic arsenic (diphenylarsinic acid) poisoning: epidemiology, clinical feature, metabolism, and toxicity]. Brain Nerve 2015;67(1):5–18.

9. Rahman M, Sohel N, Yunus M, et al. A prospective cohort study of stroke mortality and arsenic in drinking water in Bangladeshi adults. BMC Public Health 2014; 14:174.

10. Mcclintock TR, Chen Y, Parvez F, et al. Association between arsenic exposure from drinking water and hematuria: results from the Health Effects of Arsenic Longitudinal Study. Toxicol Appl Pharmacol 2014;276(1):21–7.

11. Chen CJ. Health hazards and mitigation of chronic poisoning from arsenic in drinking water: Taiwan experiences. Rev Environ Health 2014;29(1–2):13–9.

12. Bacquart T, Frisbie S, Mitchell E, et al. Multiple inorganic toxic substances contaminating the groundwater of Myingyan Township, Myanmar: arsenic, manganese, fluoride, iron, and uranium. Sci Total Environ 2015;517:232–45.

13. Lowbeer L, Clapper M, Wermer P. Clinicopathologic conference; abdominal cramps, vomiting, shock, and unexpected death. Am J Clin Pathol 1956;26(6): 645–53.

14. Mhiri C, Choyakh F, Ben Hmida M, et al. Trigeminal somatosensory evoked potentials in trichloroethylene-exposed workers. Neurosciences (Riyadh) 2004;9(2): 102–7.

15. Albee RR, Spencer PJ, Johnson KA, et al. Lack of trigeminal nerve toxicity in rats exposed to trichloroethylene vapor for 13 weeks. Int J Toxicol 2006;25(6):531–40.

16. Jalal MJ, Fernandez SJ, Menon MK. Acute toxic neuropathy mimicking guillain barre syndrome. J Family Med Prim Care 2015;4(1):137–8.

17. Kim S, Takeuchi A, Kawasumi Y, et al. A Guillain-Barré syndrome-like neuropathy associated with arsenic exposure. J Occup Health 2012;54(4):344–7.

18. Feldman RG. Approach to diagnosis: occupational and environmental neurotoxicology. Philadelphia: Lippincott-Raven; 1999.

19. Han DY, Hoelzle JB, Dennis BC, Michael Hoffmann. A brief review of cognitive assessment in neurotoxicology. Neurol Clin 2011;29(3):581–90.

20. Fiedler N, Rohitrattana J, Siriwong W, et al. Neurobehavioral effects of exposure to organophosphates and pyrethroid pesticides among Thai children. Neurotoxicology 2015;48:90–9.

21. Mason LH, Mathews MJ, Han DY. Neuropsychiatric symptom assessments in toxic exposure. Psychiatr Clin North Am 2013;36(2):201–8.

22. Ahrens CL, Manno EM. Neurotoxicity of commonly used hepatic drugs. Handb Clin Neurol 2014;120:675–82.

23. Myint AM. Inflammation, neurotoxins and psychiatric disorders. Mod Trends Pharmacopsychiatry 2013;28:61–74.

24. Mukherjee B, Bindhani B, Saha H, et al. Platelet hyperactivity, neurobehavioral symptoms and depression among Indian women chronically exposed to low level of arsenic. Neurotoxicology 2014;45:159–67.

25. Bhatia P, Singh N. Homocysteine excess: delineating the possible mechanism of neurotoxicity and depression. Fundam Clin Pharmacol 2015;29(6):522–8.

26. Ratner MH, Feldman RG, White RF. Neurobehavioral Toxicology. In: Ramachandran VS, editor. Encyclopedia of the human brain, vol. 3. New York: Elsevier Science; 2002. p. 423–39.

27. Díaz-pérez RN, Castillo-gonzález JA, Carcaño-díaz K, et al. Histopathological alterations in the striatum caused by Karwinskia humboldtiana (Buckthorn) fruit in an experimental model of peripheral neuropathy. Histol Histopathol 2016;31(4): 393–402.

28. Diaz JH. A comparative meta-analysis of tick paralysis in the United States and Australia. Clin Toxicol (Phila) 2015;53(9):874–83.

29. Pecina CA. Tick paralysis. Semin Neurol 2012;32(5):531–2.

30. Fraint A, Vittal P, Comella C. Considerations on patient-related outcomes with the use of botulinum toxins: is switching products safe? Ther Clin Risk Manag 2016; 12:147–54.

31. FDA approves pyridostigmine bromide as pretreatment against nerve gas. Available at: https://www.fda.gov/drugs/bioterrorism-and-drug-preparedness/fda-approves-pyridostigmine-bromide-pretreatment-against-nerve-gas. Accessed January 13, 2020.

32. Kermen R. Botulinum toxin for chronic pain conditions. Dis Mon 2016;62(9): 353–7.

33. Sobel J. Botulism. Clin Infect Dis 2005;41(8):1167–73.

34. Rheinboldt M, Harper D, Parrish D, et al. Nitrous oxide induced myeloneuropathy: a case report. Emerg Radiol 2014;21(1):85–8.

35. Mason LH, Harp JP, Han DY. Pb neurotoxicity: neuropsychological effects of lead toxicity. Biomed Res Int 2014;2014:840547.

36. Smith D, Strupp BJ. The scientific basis for chelation: animal studies and lead chelation. J Med Toxicol 2013;9(4):326–38.

37. Dobbs MR, editor. Clinical neurotoxicology: syndromes, substances, environments. URINE: Elsevier Health Sciences; 2009.

38. Adami H-O, Berry CL, Breckenridge CB, et al. Toxicology and epidemiology: improving the science with a framework for combining toxicological and epidemiological evidence to establish causal inference. Toxicol Sci 2011;122:223–34.

39. Swaen G, van Amelsvoort L. A weight of evidence approach to causal inference. J Clin Epidemiol 2009;62:270–7.

40. Guzelian PS, Victoroff MS, Halmes NC, et al. Evidence-based toxicology: a comprehensive framework for causation. Hum Toxicol 2005;24:161–201.

41. Hill ab. The environment and disease: association or causation? Proc R Soc Med 1965;58:295–300.

Section I
Neurotoxicology Syndromes:
Peripheral Nervous System

Toxin-Induced Neuropathies

Michel Toledano, MD

KEYWORDS

• Neurotoxicity • Peripheral neuropathy • Occupational exposure • Chemotherapy

KEY POINTS

- Neuropathies caused by occupational or environmental toxins are increasingly rare in Western countries but remain a significant problem in developing nations.
- A history of toxic exposure may not always be readily available, especially in cases of homicidal or suicidal poisoning.
- Exposure does not equal causation; familiarity with the clinical and electrophysiologic features, as well as systemic manifestations, of specific toxic neuropathies is crucial to support the diagnosis.
- Medications and chemotherapeutic agents are associated with the development of peripheral neuropathy, although causation remains difficult to establish in some cases.
- Approximately 30% to 40% of patients treated with chemotherapy go on to develop chemotherapy-induced peripheral neuropathy.

INTRODUCTION

With the exception of isolated small fiber neuropathies, the diagnosis of peripheral neuropathy (PN) is usually readily established from clinical and electrodiagnostic criteria. Efforts to identify an underlying cause are driven both by a desire to find a reversible cause and to provide prognosis. Industrial and environmental toxins, as well as medications and chemotherapeutic agents, can damage the peripheral nervous system. Acquiring a detailed history of possible occupational and home exposures is crucial to establish the diagnosis of toxic neuropathies. It is also important to review past and current medications/supplements, including past exposure to chemotherapeutic agents, as well as alcohol and recreational drug use. However, a history of exposure may not always be readily available, as can be the case with homicidal or suicidal poisoning. In contrast, exposure does not necessarily equal causation and an alternative cause may better explain what is initially suspected to arise from toxic exposure. For example, a patient presenting with pronounced sensory loss out of proportion with history, and found to have high arches and hammertoes, is more likely to have a hereditary neuropathy in spite of reported lead exposure (especially in the setting of a positive family history). In these circumstances, it is helpful to

Department of Neurology, Mayo Clinic, 200 1st Street, Rochester, MN 55905, USA
E-mail address: Toledano.michel@mayo.edu

Neurol Clin 38 (2020) 749–763
https://doi.org/10.1016/j.ncl.2020.06.002
0733-8619/20/© 2020 Elsevier Inc. All rights reserved.

neurologic.theclinics.com

have an understanding of the clinical and electrodiagnostic features of specific toxic neuropathies (**Table 1**). Multisystem involvement is common with toxic exposure, and familiarity with syndromic presentations can also facilitate recognition and support the diagnosis. In addition, whenever a toxic neuropathy is suspected, it is imperative to be able to accurately interpret results of tests currently available to verify or refute this suspicion.

Table 1
Neuropathy phenotypes associated with toxins

Type of Neuropathy	Toxin	Other Causes to Consider
Sensorimotor neuropathy without demyelinating features	Acrylamide Arsenic (chronic) Ethambutol Ethylene oxide Elemental mercury Nitrous oxide (myeloneuropathy) Phenytoin Taxanes Vinca alkaloids	HMSN II Diabetes mellitus, vitamin deficiency (B_{12}, folate, thiamin) Sarcoidosis Carcinomatosis, lymphomatosis, MGUS
Motor or mixed sensorimotor with demyelinating features	Acrylamide Amiodarone Arabinoside (ara-C) Arsenic (acute exposure) Carbon disulfide n-hexane Procainamide Suramin	HMSN I, III Diabetes mellitus CIDP, GBS MGUS, multiple myeloma (POEMS syndrome)
Motor or motor-predominant neuronopathy	Dapsone Doxorubicin Lead Organophosphate	HMSN II, V West Nile virus Porphyria MMN
Sensory-predominant neuropathy or neuronopathy	Chloramphenicol Cisplatin Colchicine Ethyl alcohol Hydralazine Isoniazid Metronidazole Platinum-based chemotherapy Proteasome inhibitors Pyridoxine Thalidomide	Amyloidosis Fabry disease Tangier disease Diabetes mellitus HIV Sjögren syndrome
Asymmetric neuropathy or mononeuritis multiplex with or without demyelinating features	Dapsone Lead	HNLPP Diabetic amyotrophy MMN Vasculitis

Abbreviations: CIDP, chronic inflammatory demyelinating polyradiculoneuropathy; GBS, Guillain-Barré syndrome; HIV, human immunodeficiency virus; HMSN, hereditary motor and sensory neuropathy; HNLPP, hereditary neuropathy with liability to pressure palsies; MGUS, monoclonal gammopathy of uncertain significance; MMN, multifocal motor neuropathy; POEMS, polyneuropathy, organomegaly, endocrinopathy, myeloma protein, and skin changes.

Data from Little AA, Albers JW. Clinical description of toxic neuropathies. Handb Clin Neurol. 2015;131. Pages 259-261; with permission.

This article reviews the clinical, laboratory, and electrodiagnostic characteristics of some of the more common or representative toxic neuropathies, including those caused by medications and chemotherapeutic agents. Although toxic neuropathies caused by heavy metals and other industrial or environmental toxins are increasingly rare in Western countries, exposure to these agents remains a significant problem in developing nations. Their rarity can make it difficult for clinicians to recognize them. Exposures to these agents should be considered when evaluating patients from immigrant populations, itinerant farm workers, or returning travelers.

ALCOHOL

Chronic alcoholism is associated with the development of a progressive, painful axonal sensorimotor neuropathy often accompanied by autonomic dysfunction. Because alcoholism is common and is often associated with malnutrition, it has been difficult to determine whether the association is caused by direct toxic effects of alcohol or secondary to multiple vitamin deficiencies.[1] In 2018, 24.5% of Americans 12 years of age or older self-reported binge alcohol use and 6.1% reported to having 5 or more drinks on each of 5 or more days in the past 30 days.[2] It is therefore important to take a careful history of alcohol use in all patients evaluated for neuropathy. Useful but nonspecific laboratory biomarkers include an aspartate aminotransferase (AST) to alanine aminotransferase (ALT) ratio of 2:1, as well as macrocytosis with or without anemia.

Treatment of alcohol-associated neuropathy requires abstinence. Early involvement of trained chemical dependency personnel may be beneficial. In addition, patients should be screened for vitamin deficiencies. Given that alcohol is a suspected neurotoxin,[3] it is reasonable to counsel moderation to all patients with neuropathy irrespective of cause.

ENVIRONMENTAL TOXINS AND INDUSTRIAL AGENTS

Exposure to environmental toxins and industrial agents, including metals, has been associated with the development of PN (**Table 2**). In many cases, the neuropathy occurs as part of a multisystem process. Knowledge of these syndromic presentations can help with diagnosis. PN caused from exposure to many of these neurotoxins is increasingly uncommon in the developed world, primarily because of restricted use and strict exposure precautions. However, they remain a problem in developing nations because of decreased oversight as well as use in traditional medicine.

Heavy Metals

Arsenic

Accidental inorganic arsenic exposure may be occupational (copper and lead smelting, mining, tanning),[4] environmental (well water or fossil fuel contamination, contact with arsenic-treated wood or arsenic-containing pesticides),[5] or through folk or herbal medicines.[6] Inorganic arsenic is also a homicidal or suicidal agent. Exposure to inorganic arsenic must be distinguished from exposure to nonneurotoxic organic arsenic, which is found in some fish and shellfish and is a frequent cause of a biologic false-positive on urine heavy metal screen.

The neurotoxic effects of arsenic differ depending on whether patients are subjected to a single massive exposure or chronic, low-level exposure. In the former, neuropathy begins 5 to 10 days after exposure and progresses over weeks even in the absence of ongoing contact with the source (a phenomenon known as coasting). In these cases, the neuropathy can evolve into a diffuse sensorimotor demyelinating

Table 2
Occupational and environmental neurotoxins

Toxin	Neuropathy Phenotype	Comments
Acrylamide (monomer not polymerized form)	Length-dependent sensorimotor axonal	Acral hyperhidrosis, dermatitis
Allyl chloride	Length-dependent sensorimotor axonal	—
Carbon disulfide	Length-dependent sensorimotor axonal	Encephalopathy, parkinsonism
Dimethylamino-propionitrile	Length-dependent sensorimotor axonal	Urogenital dysfunction and sacral sensory loss
Ethylene oxide	Length-dependent sensorimotor axonal	Encephalopathy
Heavy Metals		
Arsenic	Acute exposure: sensorimotor demyelinating polyradiculoneuropathy mimicking GBS	Nausea, vomiting, diarrhea, garlic breath. Renal insufficiency. Cardiomyopathy. Patchy alopecia/dermatitis. Brownish desquamation of palms/feet and Mees lines (late finding)
Lead	Chronic low-level exposure: painful sensory-predominant axonal. Acute: motor predominant with wrist/ankle drop. Chronic: sensorimotor axonal	Hyperpigmentation, hyperkeratosis, and mucosal irritation. Abdominal pain/constipation. Arthralgia/myalgia. Encephalopathy. Hypochromic microcytic anemia. Gingival lead line. Myalgia, fatigue, mood lability, cognitive decline
Mercury	Chronic: sensorimotor axonal	Prominent sensory ataxia, cognitive decline
Thallium	Rapidly ascending painful sensory-predominant axonal with cranial nerve involvement	Abdominal discomfort, tachycardia and hypertension early on. Encephalopathy, ataxia. Alopecia 2–3 wk after exposure, Mees lines also a late finding
Hexacarbons	Length-dependent sensorimotor axonal with electrophysiologic features of demyelination	—
Organophosphorus compounds	Motor greater than sensory	Occurs 1–3 wk after exposure. Corticospinal tract signs

Data from Staff NP, Windebank AJ. Peripheral Neuropathy Due to Vitamin Deficiency, Toxins, and Medications. Continuum (Minneap Minn). 2014 Oct;20. Pages 1301–1302.

polyradiculoneuropathy that can mimic Guillain-Barré syndrome (GBS) with cranial nerve involvement and diaphragmatic paralysis sometimes requiring ventilatory support.[7] Abdominal pain, tachycardia, and hypotension are common before the onset of neuropathy but do not help distinguish it from GBS. Nonspecific systemic manifestations of arsenic toxicity such as renal failure, anemia, cardiomyopathy, and hepatomegaly may follow and can be helpful diagnostically when present. However, more specific features of arsenic toxicity, such as brownish desquamation of the hands and feet, and Mees lines on fingernails and toenails, may not appear until a month after isolated ingestion.

Chronic low-level exposure is usually associated with the development of a painful length-dependent sensory-predominant polyneuropathy. Onset of neuropathy is often preceded by dermatologic manifestations, including hyperpigmentation, hyperkeratosis, and mucosal irritation.[4]

Although 24-hour urine arsenic sampling is a good measure of ongoing or recent (96 hours) exposure, hair and nail sampling may be necessary to detect late effects of single or repeated exposures.[8] In cases of known or suspected exposure, chelation with penicillamine or dimercaprol should be started as soon as possible; although efficacy in preventing neuropathy remains unproved.

Lead

The incidence of overt lead toxicity with PN has substantial declined in Western countries with changes in lead mining practices and decreased exposure to lead-based paint and lead-containing gasoline.

Classically, lead toxicity is associated with a motor-predominant neuropathy with subacute onset of asymmetric weakness and atrophy of the wrist and finger extensors (wrist drop). As with other heavy metal neuropathies, there is always associated systemic manifestation, including constipation (likely secondary to associated autonomic dysfunction), weight loss, hypochromic microcytic anemia with basophilic stippling on smear, renal insufficiency, and gingival lead lines.

A blood lead level (BLL) remains the primary screening method for assessing lead toxicity. Adult lead toxicity is defined as a BLL greater than or equal to 10 μg/dL but symptoms are usually associated with levels greater than or equal to 80 μg/dL. Chelation therapy can be considered in symptomatic patients with BLL greater than 50 μg/dL but should be undertaken only once exposure has been curtailed because chelation may result in enhanced absorption of lead leading to worsening of symptoms.[9]

Mercury

Elemental mercury exposure occurs frequently, but reports of toxicity are uncommon. Mercury is used in the chloralkali industry, metal plating, and tanning industry where its use by hatters led to early descriptions of mercury toxicity (mad hatter disease). It is found in thermometers, electromagnetic switches, fluorescent lights, and dental amalgam. Although poorly absorbed by skin, intoxication after topical administration of traditional Chinese medicines containing mercury has been described.[10] In contrast, mercury vapor is readily absorbed through the lungs. Acute exposure to high-level mercury vapor results in pulmonary damage and nephrotoxicity followed by agitation and postural tremor that are self-limited.[11] Chronic exposure can be associated with the development of a length-dependent primarily sensory neuropathy and with associated sensory ataxia.[12]

The onset of neuropathy is usually associated with high urine levels (>500 μg/L), a level usually associated with the development of postural tremor and dermatitis. Coexisting postural tremor and maculopapular rash support mercury intoxication as the cause of neuropathy in patients with a history of occupational exposure and increased urine levels.[11] Chelation therapy with British anti-Lewisite or penicillamine can be considered, although efficacy remains unproved.

Thallium

Thallium was previously used as a rodenticide but has since been banned in most Western countries because of accidental exposure, as well as its use in criminal poisoning. It has not been produced in the United States since 1984 but it is imported for use in the manufacture of electronics, semiconductors, optical lenses, and imitation precious jewels. However, occupational exposure rarely, if ever, results in neurotoxicity, and suicidal or homicidal poisoning should be considered when the diagnosis is established.

Thallium poisoning begins with a gastrointestinal illness associated with tachycardia and hypertension. This stage is followed by a rapidly ascending painful predominantly sensory neuropathy with associated dysautonomia and cranial neuropathies, including optic neuropathy.[13] Encephalopathy, ataxia, and nystagmus have also been reported. Alopecia, a hallmark of thallium intoxication, does not occur until 2 to 3 weeks after exposure. Mees lines are also a late finding. Alopecia and neuropathy may be the only presenting symptoms of chronic, low-level exposure.[13]

Diagnosis is via 24-hour urine sampling. Urine heavy metal screening kits do not usually include thallium, and it must be ordered separately. Prussian blue at a dosage of 250 mg/kg/d divided into 2 or 4 doses is approved for the treatment of thallium toxicity and works by promoting fecal excretion. In patients with severe constipation, Prussian blue should be administered together with a cathartic such as mannitol. When Prussian blue is not readily available, multiple-dose activated charcoal can be administered instead.[14] Hemodialysis can also be considered to expedite toxin removal but efficacy remains unproved.

Industrial Agents

Carbon disulfide

Carbon disulfide is an organic solvent absorbed by inhalation or skin contact. Occupational exposure occurs in the production of cellophane, plywood, vulcanized rubber, some pesticides, and viscose rayon.[11] Acute high-level exposure results in neuropsychiatric disturbances, parkinsonism, and polyneuropathy.[15] Chronic low-level exposure results in an indolent sensorimotor neuropathy with some electrophysiologic features of demyelination, although the neuropathy is characterized primarily by axonal degeneration with paranodal and internodal swelling.[16] An unusual feature of carbon disulfide neurotoxicity is the co-occurrence of extrapyramidal dysfunction, including bradykinesia, rest tremor, rigidity, and postural instability. Combined neuropathy and parkinsonism in the correct clinical setting should suggest carbon disulfide intoxication. Recovery is poor after cessation of exposure.

Hexacarbons

n-Hexane neuropathy has been associated with use of degreasing solvents and cleansers in electronics and press proofing (ink printing), as well as occupational exposure involving workers using glue without proper ventilation.[11] However, a substantial number cases of hexacarbon neurotoxicity in the last 2 decades have been associated with intentional abuse in the form of glue sniffing.[17]

Acute exposure to n-hexane results in central nervous system depression but repeated exposures result in a length-dependent polyneuropathy with autonomic involvement. Clinically, symptoms can progress over weeks to months and resemble GBS or chronic inflammatory demyelinating polyradiculoneuropathy (CIDP). Although primarily an axonal neuropathy, electrophysiologic demyelinating features, including conduction slowing with temporal dispersion as well as prolonged distal motor latencies and prolonged or absent F-response latencies, can occur. Focal conduction block has also been described.[18] These electrophysiologic features are thought to be a consequence of paranodal axonal swellings with myelin retraction.[18,19]

The cerebrospinal fluid protein level does not tend to be markedly increased but can be abnormal. Sural nerve biopsy shows axonal swelling supporting a toxic cause. Although n-hexane and its neurotoxic metabolite 2, 5-hexanedione can be present in the urine for a few days after exposure, urine screening is not usually part of the diagnosis. Cessation of exposure is the only treatment but prognosis is favorable, although symptoms may continue to worsen for weeks to months after the last exposure (coasting).[19]

Organophosphorus compounds

The neurotoxic effects of organophosphorus compounds, including organophosphates and carbamates, have led to their widespread use as insecticides worldwide. Toxicity generally results from accidental or intentional exposure to agricultural pesticides. In 2012, there were more than 5000 reported exposures to organophosphorus agents in the United States, with fewer than 5 deaths.[20] However, acute organophosphorus poisoning continues to be a significant cause of morbidity and mortality in developing countries, with close to 3 million cases of exposure reported worldwide.[6] Organophosphorus compounds have also been used as so-called nerve agents in bioterrorism, including the 2009 Tokyo sarin attack and the 2018 assassination attempt of a Russian dissident in the United Kingdom with a so-called novichock agent.[21,22]

Organophosphorus compounds exert their primary neurotoxic effect by inactivating acetylcholinesterase. Acute symptoms of cholinergic excess include muscarinic effects (miosis, salivation, diaphoresis, bronchorrhea, diarrhea, bradycardia), and nicotinic effects (muscle weakness, and fasciculations). Atropine reduces the muscarinic effects, and pralidoxime reactivates the phosphorylated acetylcholinesterase at the neuromuscular junction, reducing weakness.

Between 1 and 4 days, some patients develop proximal limb weakness, along with weakness of extraocular, bulbar, neck flexor, and respiratory muscles. This self-limited paresis has been termed intermediate syndrome and does not respond to atropine.[23] Intermediate syndrome most likely represents a transient depolarizing blockade of neuromuscular transmission. Organophosphate-induced delayed neurotoxicity (OPIDN) can occur between 7 and 21 days after exposure, particularly in association with triorthocresyl phosphate. OPIDN is characterized by a length-dependent axonal sensorimotor neuropathy with early foot drop and weakness of intrinsic hand muscles. Most patients go on to develop upper motor neuron signs, including spasticity suggestive of superimposed pyramidal dysfunction. No specific treatment is available to prevent OPIDN. A minority of patients make a complete recovery but most experience modest recovery of symptoms.[6]

MEDICATIONS

Medications, including chemotherapeutic agents, are a known to be associated with the development of toxic neuropathies (**Table 3**). However, causation remains controversial in some instances, as is the case with fluoroquinolones.

Dapsone

Dapsone is an antiparasitic and antimycobacterial agent used to treat leprosy. It is also a second-line agent in the treatment or prevention of pneumocystis pneumonia or

Table 3
Medications and chemotherapeutic agents

Class and Drug	Type of Neuropathy	Comments
Anesthetics		
Nitrous Oxide	Myeloneuropathy	Causes myeloneuropathy syndrome (including subacute combined degeneration), seen in vitamin B12 deficiency, by irreversibly oxidizing cobalamin
Antialcoholism		
Disulfiram	Sensorimotor axonal	
Antiarrhythmic		
Amiodarone	Sensorimotor axonal/ demyelinating	
Procainamide	Sensorimotor demyelinating	Can mimic chronic inflammatory polyradiculoneuropathy (CIDP)
Antigout		
Colchicine	Mild sensory-predominant axonal	Myopathy usually more prominent; disrupts microtubules; risk is high in patients with renal disease
Antihypertensive		
Hydralazine	Sensory-predominant axonal	Rare except with prolonged high doses; prevented with pyridoxine treatment
Antimicrobial		
Chloramphenicol	Mild painful sensory-redominant axonal	
Dapsone	Motor-predominant axonal	May mimic mononeuritis multiplex
Ethambutol	Sensory-predominant axonal	May also cause retrobulbar optic neuropathy
Fluoroquinolones	Sensorimotor axonal	Still controversial as to whether it represents it causes peripheral neuropathy
Metronidazole	Sensory-predominant axonal	May also cause encephalopathy
Nitrofurantoin	Sensorimotor axonal	Can be severe, mimicking Guillain-Barre syndrome; usually occurs in patients with renal impairment
Antineoplastic		
Ado-trastuzumab emtansine	Sensorimotor axonal	Antibody-drug conjugate
Brentuximab vedotin	Sensorimotor axonal	

(continued on next page)

Table 3
(continued)

Class and Drug	Type of Neuropathy	Comments
Epothelones (eg, ixabepilone)	Sensorimotor axonal	
Eribulin mesylate	Sensorimotor axonal	
Etoposide and teniposide	Sensorimotor axonal	
Platinum-based (cisplatin, oxaliplatin, carboplastin)	Sensory axonal/ neuronopathy	Cold-induced dysesthesia with oxiplatin
Proteasome inhibitors (bortezomib, carfilzomib)	Sensory-predominant axonal	Carfilzomib less commonly causes peripheral neuropathy; occasionally mimics mononeuritis multiplex
Suramin	Sensorimotor axonal/ demyelinating	
Taxane (paclitaxel, docetaxel)	Sensorimotor axonal	
Thalidomide, lenalidomide	Sensorimotor axonal	
Vinca alkaloids (vincristine, Vinblastine)	Sensorimotor axonal	
Antiseizure		
Phenytoin	Mild sensorimotor axonal	Chronic use
Antituberculosis		
Isoniazid	Sensory-predominant axonal	Prevented with pyridoxine treatment
Immunosuppressant		
Chloroquine	Sensorimotor axonal/ demyelinating	Myopathy usually more prominent
Gold salts	Sensorimotor axonal/ demyelinating	
Leflunomide	Painful sensory predominant axonal	
Nucleoside analogue reverse transcriptase inhibitors		
Zalcitabine (ddC), Didanosine (ddl), Stavudine (d4T)	Painful sensory axonal	May have coasting; associated with elevated lactate

From Staff NP, Windebank AJ. Peripheral Neuropathy Due to Vitamin Deficiency, Toxins, and Medications. Continuum (Minneap Minn). 2014 Oct;20. Pages 1301-1302; with permission.

toxoplasmosis, and is also used in the treatment of dermatitis herpetiformis and refractory cutaneous lupus erythematosus.

Dapsone-associated neuropathy usually develops with chronic use. Most patients present with an asymmetric motor-predominant neuropathy, although a minority develop a length-dependent sensorimotor neuropathy.[24] Prognosis is good following cessation of the drug, but most patients experience coasting.

Fluoroquinolones

Fluoroquinolones are among the most widely used antibiotics given their broad-range coverage and favorable adverse-effect profile. Shortly after their introduction, several reports were published suggesting an association between their use and the onset of neuropathy.[25] Most of the initial data linking the two came from pharmacovigilance studies and case reports, making it difficult to establish the veracity of the association. More recent publications, including a study using US health claims data, as well as a population-based nested case-control study using data from the United Kingdom, have provided statistical rigor to support a true association.[26,27]

Detailed clinical descriptions of fluoroquinolone-associated neuropathy are lacking, with most reports describing length-dependent primarily axonal sensorimotor neuropathies of varying severity. No definitive predisposing factors have been identified. Reported recovery following discontinuation has been variable.[28]

Nitrous Oxide

Nitrous oxide (N_2O) is an anesthetic commonly used in surgical and dental procedures. Because of its euphorigenic properties (it is also known as laughing gas), it has been used as a drug of abuse. It is available commercially in aerosol delivery systems for whipped cream. N_2O leads to irreversible oxidation of cobalamin (vitamin B_{12}), rendering it inactive. Vitamin B_{12} is needed for the conversion of homocysteine to methionine. Reduced levels of methionine prevent methylation of myelin proteins, resulting in central and peripheral nervous system demyelination.[29] As expected, N_2O neurotoxicity results in myelopathy, typically presenting as a myeloneuropathy with predominant posterior column involvement, indistinguishable from that seen with cobalamin deficiency. It may also rarely present with an isolated sensorimotor neuropathy with demyelinating features.[24]

MRI spine may show T2 hyperintensity in the posterior and lateral columns. Vitamin B_{12} levels may be normal but homocysteine and methylmalonic acid levels (both substrates of reactions catalyzed by cobalamin) may be increased, indicating functional vitamin B_{12} deficiency. Treatment is with intramuscular high-dose cobalamin replacement.

Pyridoxine

Vitamin B_6 (pyridoxine) is converted in the liver to its active form, pyridoxine 5-phosphate (PLP). Overt nutritional deficiency is rare, but certain drugs can interfere with pyridoxine metabolism, including isoniazid, penicillamine, hydralazine, and carbidopa/levodopa. Pyridoxine deficiency has been associated with seborrheic dermatitis, microcytic anemia, and seizures. In spite of a reported link, there is insufficient evidence to support an association between PN and pyridoxine deficiency.[30] In contrast, excessive pyridoxine intake is likely associated with the development of a painful small fiber neuropathy, although large fiber neuronopathy has also been described.[30] Associated dermatoses, photosensitivity, nausea, and dizziness can occur.

The emergence of neuropathy seems to be both dose and duration dependent. Risk is highest in people taking pyridoxine for longer than 6 months at dosages greater than

50 mg/d. Pyridoxine given at a dose of 6 mg daily is likely adequate and safe in cases where there is concern for deficiency, such as in patients with malnutrition or those taking isoniazid.[30] The mean plasma PLP concentration can be measured to assess for both deficiency and toxicity.[31]

Chemotherapy-induced peripheral neuropathy

Approximately 30% to 40% of patients treated with neurotoxic chemotherapies go on to develop chemotherapy-induced PN (CIPN), a common dose-limiting side effect of these therapies.[32] However, before making a diagnosis of CIPN, it is important to consider alternative causes. Although patients with diabetes may be at increased risk of developing CIPN, metabolic and endocrine disorders are not a common cause of PN in patients with cancer. Paraneoplastic neuropathies usually develop before or at the time that cancer is discovered but can rarely occur during treatment, as in lymphoma-associated dysimmune polyneuropathies.[33] Carcinomatous, or more commonly lymphomatous, involvement of the peripheral nerves can mimic inflammatory polyradiculoneuropathies,[34] and paraproteinemias are associated with several different types of neuropathies,[35] including amyloid-associated neuropathy.[36]

However, there are no effective preventive treatments of CIPN, and, although recent studies have revealed genetic variants associated with neurotoxic susceptibilities to specific agents, currently no test is available that can predict the likelihood of CIPN developing in an individual patient.[32] Most CIPN develops in a dose-dependent fashion and treatment relies on reducing or discontinuing the offending agent when possible. The recent American Society of Clinical Oncology for CIPN (48 phase III trials reviewed) only recommends duloxetine for the treatment of CIPN-associated neuropathic pain, although many other agents are still used in an off-label fashion.[37] A recent systematic review of these trials identified significant design flaws and concluded that internal validity threats may have resulted in type II error and premature dismissal of potentially effective interventions.[38] Novel electrostimulation techniques (eg, scrambler therapy) have shown some promise but larger randomized control trials are needed to confirm benefit.[39]

Antimicrotubule Agents

Taxanes (paclitaxel, docetaxel, cabazitaxel) typically cause a painful length-dependent sensory-predominant neuropathy. Cabazitaxel seems to have less cumulative toxicity but can be associated with dysgeusia.[40] Paclitaxel is associated with an acute, transient musculoskeletal pain syndrome that, although not clearly neuropathic, may correlate with the development of paclitaxel-induced CIPN.[41]

Vinca alkaloids (vincristine, vinblastine), which are used primarily to treat hematological malignancies, are associated with the development of a length-dependent sensorimotor neuropathy.[42] Rarely, vasomotor phenomena such as Raynaud as well as cranial neuropathies can occur.[43,44]

Newer chemotherapeutic agents that also affect microtubule dynamics, such as eribulin and ixabepilone, can also cause a sensorimotor neuropathy.[45] A novel therapeutic strategy has been to conjugate tumor-specific antibodies with chemotherapeutic agents as used in brentuximab vedotin, where an antibody to CD30 (cluster of differentiation 30; present in lymphoma) is conjugated to a microtubule toxin (monomethyl auristatin E). Similarly, ado-trastuzumab emtasine combines an antibody against HER2 (found in breast cancer) and the microtubule toxin emtasine. Despite the attempted targeting of tumor antigens, both these agents are associated with a high frequency of PN.[46,47]

Platinum Compounds

Platinum-based compounds (cisplatin, carboplatin, and oxaliplatin) primarily produce a sensory neuronopathy via damage to the sensory dorsal root ganglia.[48] The parent compound cisplatin produces ototoxicity, nephropathy, and myelosuppression in addition to the neuropathy. Both CIPN and hearing loss are dose related and occur concurrently. Carboplatin and oxaliplatin are considered less neurotoxic than cisplatin but are still associated with the development of sensory neuropathy in 30% to 40% of exposed patients.[49]

As with many toxic neuropathies, platinum-based CIPN is associated with coasting, and symptoms usually worsen for weeks to months after discontinuation of therapy. In addition to sensory neuronopathy, oxaliplatin is also associated with a distinct neuropathic syndrome characterized by the development of temporary, cold-induced dysesthetic pain in the hands and face.[50] These symptoms usually arise after the second or third cycle of treatment and last for only 2 to 4 days following the infusion.

Proteasome Inhibitors

Proteasome inhibitors (bortezomib, carfilzomib, ixazomib) are associated with the development of a painful length-dependent small fiber–predominant axonal sensory neuropathy with autonomic involvement. Carfilzomib and ixazomib are associated with lower incidence of CIPN compared with bortezomib. Subcutaneous delivery of bortezomib is associated with lower incidence and severity of neuropathy.[51] Rarely, patients receiving bortezomib can develop a severe polyradiculoneuropathy, which is likely immune mediated and can respond to immunotherapy.[52]

Thalidomide

Thalidomide is associated with the development of a sensory-predominant neuropathy with prolonged use.[53] In contemporary practice, thalidomide is used primarily in the treatment of multiple myeloma, although the drug was introduced in the 1960s as a sedative. Lenalidomide and pomalidomide are newer formulations and associated with decreased neurotoxicity.[54,55]

SUMMARY

When evaluating patients presenting with signs and symptoms of PN, toxic neuropathies should be considered as part of the differential. A thorough review of medications, supplements, and recreational drug use, as well as possible occupational or environmental exposures, is crucial to establish the diagnosis. A history of exposure may not always be evident. In contrast, exposure does not necessarily entail causation. Familiarity with the neuropathy phenotypes of specific toxic neuropathies, as well as associated systemic manifestations, can help support the diagnosis in cases where ambiguity remains.

REFERENCES

1. Mellion M, Gilchrist JM, de la Monte S. Alcohol-related peripheral neuropathy: nutritional, toxic, or both? Muscle Nerve 2011;43(3):309–16.
2. Substance Abuse and Mental Health Services Administration. Key substance use and mental health indicators in the United States: results from the 2018 national Survey on drug use and health (HHS publication No. PEP19-5068, NSDUH Series H-54). Rockville, MD: Center for Behavioral Health Statistics and Quality, Substance Abuse and Mental Health Services Administration; 2019. Available at: https://www.samhsa.gov/data/.

3. Mellion ML, Nguyen V, Tong M, et al. Experimental model of alcohol-related peripheral neuropathy. Muscle Nerve 2013;48(2):204–11.

4. Feldman RG, Niles CA, Kelly-Hayes M, et al. Peripheral neuropathy in arsenic smelter workers. Neurology 1979;29(7):939–44.

5. Trivedi S, Pandit A, Ganguly G, et al. Epidemiology of peripheral neuropathy: an Indian perspective. Ann Indian Acad Neurol 2017;20(3):173–84.

6. Chakraborti D, Mukherjee SC, Saha KC, et al. Arsenic toxicity from homeopathic treatment. J Toxicol Clin Toxicol 2003;41(7):963–7.

7. Greenberg SA. Acute demyelinating polyneuropathy with arsenic ingestion. Muscle Nerve 1996;19(12):1611–3.

8. Choucair AK, Ajax ET. Hair and nails in arsenical neuropathy. Ann Neurol 1988;23(6):628–9.

9. Kosnett MJ, Wedeen RP, Rothenberg SJ, et al. Recommendations for medical management of adult lead exposure. Environ Health Perspect 2007;115(3):463–71.

10. Wu ML, Deng JF, Lin KP, et al. Lead, mercury, and arsenic poisoning due to topical use of traditional Chinese medicines. Am J Med 2013;126(5):451–4.

11. Little AA, Albers JW. Clinical description of toxic neuropathies. Handb Clin Neurol 2015;131:253–96.

12. Franzblau A, d'Arcy H, Ishak MB, et al. Low-level mercury exposure and peripheral nerve function. Neurotoxicology 2012;33(3):299–306.

13. Zhao G, Ding M, Zhang B, et al. Clinical manifestations and management of acute thallium poisoning. Eur Neurol 2008;60(6):292–7.

14. Hoffman RS, Stringer JA, Feinberg RS, et al. Comparative efficacy of thallium adsorption by activated charcoal, prussian blue, and sodium polystyrene sulfonate. J Toxicol Clin Toxicol 1999;37(7):833–7.

15. Liu CH, Huang CY, Huang CC. Occupational neurotoxic diseases in taiwan. Saf Health Work 2012;3(4):257–67.

16. Gottfried MR, Graham DG, Morgan M, et al. The morphology of carbon disulfide neurotoxicity. Neurotoxicology 1985;6(4):89–96.

17. Huang CC. Polyneuropathy induced by n-hexane intoxication in Taiwan. Acta Neurol Taiwan 2008;17(1):3–10.

18. Chang AP, England JD, Garcia CA, et al. Focal conduction block in n-hexane polyneuropathy. Muscle Nerve 1998;21(7):964–9.

19. Misirli H, Domac FM, Somay G, et al. N-hexane induced polyneuropathy: a clinical and electrophysiological follow up. Electromyogr Clin Neurophysiol 2008;48(2):103–8.

20. Mowry JB, Spyker DA, Cantilena LR Jr, et al. 2012 annual report of the American Association of Poison Control Centers' National Poison Data System (NPDS): 30th Annual Report. Clin Toxicol (Phila) 2013;51(10):949–1229.

21. Chai PR, Hayes BD, Erickson TB, et al. Novichok agents: a historical, current, and toxicological perspective. Toxicol Commun 2018;2(1):45–8.

22. Hoffman A, Eisenkraft A, Finkelstein A, et al. A decade after the Tokyo sarin attack: a review of neurological follow-up of the victims. Mil Med 2007;172(6):607–10.

23. Senanayake N, Karalliedde L. Neurotoxic effects of organophosphorus insecticides. An intermediate syndrome. N Engl J Med 1987;316(13):761–3.

24. Thompson AG, Leite MI, Lunn MP, et al. Whippits, nitrous oxide and the dangers of legal highs. Pract Neurol 2015;15(3):207–9.

25. Aoun M, Jacquy C, Debusscher L, et al. Peripheral neuropathy associated with fluoroquinolones. Lancet 1992;340(8811):127.

26. Etminan M, Brophy JM, Samii A. Oral fluoroquinolone use and risk of peripheral neuropathy: a pharmacoepidemiologic study. Neurology 2014;83(14):1261–3.
27. Morales D, Pacurariu A, Slattery J, et al. Association between peripheral neuropathy and exposure to oral fluoroquinolone or amoxicillin-clavulanate therapy. JAMA Neurol 2019;76(7):827–33.
28. Staff NP, Dyck PJB. On the association between fluoroquinolones and neuropathy. JAMA Neurol 2019;76(7):753–4.
29. Sanders RD, Weimann J, Maze M. Biologic effects of nitrous oxide: a mechanistic and toxicologic review. Anesthesiology 2008;109(4):707–22.
30. Ghavanini AA, Kimpinski K. Revisiting the evidence for neuropathy caused by pyridoxine deficiency and excess. J Clin Neuromuscul Dis 2014;16(1):25–31.
31. Leklem JE. Vitamin B-6: a status report. J Nutr 1990;120:1503–7. Suppl 11(4).
32. Staff NP, Grisold A, Grisold W, et al. Chemotherapy-induced peripheral neuropathy: A current review. Ann Neurol 2017;81(6):772–81.
33. Stubgen JP. Lymphoma-associated dysimmune polyneuropathies. J Neurol Sci 2015;355(1–2):25–36.
34. Tomita M, Koike H, Kawagashira Y, et al. Clinicopathological features of neuropathy associated with lymphoma. Brain 2013;136(Pt 8):2563–78.
35. Bayat E, Kelly JJ. Neurological complications in plasma cell dyscrasias. Handb Clin Neurol 2012;105:731–46.
36. Shin SC, Robinson-Papp J. Amyloid neuropathies. Mt Sinai J Med 2012;79(6):733–48.
37. Hershman DL, Lacchetti C, Dworkin RH, et al. Prevention and management of chemotherapy-induced peripheral neuropathy in survivors of adult cancers: American Society of Clinical Oncology clinical practice guideline. J Clin Oncol 2014;32(18):1941–67.
38. Lee D, Kanzawa-Lee G, Knoerl R, et al. Characterization of internal validity threats to phase III clinical trials for chemotherapy-induced peripheral neuropathy management: a systematic review. Asia Pac J Oncol Nurs 2019;6(4):318–32.
39. Loprinzi C, Le-Rademacher JG, Majithia N, et al. Scrambler therapy for chemotherapy neuropathy: a randomized phase II pilot trial. Support Care Cancer 2019;28(3):1183–97.
40. Omlin A, Sartor O, Rothermundt C, et al. Analysis of side effect profile of alopecia, nail changes, peripheral neuropathy, and dysgeusia in prostate cancer patients treated with docetaxel and cabazitaxel. Clin Genitourin Cancer 2015;13(4):e205–8.
41. Reeves BN, Dakhil SR, Sloan JA, et al. Further data supporting that paclitaxel-associated acute pain syndrome is associated with development of peripheral neuropathy: North Central Cancer Treatment Group trial N08C1. Cancer 2012;118(20):5171–8.
42. Lavoie Smith EM, Li L, Chiang C, et al. Patterns and severity of vincristine-induced peripheral neuropathy in children with acute lymphoblastic leukemia. J Peripher Nerv Syst 2015;20(1):37–46.
43. Atas E, Korkmazer N, Artik HA, et al. Raynaud's phenomenon in a child with medulloblastoma as a late effect of chemotherapy. J Cancer Res Ther 2015;11(3):666.
44. Rosenthal S, Kaufman S. Vincristine neurotoxicity. Ann Intern Med 1974;80(6):733–7.
45. Carlson K, Ocean AJ. Peripheral neuropathy with microtubule-targeting agents: occurrence and management approach. Clin Breast Cancer 2011;11(2):73–81.

46. Gopal AK, Ramchandren R, O'Connor OA, et al. Safety and efficacy of brentuximab vedotin for Hodgkin lymphoma recurring after allogeneic stem cell transplantation. Blood 2012;120(3):560–8.
47. Krop IE, Modi S, LoRusso PM, et al. Phase 1b/2a study of trastuzumab emtansine (T-DM1), paclitaxel, and pertuzumab in HER2-positive metastatic breast cancer. Breast Cancer Res 2016;18(1):34.
48. Gill JS, Windebank AJ. Cisplatin-induced apoptosis in rat dorsal root ganglion neurons is associated with attempted entry into the cell cycle. J Clin Invest 1998;101(12):2842–50.
49. Johnson C, Pankratz VS, Velazquez AI, et al. Candidate pathway-based genetic association study of platinum and platinum-taxane related toxicity in a cohort of primary lung cancer patients. J Neurol Sci 2015;349(1–2):124–8.
50. Lehky TJ, Leonard GD, Wilson RH, et al. Oxaliplatin-induced neurotoxicity: acute hyperexcitability and chronic neuropathy. Muscle Nerve 2004;29(3):387–92.
51. Moreau P, Pylypenko H, Grosicki S, et al. Subcutaneous versus intravenous bortezomib in patients with relapsed multiple myeloma: subanalysis of patients with renal impairment in the phase III MMY-3021 study. Haematologica 2015;100(5): e207–10.
52. Mauermann ML, Blumenreich MS, Dispenzieri A, et al. A case of peripheral nerve microvasculitis associated with multiple myeloma and bortezomib treatment. Muscle Nerve 2012;46(6):970–7.
53. Grover JK, Uppal G, Raina V. The adverse effects of thalidomide in relapsed and refractory patients of multiple myeloma. Ann Oncol 2002;13(10):1636–40.
54. Dalla Torre C, Zambello R, Cacciavillani M, et al. Lenalidomide long-term neurotoxicity: Clinical and neurophysiologic prospective study. Neurology 2016;87(11): 1161–6.
55. Siegel DS, Weisel KC, Dimopoulos MA, et al. Pomalidomide plus low-dose dexamethasone in patients with relapsed/refractory multiple myeloma and moderate renal impairment: a pooled analysis of three clinical trials. Leuk Lymphoma 2016;57(12):2833–8.

Toxin-Induced Channelopathies, Neuromuscular Junction Disorders, and Myopathy

Jacqueline Janecek, MD[a], Hani Kushlaf, MD[b,c],*

KEYWORDS

- Ciguatera • Tetrodotoxin • Botulism • Toxin-induced rhabdomyolysis
- Medication-induced myopathy • HMGCR antibody myopathy
- Immune checkpoint inhibitor myopathy

KEY POINTS

- Ciguatera fish poisoning is the most common marine food poisoning. The clinical presentation includes paresthesia and cold allodynia. Neurologic examination shows findings of a sensory length–dependent polyneuropathy with greater involvement of small fiber modalities.
- Tetrodotoxicity is the most severe known marine poisoning. The clinical presentation is dependent on the severity and includes sensory and motor manifestations. Respiratory failure can occur in severely affected patients.
- Botulism can clinically resemble acute presentations of neuromuscular junction disorders, such as myasthenia gravis and Lambert-Eaton myasthenic syndrome; however, a search for symptoms and signs of cholinergic blockade, such as dilated pupils, dry eyes, dry mouth, anhidrosis, and constipation, is diagnostically helpful.
- Statin-induced immune-mediated necrotizing myopathy presents with progressive muscle weakness and a markedly elevated creatine kinase (CK) that does not improve and continues to progress even with statin discontinuation. HMGCR antibodies are diagnostic. Immunotherapy is needed to prevent disability.
- Immune checkpoint inhibitors are a newer class of anticancer drugs. Inflammatory myopathy and myasthenia gravis are recognized complications. Marked elevation of CK in this setting indicates inflammatory myopathy. Prompt recognition and therapy are needed to prevent significant complications.

---

[a] Department of Neurology and Rehabilitation Medicine, University of Cincinnati, Cincinnati, OH, USA; [b] Department of Neurology and Rehabilitation Medicine, University of Cincinnati, 260 Stetson Street Suite 2300, Cincinnati, OH 45219, USA; [c] Department of Pathology and Laboratory Medicine, University of Cincinnati, 234 Goodman Street, LMB, Suite 110, Cincinnati, OH 45219, USA
* Corresponding author. Department of Neurology and Rehabilitation Medicine, University of Cincinnati, 260 Stetson Street Suite 2300, Cincinnati, OH 45219.
E-mail address: Hani.Kushlaf@uc.edu
Twitter: @hanikushlaf (H.K.)

Neurol Clin 38 (2020) 765–780
https://doi.org/10.1016/j.ncl.2020.07.001
0733-8619/20/© 2020 Elsevier Inc. All rights reserved.

neurologic.theclinics.com

INTRODUCTION

Several toxins can lead to neurotoxicity through toxin-induced channelopathies, neuromuscular junction disorders, and myopathies. This article discusses various toxins—ranging from common medications to rare venomous snake bites—that can affect the peripheral nervous system through multiple mechanisms. These toxins are important to be aware of because they can lead to serious neurologic disease or even death, and many can be treated and reversed if recognized early.

CIGUATOXIN

- Ciguatera fish poisoning is the commonest marine poisoning and occurs as a result of the consumption of ciguateric reef fish (mackerel, coral trout, grouper, snapper, barracuda, and moray eels, to name a few), which contain ciguatoxins in their flesh and viscera.[1,2] The dinoflagellate *Gambierdiscus toxicus* ingested by fish produces ciguatoxins that are tasteless and odorless and can survive temperatures of cooking and commercial freezing for up to 6 months.[1]
- The incidence of ciguatera fish poisoning approaches 10% in the Caribbean and Pacific regions, with an estimation of 10,000 to 50,000 contracting the disease annually.[1] Cases also have been reported in the United States, Europe, and Hong Kong, perhaps as a result of fish transportation.[1,2]
- Ciguatoxin binds to and activates sodium channels of both somatic and autonomic nerves, leading to the spontaneous firing of neurons.[1,3] Water follows the influx of sodium ions, leading to swelling of nodes of Ranvier and perisynaptic Schwann cells.[1,3]
- Ciguatera fish poisoning is characterized by nausea, diarrhea, and abdominal pain within 30 minutes to 12 hours after consumption of fish and can last for 1 day to 7 days.[3] As the gastrointestinal (GI) symptoms improve, the neurologic symptoms emerge, with paresthesia (perioral and distal), cold allodynia (pain when touching cold objects), myalgias, pruritus, bradycardia, and, rarely, hypotension and transient cerebellar symptoms (ataxia and tremor).[3,4] Cold allodynia is almost pathognomonic of ciguatera poisoning. Reported chronic symptoms after ciguatera poisoning are unlikely related to a pathophysiologic effect of toxin ingestion. Anxiety and depression should be considered in cases labeled as chronic ciguatera poisoning.
- The neurologic examination typically shows findings of length-dependent sensory polyneuropathy, with small fiber greater than large fiber sensory involvement. There is no cranial nerve involvement, muscle weakness, or Romberg sign.
- The differential diagnosis includes neurotoxic shellfish poisoning, paralytic shellfish poisoning, pufferfish poisoning, botulism, and Guillain-Barré syndrome (**Table 1**).[2] The diagnosis is clinical and depends on eliciting a history of ingestion of reef fish and recognizing typical symptoms. There is no current test to detect the toxin or biomarkers in humans; however, the Food and Drug Administration can perform analysis on the remainders of the implicated fish, but results are not available promptly.[2] Nerve conduction study findings range from normal in mildly affected patients to slowing of sensory and motor nerve conduction velocities, without a reduction in amplitudes in other more severely affected patients; however, these electrodiagnostic findings are not specific to ciguatoxin exposure.[5]
- Treatment of ciguatera poisoning is symptomatic and supportive. Mannitol was not superior to normal saline in a double-blind randomized trial.[6] Mortality of ciguatera fish poisoning is less than 0.5% and is related to severe dehydration

Table 1
Comparison of neurotoxicity from ciguatoxin, tetrodotoxin and Botulinum Toxin

	Ciguatoxin	Tetrodotoxin	Botulinum Toxin (Foodborne)
Exposure	Consumption of reef fish	Consumption of pufferfish, shellfish	Consumption of improperly canned or refrigerated food
Molecular target	Sodium channels	Fast-type sodium channels	Presynaptic proteins (SNAP-25, synabtoprevin, syntaxin)
Generalized symptoms	Nausea, diarrhea, abdominal pain, hypotension, bradycardia	Vomiting, diarrhea, dermatologic changes, hypotension, bradycardia	Dry mouth, nausea, vomiting, dysphagia, fatigue, dilated pupils
Neurologic symptoms	Headache, paresthesia, cold allodynia, transient ataxia	Paresthesia, dysesthesias, quadriparesis	Diplopia, symmetric cranial nerve involvement with rapid descending paralysis
Treatment	Supportive care	Supportive care	Heptavalent botulinum antitoxin, supportive care

secondary to the GI symptoms or hypotension/bradycardia from the autonomic symptoms.[2]

TETRODOTOXIN

- Tetrodotoxin is a neurotoxin found in many pufferfish species and rarely in shellfish, snails, octopus, mollusks, and frogs.[7,8] The toxin is produced by bacteria, mainly *Vibrio* species, that bioaccumulates in the pufferfish.[9] The liver, intestines, muscles, ovaries, and skin of the pufferfish contain the toxin.[8] Oral consumption of this heat-stable toxin at cooking temperatures produces the symptoms in humans.
- The incidence is 30 to 50 cases per year[8] and is seen mainly throughout the Pacific Ocean (Japan), where pufferfish is a culinary delicacy and the Baja California coastal region.[9] Tetrodotoxin is a fast-type sodium channel blocker that depresses action potential generation in neurons and skeletal muscles. It affects sensory neurons more rapidly than motor neurons.[10]
- The onset of symptoms of pufferfish poisoning is variable and depends on the amount of the ingested tetrodotoxin; it is typically 5 minutes to several hours after ingestion. Systemic symptoms include vomiting, diarrhea, bradycardia, hypotension, dermatologic abnormalities (blistering and petechiae), and hypersalivation.[8,10] The neurologic manifestations include dysesthesias and paresthesia (trunk and extremities) and can progress to flaccid quadriparesis, bulbar, and facial weakness. There are 4 grades of clinical severity (**Table 2**).[10] The differential diagnosis includes Guillain-Barré syndrome, botulism, and ciguatera fish poisoning. Nerve conduction studies show prolongation of the latency and decrease in the amplitude of the sensory responses and prolongation of the distal latency and F-wave latency and decrease in the amplitude and conduction velocity of the motor responses without conduction blocks or temporal dispersion.[11] Increases in stimulus intensity needed to elicit sensory and motor responses also occur. These abnormalities resolve as symptoms improve.

Table 2
Clinical grading of tetrodotoxication

Grade 1	Perioral numbness and paresthesia (sensation of tingling, tickling, prickling, pricking, or burning of a person's skin), with or without GI symptoms
Grade 2	Lingual numbness (numbness of face and other areas), early motor paralysis and incoordination, slurred speech with normal reflexes
Grade 3	Generalized flaccid paralysis (reduced muscle tone without other obvious cause), respiratory failure, aphonia (the inability to produce voice due to disruption of the recurrent laryngeal nerve), and fixed/dilated pupils (conscious patient)
Grade 4	Severe respiratory failure and hypoxia (inadequacy of oxygen), hypotension (low blood pressure), bradycardia (resting heart rate of under 60 beats per minute), cardiac dysrhythmias (irregular heartbeat), and unconsciousness may occur

- The diagnosis is clinical and depends on eliciting a history of puffer fish ingestion in the appropriate clinical context. Testing for tetrodotoxin in human urine and blood is possible but does not give timely results.
- Supportive care is the primary mode of treatment. The symptoms are transient and typically resolve in 24 hours.[10] Patients with severe symptoms should be admitted to an intensive care unit for observation in case respiratory failure or cardiac effects occur.
- The mortality rate is low. Fatalities can occur as a result of respiratory failure.[7] Regulatory limits for tetrodotoxin in food have been established in Japan as a method of prevention.[10]

BOTULISM

- Botulism is a nationally reportable disease caused by botulinum toxin. Botulinum toxin is produced by *Clostridium botulinum*—an anaerobic gram-positive spore-forming bacillus.[12] There are 7 subtypes of botulinum toxin (A through G) that cause 5 distinct forms of botulism—infantile, foodborne, wound, adult intestinal colonization, and iatrogenic disease (**Table 3**).[12–14] Subtypes A, B, E, and F are the commonest causes of human botulism; types C and D predominantly affect animals; and type G is not known to cause disease at this time.[12] The toxin acts at the presynaptic terminals of the neuromuscular junction and inhibits acetylcholine release through interference with proteins involved in neurotransmitter vesicle fusion (**Table 4**). This results in decreased and/or blocking neural transmission in both autonomic and motor peripheral nerves.[12]
- Infantile botulism is the most common form of botulism and occurs as a result of subtype A (83%) or B (11%) botulinum toxin. Ingestion of honey is the most common cause, but it also has been linked to the ingestion of spores from dust and the environment.[12] The incidence is 2.1 cases per 100,000 live births or on average 105 cases per year. The median age of affected infants is 4 months.[12] The symptoms include constipation, weak cry, weak suck, hypotonia, ptosis, and respiratory distress. Neurologic examination reveals absent/decreased gag reflex, preserved reflexes, dilated pupils, and ophthalmoplegia. Approximately half of affected infants require intubation within 24 hours of presentation.[12] Treatment of infantile botulism includes the human-derived botulism immunoglobulin along with supportive treatment. Recovery occurs over weeks to months and most patients make a complete recovery. Mortality is 1.1% worldwide.[12]

Table 3
Comparison of the types of botulism

	Infantile Botulism	Foodborne Botulism	Wound Botulism	Adult Intestinal Botulism	Iatrogenic Botulism
Subtype involved	A (83%) or B (11%)	A (50%), E (37%), or B (10%)	A or B	A, B, or F	A or B
Exposure	Ingestion of honey, environmental spores (dust)	Improperly canned or refrigerated food	IV drug use, intranasal cocaine	Altered GI flora (instrumentation, recent antibiotic treatment)	Therapeutic/cosmetic use of botulinum toxin
Symptoms	Constipations, weak cry/suck, respiratory distress, hypotonia, ptosis	Dry mouth, nausea, vomiting, dysphagia, diplopia, paresthesia, rapid descending paralysis	Fever, dry mouth, diplopia, paresthesia, rapid descending paralysis	Dry mouth, nausea, vomiting, dysphagia, diplopia, paresthesia, rapid descending paralysis	Dry mouth, diplopia, paresthesia, rapid descending paralysis
Exam	Preserved muscle stretch reflexes, absent gag, dilated pupils, ophthalmoplegia	Fixed dilated pupils, cranial nerve abnormalities, weakness	Fixed dilated pupils, cranial nerve abnormalities, weakness	Fixed dilated pupils, cranial nerve abnormalities, weakness	Fixed dilated pupils, cranial nerve abnormalities, weakness
Treatment	Human-derived botulism immunoglobulin, supportive	Heptavalent botulinum antitoxin, supportive care	Heptavalent botulinum antitoxin, antibiotics, supportive care	Heptavalent botulinum antitoxin, supportive care	Heptavalent botulinum antitoxin, supportive care

- The foodborne type of botulism occurs from ingestion of improperly refrigerated, cooked, or canned food. Botulinum toxin subtypes A (50%), E (37%), and B (10%) cause foodborne botulism in decreasing order of frequency. Foodborne botulism due to subtype E is seen mostly in Alaska and is associated with consumption of seal oil, fermented whale/seal/fish, and fish eggs.[15] The incidence is 1 per 10 million people or an average of 19 cases per year.[12] Clinical manifestations include ptosis, diplopia, fixed dilated pupils, blurred vision, dysarthria, dysphagia, and dry mouth, which are followed by a rapidly progressive descending paralysis that involves the cranial nerves.[12,15] Abdominal pain, nausea, vomiting, and diarrhea, thought to be due to food contaminants, precede neurologic manifestations. Botulism due to subtype A botulinum toxin is associated with a more severe illness and higher mortality rate. Treatment of adults includes the heptavalent botulinum antitoxin and supportive care. The mortality for botulism due to subtype A is 5%, subtype B is 4%, and subtype E is 3%. Poor prognostic factors include older age, history of congestive heart failure or coronary artery disease, shortness of breath or dysphagia at the time of presentation, and the need for mechanical ventilation.
- The wound botulism type occurs in IV drug users, specifically subcutaneous infiltration of black tar heroin, known as skin popping, but also can occur with sinusitis due to intranasal use of cocaine. The underlying botulinum toxin subtypes are A and B. The average incidence in the United States is 20 cases per year. The symptoms are similar to foodborne botulism (dry mouth, dysphagia, diplopia, and rapidly progressive descending paralysis) but there are no GI symptoms. The incubation period (4–14 days) is longer than foodborne botulism, likely reflecting the time needed for colonization, growth, and adequate toxin production by Clostridium botulinum. Treatment consists of antitoxin administration, antibiotics, wound débridement, and supportive care.
- The adult intestinal colonization type of botulism occurs due to subtype A, B, or F in patients with altered GI flora due to GI disease, instrumentation, or recent antibiotics. The average incidence in the United States is 1 case per year.[12] The symptoms are similar to foodborne botulism—dry mouth, nausea/vomiting, dysphagia, diplopia, and fixed dilated pupils, which are followed by a rapidly progressive descending paralysis that involves the cranial nerves.[12] The treatment is antitoxin administration and supportive care.
- Iatrogenic botulism is due to an adverse event after therapeutic or cosmetic use of botulinum toxin. Symptoms are similar to foodborne botulism, but patients do not have GI symptoms. The treatment includes antitoxin administration and supportive care. The prognosis is good.

Table 4
Botulinum toxin types and site of action

Botulinum Toxin Type	Site of Action	Other Characteristics
A	SNAP-25	Most toxic botulinum toxin serotype
B	Synaptobrevin	Less toxic than type A
C	Syntaxin and SNAP-25	Mainly cause animal disease
D	Synaptobrevin	Mainly cause animal disease
E	SNAP-25	Produced by Clostridium butyricum
F	Synaptobrevin	Produced by Clostridium baratii
G	Synaptobrevin	Not known to cause human disease

- The differential diagnosis of botulism includes Guillain-Barré syndrome, myasthenia gravis, or even acute brainstem infarct due to the involvement of cranial nerves.[12,13,15] The presence of any to all of the effects of botulinum toxin cholinergic blockade (dilated pupils, dry mouth, dry eyes, palmoplantar anhidrosis, and constipation) helps differentiate acute presentations of autoimmune neuromuscular junction disorders from botulism. A diagnosis is confirmed by botulinum toxin identification (ELISA or polymerase chain reaction) in serum, stool, or the food source.[12,13] Electrodiagnostic testing shows variable findings, depending on the severity of the symptoms, but commonly shows decreased compound muscle action potential amplitudes with normal velocities and latencies, post-tetanic facilitation (30%–100%), and short duration low-amplitude motor unit action potentials. Single-fiber electromyography shows increased jitter with blocking and can be the only abnormality in patients with mild botulism.[16] Repetitive nerve stimulation can be used to distinguish between Guillain-Barré syndrome and botulism—a decremental response to low-frequency repetitive nerve stimulation and incremental response to high-frequency repetitive stimulation is seen in botulism.[16]

BLACK WIDOW SPIDER VENOM

- The black widow spider venom contains the neurotoxin α-latrotoxin and is found in 5 species of widow spiders in North America.[17] Exposures rise in the spring and continue to increase throughout the summer, with peak exposures in September.[18] Widow spiders prefer dark and damp areas to live, like garages and storage/outdoor areas, and make their webs near ground level. They also tend to hide in boots/gloves that have been in storage; therefore, most bites are on the extremities.
- α-Latrotoxin binds to the presynaptic neuronal receptor and inserts itself into the neuronal membrane, becoming a transmembrane channel that leads to an independent influx of extracellular calcium.[19,20] Presynaptic calcium entry triggers uncontrolled exocytosis of neurotransmitters with resultant acetylcholine release at the neuromuscular junction that causes muscle contraction. The toxin also causes the release of other neurotransmitters (norepinephrine, glutamate, dopamine, and γ-aminobutyric acid) and prevents neurotransmitter reuptake, which leads to prolonged stimulation of the muscles and sustained painful muscle contractions.
- Symptoms of a black widow spider bite include erythema and edema around the bite site 1 hour after exposure along with generalized muscle pain, abdominal cramps with abdominal muscle rigidity, and autonomic disturbances (diaphoresis, hypertension, and tachycardia). Pain develops at the site of the bite and progresses throughout the body, with muscle contractions that range from mild aching to debilitating pain. Differential diagnosis includes any medical or surgical condition that produces acute abdomen due to the amount of rigidity seen in the abdomen. Target skin lesion at the bite site and diaphoresis of the bitten limb are suggestive of a black widow spider bite. Rhabdomyolysis and renal failure can occur as a result of prolonged muscle rigidity and compartment syndrome, but this is exceedingly rare.
- Treatment includes wound care and tetanus prophylaxis. Opioids and benzodiazepines are used for pain control and muscle relaxation.[21] Antivenom is recommended for moderate to severe latrodectism but is rarely used (4% of exposures) due to concerns for anaphylaxis, as it is derived from horse serum. The symptoms typically are self-limited and resolve 24 hours to 72 hours after exposure.

RHABDOMYOLYSIS

- Rhabdomyolysis indicates the dissolution of skeletal muscle. The term is used interchangeably with myoglobinuria. Patients with rhabdomyolysis present with muscle pain, weakness, swelling, and dark urine.[22] Creatine kinase (CK) is typically elevated more than 1000. A large proportion of patients with rhabdomyolysis are asymptomatic and present only with elevated CK.[22] The annual incidence is approximately 26,000 cases in the United States. Laboratory evaluation reveals elevated CK, electrolyte abnormalities depending on the severity, and heme-positive urine without hematuria on urine dipstick in patients with myoglobinuria.
- General management of rhabdomyolysis involves stopping the offending drug or toxin, paying particular attention to circulatory volume, urine output, electrolyte abnormalities, and possible complications of rhabdomyolysis.[23] Multiple severe complications that portend poor prognosis include disseminated intravascular coagulation, extreme hyperkalemia, acute renal failure, and cardiac arrhythmias (**Box 1**). Mortality in patients with rhabdomyolysis is variable according to the cause and complications and ranges from 3.4% to 59%.[23] There are numerous causes of rhabdomyolysis, including myriad genetic muscle disorders; however, this discussion is limited to toxin-induced immobility or excess activity, toxin-induced hypokalemia, metabolic poisons, medication-induced myopathy, and direct-acting myotoxins.

Toxin-Induced Immobility or Excess Activity

- Toxins and drugs are the most common cause of rhabdomyolysis and can induce rhabdomyolysis by various mechanisms.[22] One of these mechanisms is immobility or excess activity of muscles, which in turn causes muscle injury. Once the muscle fibers are injured, intracellular contents leak from myocytes into the circulation, which leads to further complications.
- Central nervous system depression with loss of consciousness is common and can be associated with extended periods of immobility with sustained pressure on large muscle groups, which leads to ischemic muscle injury.[22] Compression neuropathies can occur in this subset of patients. Drugs that induce central nervous system depression include narcotics, general anesthetics, benzodiazepines, tricyclic antidepressants, antihistamines, barbiturates, and ethanol.[22] Because of the mental status changes that occur with these medications, patients do not report symptoms of rhabdomyolysis, making acute renal failure the first manifestation of rhabdomyolysis in these patients.

Box 1
Complications of rhabdomyolysis

Local complications
  Compartment syndrome
  Compression neuropathies

Systemic complications
  Acute renal failure
  Electrolyte abnormalities (hyperkalemia, hyperphosphatemia, and hypocalcemia)
  Cardiac arrhythmia
  Disseminated intravascular coagulation

- Toxins also can cause extreme muscle activity (such as seizures, choreoathetosis, and dystonia), which causes excessive energy demands on muscles, leading to muscle injury.[22] Drugs that induce increased activity include cocaine, amphetamines, phencyclidine, lysergic acid diethylamide (LSD), and succinylcholine **(Table 5)**.

Toxin-Induced Hypokalemia

Hypokalemia is a known cause of rhabdomyolysis.[22] Several drugs and toxins can lead to hypokalemia, including diuretics, amphotericin B, chronic ingestion of licorice, barium poisoning, and insulin. The precise mechanism of hypokalemia-induced rhabdomyolysis is unknown but possible mechanisms include abnormally low blood flow with exercise, suppression of glycogenesis and glycogen storage, and altered ion transport.[24] Symptoms of hypokalemia can range from asymptomatic to paralysis. Acute hypokalemic myopathy usually occurs when serum potassium levels are less than 2 mEq/L. The clinical presentation includes proximal or generalized muscle weakness and elevated CK. Tendon reflexes can be absent. Vacuolar dilatation of T tubules can be seen in patients who undergo muscle biopsy. Fasting and exercise are known precipitants of rhabdomyolysis in the presence of hypokalemia.

Metabolic Poisons

Some toxins interfere with metabolic processes, such as the cellular production of adenosine triphosphate (ATP). Most metabolic toxins—hydrogen sulfide, phosphine, salicylate, chlorophenoxy herbicides, iodoacetate, and sodium fluoroacetate—are not common and are not discussed further. Cyanide and carbon monoxide (CO) are discussed further.

- Exposure to cyanide occurs via inhalation of smoke in house fires (combustion of fabrics) or through contaminated food or water or the use of antihypertensive medication sodium nitroprusside.[25] Cyanide disrupts the metabolism by binding to cytochrome c oxidase and blocks the mitochondrial electron transport chain, with subsequent inhibition of aerobic respiration in tissues. Acute cyanide poisoning manifests with headache, confusion, seizures, vomiting, cherry red coloring of the skin, and bitter almond breath.[26] Diagnosis of cyanide poisoning is suggested by the finding of high anion gap metabolic acidosis, elevated lactate level, and mixed venous oxygen saturation and confirmed by elevated blood cyanide levels.[26] Treatment of acute cyanide poisoning includes the antidote hydroxocobalamin followed by thiosulfate with supportive management. Prolonged exposure to cyanide can lead to spastic paraparesis, known as konzo, which is seen mostly in Africa. Konzo occurs as a result of the consumption of

Table 5
Classes of drugs associated with rhabdomyolysis due to hyperactivity or immobility of muscles

Mechanism	Drug List
Increased muscle activity leading to rhabdomyolysis	Cocaine, amphetamines, phencyclidine, sympathomimetics, LSD, succinylcholine
Immobility leading to rhabdomyolysis	Narcotics, general anesthetics, benzodiazepines, tricyclic antidepressants, antihistamines, ethanol, glutethimide, barbiturates

cyanogenic cassava. This is characterized by an acute/subacute onset of symmetric spastic paraparesis or tetraparesis along with paresthesia. Signs of severe disease include dysarthria and dysphagia. Neurophysiologic studies in a patient with konzo show inability to elicit motor evoked potentials, prolonged central motor conduction time with normal motor and sensory nerve conduction, and increased amplitudes of F waves.[25] Symptomatic treatment of konzo includes botulinum toxin injections for spasticity.[25] Konzo is a nonprogressive disease after the initial subacute onset.

- CO is a tasteless and odorless gas. Exposure occurs through house fires, malfunctioning heating systems, fuel-burning devices, and motor vehicles in poorly ventilated areas.[27] Incidence of CO poisoning peaks in the winter months. CO affects ATP production by competing with the binding of oxygen to hemoglobin and mitochondrial inhibition. Symptoms include headache, dizziness, generalized weakness, shortness of breath, and confusion. Characteristic findings include cherry red lips, cyanosis, and retinal hemorrhages. Severe symptoms, including seizures, cerebral edema, cardiac arrythmias, and pulmonary edema, can lead to death. Elevated venous blood carboxyhemoglobin levels in most cases confirm the diagnosis. Treatment includes high-flow normobaric oxygen or hyperbaric oxygen for very severe cases; however, consultation with a toxicologist is recommended.

Medication-Induced Myopathy

Medications can produce muscle damage in several ways—directly acting on muscle cells, damage secondary to electrolyte disturbances, immunologic reaction, excessive energy requirements, or inadequate oxygen delivery. Numerous medications can cause myopathy, but only a few of significant clinical importance are discussed.

- Statins: statins are 3-hydroxy-3-methyl-glutaryl-CoA reductase (HMG-CoA reductase) inhibitors that inhibit cholesterol synthesis. A variety of muscle symptoms can occur in patients taking statins. These include muscle pain, muscle cramps, hyperCKemia (asymptomatic or with muscle pain), hyperCKemia with muscle weakness, rhabdomyolysis, and immune-mediated necrotizing myopathy. There are tools to determine the relevance of statins to muscle symptoms in patients. These include the American College of Cardiology Statin Intolerance tool and The Statin-Associated Muscle Symptom Clinical Index.[28,29] The mechanism of direct myofiber injury due to statins remains unknown; however, the risk is increased in patients taking medications known to increase the risk of statin-related muscle symptoms. The immune-mediated necrotizing myopathy due to statins is known to be caused by antibodies directed against HMG-CoA reductase. These HMGCR antibodies are detectable in the serum.[30] Patients with HMGCR antibodies due to statins develop hyperCKemia and insidious weakness while on a statin. CK level of 40,000 U/L can occur. The duration of statin exposure before developing immune-mediated necrotizing myopathy ranges from weeks to years. Electrodiagnostic studies show myopathy with spontaneous activity in the form of fibrillation potentials and positive sharp waves. Myotonic discharges are not uncommon. Muscle biopsy demonstrates scattered myofiber necrosis with no to mild endomysial inflammation (**Fig. 1**). There also is a sarcolemmal up-regulation of the major histocompatibility complex (MHC)-1 and a sarcolemmal deposition of the membrane attack complex (MAC) on non-necrotic myofibers. Treatment of all muscle symptoms related to statins includes statin discontinuation as the first step. In patients with rhabdomyolysis,

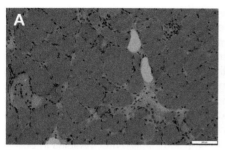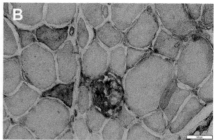

Fig. 1. (*A*) Hematoxylin-eosin section, original magnification x 40, displays an excessive variation of fiber size, an increase in internal nuclei, necrotic fibers replaced by macrophages, and regenerating fibers. (*B*) MHC-1 immunostained section, original magnification x 40, displays up-regulation of MHC-1 in macrophages replacing a necrotic fiber and sarcolemmal as well as sarcoplasmic up-regulation of MHC-1 in a regenerating fiber.

hyperCkemia, or myalgia, the symptoms improve within 2 months to 3 months after statin cessation; in immune-mediated necrotizing myopathy, however, statin discontinuation is not sufficient and immunosuppressive therapy is started. Typically, prednisone or intravenous (IV) solumedrol is used but in patients with a high risk of steroid side effects, IV immunoglobulin (IVIG) is considered. There are reports of IVIG monotherapy in HMGCR antibody necrotizing myopathy. Rituximab is a third line of treatment. Proprotein convertase subtilisin/kexin type 9 (PCSK9) inhibitors are safe when used instead of statins in patients with HMGCR antibody myopathy.[31]

- Corticosteroids: corticosteroid myopathy may occur with prednisone (or equivalent) doses greater than 10 mg daily and is dose-dependent. The mechanism of steroid myopathy appears to be interference with messenger RNA synthesis and, in turn, muscle protein synthesis. Patients present with progressive proximal limb-girdle weakness and atrophy. CK is normal or decreased. Elevated CK while on prednisone should suggest another myopathic process causing myofiber necrosis. Electrodiagnostic studies are normal in steroid myopathy. Muscle biopsy demonstrates type 2 fiber atrophy. The symptoms improve as the prednisone is decreased or stopped.
- Zidovudine: zidovudine is a nucleoside analog used in the management of human immunodeficiency virus (HIV). It causes a reversible, dose-dependent myopathy in 20% of patients on the medication.[24] Mitochondrial dysfunction due to zidovudine-induced inhibition of mitochondrial DNA polymerase is the mechanism by which zidovudine causes myopathy. Patients present with myalgias, fatigue, and limb-girdle weakness associated with mildly elevated CK. The symptoms improve with medication withdrawal. Myopathy due to zidovudine is difficult to distinguish from HIV myopathy; however, muscle biopsy in zidovudine myopathy shows ragged-red fibers and cytochrome-c oxidase–negative fibers without the inflammatory cell infiltrates seen in patients with HIV myopathy.
- Chloroquine and hydroxychloroquine: these medications are used for malaria treatment. Hydroxychloroquine is now more commonly used for the treatment of autoimmune diseases, such as systemic lupus erythematosus. The annual incidence of antimalarial myopathy is 1.2% in patients on chloroquine/hydroxychloroquine; however, only 8 of the 119 patients were on hydroxychloroquine in the studied cohort.[32] Autophagic myopathy due to hydroxychloroquine is less frequent and severe. Both medications are amphiphilic compounds with

hydrophilic and hydrophobic components. They interfere with lysosomal function and cause neuromyopathy. Patients develop a painless, slowly progressive proximal lower extremity weakness that eventually involves the upper extremities and sometimes facial muscles. Concurrently, patients have distal sensory loss and areflexia. CK levels are normal or slightly elevated. Electrodiagnostic studies show fibrillation potentials and myotonic discharges along with slowing on nerve conduction studies and myopathic motor unit action potentials. Muscle biopsy shows autophagic vacuoles that affect primarily type 1 fibers.[24] The prognosis is good with improvement after medication cessation.

- Colchicine: myopathy can develop with long-term colchicine use. Colchicine is most used to treat gout. Colchicine myopathy occurs most frequently in older patients who have mild chronic renal insufficiency. The mechanism of myopathy is related to colchicine's antimicrotubular activity that disrupts the cytoskeletal network, which results in intracellular accumulation of autophagic vacuoles.[24] Patients present with subacute proximal weakness and peripheral neuropathy.[24] Symptoms tend to resolve within 3 weeks to 4 weeks after medication cessation.

- Cyclosporine: cyclosporine is an immunosuppressive drug that is commonly used in transplant patients. Myopathy due to cyclosporine typically occurs in the context of concurrent colchicine or statin treatment. Patients develop myalgias and proximal weakness within months of starting the medication. Elevated CK and myoglobinuria can occur.[24] Electrodiagnostic studies demonstrate normal nerve conductions studies, fibrillations, positive sharp waves, occasional myotonic potentials, and myopathic motor unit potentials. Muscle biopsy shows myofiber necrosis and type 2 myofiber atrophy. Symptoms improve with reduction or cessation of cyclosporine.

- Labetalol: labetalol is a β-blocker commonly used for the treatment of hypertension. It rarely can result in pain proximal weakness with significant hyperCKemia. The authors encountered labetalol necrotizing myopathy in a patient treated with labetalol for preeclampsia. The pathogenesis is unknown, but muscle pathology typically shows necrotic and regenerating fibers. Symptoms improve with medication cessation.

- Amiodarone: amiodarone is used to treat cardiac arrhythmia. Rarely, it can lead to the development of neuromyopathy. The neuropathy component typically predominates the clinical picture. Amiodarone is an amphiphilic drug that interacts with components of the cell membrane and organelles and can interfere with lysosomal function. Patients present with proximal and distal muscle weakness along with distal sensory loss and areflexia representative of the polyneuropathy component. The muscle weakness is more severe in the legs. CK can be normal or elevated. Electrodiagnostic studies show reduced amplitudes and slow conduction velocities, distal neurogenic changes, and proximal myopathic changes with spontaneous activity in the form of fibrillation potentials and positive sharp waves. Muscle biopsy reveals autophagic vacuoles and myofiber necrosis. The weakness improves over months after stopping amiodarone, but the improvement can be partial.

- Immune checkpoint inhibitors
  ○ Immune checkpoint inhibitors represent a newer class of anticancer drugs used to treat various cancers, including melanoma, renal cell carcinoma, and small cell lung cancer. These medications prevent negative regulation of T cells by interacting with cell membrane receptors, in turn, enhancing the immune response against cancer cells. Ipilimumab inhibits cytotoxic T-lymphocyte–associated protein 4 (CTLA-4), pembrolizumab and nivolumab inhibit

programmed cell death protein 1 (PD-1), and avelumab and atezolizumab inhibit programmed cell death protein ligand 1 (PD-L1).

o The neurologic complications of immune checkpoint inhibitors include myasthenia gravis with or without myopathy, encephalopathy, polyradiculoneuropathy mimicking Guillain-Barré syndrome, autonomic neuropathy, aseptic meningitis, and transverse myelitis.

o Patients with immune checkpoint inhibitor myopathy develop symptoms of myalgia and muscle weakness in limb-girdle, axial, and oculobulbar weakness. These symptoms start in 2 months from treatment onset and progressively worsen. Associated myocarditis and myasthenia gravis can occur with positive acetylcholine receptor antibodies and a decremental response on slow repetitive nerve stimulations.

o CK is elevated in the thousands.[33] Electrodiagnostic findings include myopathic motor unit potentials with spontaneous activity in the form of fibrillations and positive sharp waves. Muscle biopsy demonstrates myophagocytosis, endomysial inflammatory exudate consisting of $CD68^+$ $PD-L1^+$ and $PD-L2^+$ macrophages and $CD8^+$ $PD-1^+$ T lymphocytes, and sarcolemmal MHC-1 up-regulation.

o The American College of Clinical Oncology published a guideline for the treatment of immune checkpoint inhibitor myopathy (**Table 6**).[34] Management depends on the grade of toxicity and may include continuing the immune checkpoint inhibitor with monitoring to discontinuing the immune checkpoint inhibitor and starting immunosuppression. The weakness improves and CK trends down with these measures.

o Rechallenge with the same agent that caused the myopathy can be considered on an individual basis and can be successful.[35]

- Direct-acting myotoxins

Few toxins act directly on muscles to cause muscle injury. These include myotoxin a, crotamine, and phospholipase A2, which are found in snake venoms. The average annual number of native US venomous snakebites is 4735.[36] Up to 25% of snakebites are dry bites without venom injection. Myotoxins are components of the venom of sea

Table 6	
Management of immune checkpoint inhibitor myopathy	
Severity	**Management**
Mild weakness with or without pain, no CK elevation	• Can continue immune checkpoint inhibitor with continued monitoring • Analgesia
Moderate weakness limiting age-appropriate instrumental activities of daily living with or without pain	• Hold immune checkpoint inhibitor temporarily with continued monitoring • Analgesia • Prednisone <10 mg per day, but if the patient worsens treat as in severe weakness
Severe weakness limiting self-care activities of daily living and/or CK higher than 3 times	• Hold immune checkpoint inhibitor • Analgesia • Start oral prednisone • Consider IV solumedrol if there is associated dysphagia, respiratory muscle weakness, or myocarditis • Consider IVIG, plasmapheresis, and other oral immunosuppressive medications

snakes, Australian tiger snakes, and north/south American rattlesnakes. Rattlesnakes are found in much of the United States; however, a majority of rattlesnake bites occur in warmer climate states, such as California, Arizona, New Mexico, Texas, and Florida.[34] These myotoxins produce myonecrosis. Rattlesnake poisoning presents with initial local tissue effects, such as swelling, blister formation, erythema, and pain, within 30 minutes to 2 hours of a bite. Bullae, ecchymosis, and necrosis then develop over time and can lead to autoamputation, particularly with bites to the distal extremities. Systemic symptoms also can occur and include nausea, vomiting, diaphoresis, hypotension, tachycardia, coagulopathies, and anaphylaxis.[34] In rare circumstances, compartment syndrome can occur due to swelling from significant myonecrosis. Treatment consists of antivenom and symptomatic treatment. There are 2 antivenoms available: crotalidae polyvalent immune Fab (CPIF) and crotalidae immune Fab2 (CIF). CIF was developed more recently and made available in 2018 and has a longer half-life than CPIF. Dry bites without venom injection do not need the antivenom. Clinical improvement usually occurs after antivenom dosing if needed; however, 50% of patients may have a recurrence of symptoms and need to be monitored. Prognosis is good as deaths due to rattlesnake bites are rare (average of 5–6 per year) and are seen mostly in children and the elderly.

SUMMARY

Toxic and medication-induced channelopathies, neuromuscular junction disorders, and myopathies are not uncommon. The mechanisms of toxicity can be direct action on a sodium channel or immunologic. These drug-mediated and toxic syndromes are rarely thought of in the daily practice of medicine. Immediate recognition and rapid institution of specific therapeutic measures are needed for reversal or amelioration of symptoms.

CLINICS CARE POINTS

- Inquiring about history of sea food ingestion in the emergency department, in a patient with GI symptoms followed by acute paresthesia and myalgia, is essential in leading to the diagnosis of ciguatera fish poisoning.
- Botulism is commonly mistaken for myasthenic crisis due to the acute onset of rapidly progressive craniobulbar weakness followed by descending weakness. A high index of suspicion is important to avoid immunotherapy.
- Black widow spider venom rarely causes rhabdomyolysis. It is important to consider other potential etiologies before attributing rhabdomyolysis to the spider bite.
- Eliciting a history of statin use in a patient with progressive weakness and significant hyperCKemia should prompt testing for HMGCR antibodies.
- Weakness and significant hyperCKemia in the setting of treatment of an underlying cancer with immune checkpoint inhibitors should prompt urgent neuromuscular evaluation and treatment

DISCLOSURE

J. Janecek has nothing to disclose. H. Kushlaf served as a consultant on advisory boards for Alexion, Catalyst Pharmaceuticals, and PTC therapeutics and is on the speakers bureau of Akcea, Catalyst Pharmaceuticals, and Sanofi Genzyme.

REFERENCES

1. Pearn J. Neurology of ciguatera. J Neurol Neurosurg Psychiatry 2001;70(1):4–8.

2. Friedman MA. Ciguatera fish poisoning: treatment, prevention and management. Mar Drugs 2008;6(3):456–79.

3. Zhang X, Cao B, Wang J, et al. Neurotoxicity and reactive astrogliosis in the anterior cingulate cortex in acute ciguatera poisoning. Neuromolecular Med 2013; 15(2):310–23.

4. Dickey RW, Plakas SM. Ciguatera: A public health perspective. Toxicon 2010; 56(2):123–36.

5. Cameron J, Flowers AE, Capra MF. Electrophysiological studies on ciguatera poisoning in man (Part II). J Neurol Sci 1991;101:93–7.

6. Schnorf H, Taurarii M, Cundy T. Ciguatera fish poisoning:a double-blind randomized trial of mannitol therapy. Neurology 2002;58:873–80.

7. Lorentz MN, Stokes AN, Rößler DC, et al. Tetrodotoxin. Curr Biol 2016;26(19): R870–2.

8. Lago J, Rodríguez L, Blanco L, et al. Tetrodotoxin, an extremely potent marine neurotoxin: distribution, toxicity, origin and therapeutical uses. Mar Drugs 2015; 13(10):6384–406.

9. Liu S-H, Tseng C-Y, Lin C-C. Is neostigmine effective in severe pufferfish-associated tetrodotoxin poisoning? Clin Toxicol 2014;53(1):13–21.

10. Bane V, Lehane M, Dikshit M, et al. Tetrodotoxin: chemistry, toxicity, source, detection. Toxins 2014;6(2):693–755.

11. Oda K, Araki K, Totoki T, et al. Nerve conduction study of human tetrodotoxication. Neurology 1989;39:743–5.

12. Berkowitz AL. Tetanus, botulism, and diphtheria. Continuum (Minneap Minn) 2018;24(5):1459–88.

13. Sobel J. Botulism. Clin Infect Dis 2005;41(8):1167–73.

14. Austin JW, Leclair D. Botulism in the north: a disease without borders. Clin Infect Dis 2011;52(5):593–4.

15. Rao AK, Lin NH, Jackson KA, et al. Clinical Characteristics and Ancillary Test Results Among Patients with Botulism—United States, 2002–2015. Clin Infect Dis 2017;66(suppl_1):S4–10.

16. Padua L, Aprile I, Monaco ML, et al. Neurophysiological assessment in the diagnosis of botulism: Usefulness of single-fiber EMG. Muscle Nerve 1999;22(10):1388–92.

17. Saibil HR. The black widow's versatile venom. Nat Struct Biol 2000;7(1):3–4.

18. Monte AA, Bucher-Bartelson B, Heard KJ. A US perspective of symptomatic latrodectus spp. envenomation and treatment: a national poison data system review. Ann Pharmacother 2011;45(12):1491–8.

19. Garb JE, Hayashi CY. Molecular evolution of α-latrotoxin, the exceptionally potent vertebrate neurotoxin in black widow spider venom. Mol Biol Evol 2013;30(5):999–1014.

20. Südhof TC. α-latrotoxin and its receptors: neurexins and CIRL/latrophilins. Annu Rev Neurosci 2001;24(1):933–62.

21. Clark RF, Wethern-Kestner S, Vance MV, et al. Clinical presentation and treatment of black widow spider envenomation: A review of 163 cases. Ann Emerg Med 1992;21(7):782–7.

22. Warren JD, Blumbergs PC, Thompson PD. Rhabdomyolysis: a review. Muscle Nerve 2002;25:332–47.

23. Bosch X, Poch E, Grau JM. Rhabdomyolysis and acute kidney injury. N Engl J Med 2009;361:62-72.

24. Sieb JP, Gillessen T. Iatrogenic and toxic myopathies. Muscle Nerve 2003;27(2): 142–56.

25. Tshala-Katumbay DD, Ngombe NN, Okitundu D, et al. Cyanide and the human brain: perspectives from a model of food (cassava) poisoning. Ann N Y Acad Sci 2016;1378(1):50–7.

26. Henretig FM, Kirk MA, Mckay CA. Hazardous chemical emergencies and poisonings. N Engl J Med 2019;380(17):1638–55.

27. Ernst A, Zibrak JD. Carbon monoxide poisoning. N Engl J Med 1998;339:1603–8.

28. American College of Cardiology. Statin intolerance. Available at: tools.acc.org/statinintolerance/#!/content/home. Accessed January 31, 2020.

29. Rosenson RS, Miller K, Bayliss M, et al. The Statin-associated Muscle Symptom Clinical Index (SAMS-CI): revision for clinical use, content validation, and inter-rater reliability. Cardiovasc Drugs Ther 2017;31(2):179–86.

30. Mammen AL, Chung T, Christopher-Stine L, et al. Autoantibodies against 3-hydroxy-3-methylglutaryl-coenzyme A reductase in patients with statin-associated autoimmune myopathy. Arthritis Rheum 2011;63:713–21.

31. Tiniakou E, Rivera E, Mammen AL, et al. Use of proprotein convertase subtilisin/kexin type 9 inhibitors in statin-associated immune-mediated necrotizing myopathy: a case series. Arthritis Rheumatol 2019;71(10):1723–6.

32. Casado E, Gratacós J, Tolosa C, et al. Antimalarial myopathy: an underdiagnosed complication? Prospective longitudinal study of 119 patients. Ann Rheum Dis 2006;65(3):385–90.

33. Touat M, Maisonobe T, Knauss S, et al. Immune checkpoint inhibitor-related myositis and myocarditis in patients with cancer. Neurology 2018;91(10):e985–94.

34. Brahmer JR, Lacchetti C, Schneider BJ, et al. Management of immune-related adverse events in patients treated with immune checkpoint inhibitor therapy: American Society of Clinical Oncology clinical practice guideline. J Clin Oncol 2018;36(17):1714–68.

35. Delyon J, Brunet-Possenti F, Leonard-Louis S, et al. Immune checkpoint inhibitor rechallenge in patients with immune-related myositis. Ann Rheum Dis 2019;78(11):e129.

36. Gold BS, Dart RC, Barish RA. Bites of venomous snakes. N Engl J Med 2002;347(5):347–56.

Section II
Neurotoxicology Syndromes: Central Nervous System

Toxin-Induced Acute Delirium

Alice Cai, MD[a,1], Xuemei Cai, MD[b,c,*]

KEYWORDS

- Delirium • Toxidrome • Anticholinergic • Sympathomimetic • Hallucinogen
- GABA withdrawal • Wernicke

KEY POINTS

- The differential of an acute mental status change includes toxic effects from commonly prescribed medications and drugs of abuse.
- Specific toxidromes present with a constellation of neurologic, psychiatric, and systemic effects that can lead to the diagnosis.
- Diagnosis must be made clinically, because drug screens do not include all substances, and there may be no specific laboratory or imaging findings.
- Certain drugs act on multiple receptors and can produce overlapping toxidrome effects.
- Toxidromes are treated with cessation of the offending drug, supportive care, and antidotal therapy.

INTRODUCTION

Delirium is an acute alteration of mental status triggered by a systemic illness or other underlying condition. The defining features are acute onset, fluctuating course, and inattention, often accompanied by disorganized thinking, hallucinations, and altered level of consciousness.[1] The key to resolving delirium is identifying and correcting the underlying cause.

The approach to patients with altered mental status is first to determine the time course of change from the patient's baseline. Encephalopathy with a time course of hours to days is strongly suggestive of a toxic, metabolic, or infectious cause. The differential broadly includes postoperative or hospital delirium, central nervous system (CNS) injury, infection, hyperammonemia, uremia, hypercarbia, hypernatremia or hyponatremia, hypercalcemia, carbon monoxide or other toxic poisoning, and polypharmacy. History of medication or drug exposures should be gathered from caregivers or pharmacies. Laboratory testing, including urine drug screen (UDS), serum

[a] Department of Neurology, University of Pennsylvania, Philadelphia, PA 19104, USA; [b] Department of Neurology, Tufts Medical Center, Boston, MA 02111, USA; [c] Department of Neurosurgery, Tufts Medical Center, Boston, MA 02111, USA
[1] Present address: 3400 Spruce Street, Gates 3, Philadelphia, PA 19103.
* Corresponding author. 800 Washington Street #314, Boston, MA 02111.
E-mail address: xcai@tuftsmedicalcenter.org

Neurol Clin 38 (2020) 781–798
https://doi.org/10.1016/j.ncl.2020.07.005
0733-8619/20/© 2020 Elsevier Inc. All rights reserved.

neurologic.theclinics.com

acetaminophen, salicylate, and ethyl alcohol (ETOH) levels, and electrolyte levels for anion gap, hyponatremia, renal dysfunction, liver function test increase, ammonia level increase, and glucose analysis, are essential in evaluation. An electrocardiogram (ECG) and cardiac monitoring is necessary in many cases, and head imaging with computed tomography (CT) or MRI should be considered.

This article focuses on the presentations of several toxidromes that result in acute delirium: anticholinergic syndrome, sympathomimetic syndrome, serotonin syndrome, hallucinogen intoxication, γ-aminobutyric acid (GABA) agonist withdrawal syndromes, and Wernicke encephalopathy. **Table 1** summarizes distinguishing features of each toxidrome and its antidote. Identifying the correct syndrome with cessation of the perpetrating agents and administration of the proper treatment can reverse potentially lethal toxicity.

Anticholinergic Syndrome

Anticholinergic syndrome is caused by compounds that competitively block cholinergic transmission in parasympathetic and some sympathetic sites. Certain medications are used primarily for these effects, but some anticholinergic symptoms are side effects of drugs with other targets.

Mechanism

Acetylcholine is the main excitatory neurotransmitter in the CNS and skeletal muscle. There are 2 types of acetylcholine receptors: nicotinic receptor (in the neuromuscular junction and autonomic ganglia) and muscarinic receptor. Classic anticholinergic drugs causing delirium act on muscarinic receptors and do not affect skeletal muscle, which expresses nicotinic receptors. These agents can be termed antimuscarinics.[2]

Muscarinic receptors have 5 subtypes. Different subtypes are expressed throughout the body to receive acetylcholine that is released preganglionically in sympathetic and parasympathetic synapses.

In the brain, acetylcholine controls higher cognitive processes, such as learning and memory. CNS acetylcholine levels have an impact on multiple neurodegenerative diseases. For example, cholinergic deficit and loss of cholinergic neurons in the basal forebrain are central to cognitive impairment in Alzheimer disease.[3] M4 and M5 receptors are involved in Parkinson's disease and schizophrenia.[4] Antimuscarinic compounds that bind to the M1 receptor subtype produce the most cognitive dysfunction, and those more selective against M3 (as in the case of certain overactive bladder medications) may produce the least.[4] Penetrability of the blood-brain barrier, administration of multiple drugs, and rate of CNS metabolism also contribute to severity of CNS toxicity. Toxicity is amplified in the setting of blood-brain barrier breakdown, such as in the case of older age, infection, multiple sclerosis, and diabetes.[5] Patients with baseline cognitive dysfunction and dementia are also at highest risk of developing delirium.

Clinics Care Points

- Identifying a cholinergic toxidrome can determine the over or under treatment of a disease such as myasthenia gravis. A patient with myasthenia presenting with weakness and respiratory distress is either in myasthenic crisis from under treatment, or in cholinergic crisis from overdosing of acetylcholinesterase inhibitors.

- The cholinergic crisis features lacrimation, emesis, diarrhea, and miosis. Excessive salivation occurs, but is also seen in myasthenic crisis due to dysphagia.

- A high dose of pyridostigmine is suggestive of cholinergic crisis. A detailed drug history with timing of administered or missed doses should be obtained.

Table 1
Distinguishing features of delirogenic toxidromes

Toxidrome	Classic Symptoms	Testing to Confirm Diagnosis	Antidote
Anticholinergic	Delirium, tachycardia, urinary retention, flushing, mydriasis. Distinguishing features: dry skin, hypoactive bowel sounds, lilliputian or Alice-in-Wonderland–type hallucinations	Clinical diagnosis	Physostigmine
Sympathomimetic	Euphoria, agitation, mydriasis, hypertension, tachycardia, diaphoresis	UDS	Benzodiazepines
Serotonin syndrome	AMS, anxiety, agitation. Distinguishing features: hyperreflexia and clonus, ocular clonus. Autonomic hyperactivity: tachycardia, hypertension, hyperthermia, diaphoresis. Distinguishing features: hyperactive bowel sounds	Clinical diagnosis	Cyproheptadine
Hallucinogen	Euphoria, altered perceptions, and hallucinations. Distinguishing features: feeling of boundlessness, dreamlike, dissociation	UDS	Benzodiazepines
GABA-A agonist withdrawal	AMS, hallucinations, anxiety, insomnia, delirium tremens (autonomic instability). Distinguishing features: seizures/status epilepticus	UDS, ETOH level	Benzodiazepines
Wernicke encephalopathy	AMS, ataxia. Distinguishing features: ophthalmoparesis, ocular cranial nerve deficits, confabulation	Lactate, pyruvate, thiamine levels, MRI brain	IV thiamine

Abbreviations: AMS, altered mental status; IV, intravenous.

Presentation

A well-known mnemonic for the anticholinergic toxidrome is mad as a hatter, for delirium; blind as a bat, for mydriasis; red as a beet, for flushing; hot as a hare, for fever; dry as a bone, for dry skin and mucus membranes; and full as a flask, for urinary retention. The delirium may be accompanied by anxiety, agitation, and paranoia. Hallucinations are specifically described as lilliputian type, or Alice-in-Wonderland type, where people appear to be larger and smaller. Outside of the mnemonic, bowel sounds are decreased or absent. Wide complex tachycardia with a prolonged QRS interval are reported with diphenhydramine and tricyclic antidepressant (TCA) overdoses.[6] Seizures and status epilepticus have also been reported. In some cases, central symptoms may persist after resolution of peripheral symptoms.

Lack of sweating and hypoactive bowel sounds differentiate this toxidrome from sympathomimetic toxicity. Drugs can have anticholinergic effects in addition to other receptor effects, causing a combination of poisonings. For example, sedatives with strong antihistamine effects (eg, TCAs) may have sedation and hypotension as the predominating symptoms.

Responsible medications

Atropine, hyoscyamine, and scopolamine are the typical antimuscarinics with potent effects. Antimuscarinics are prescribed widely across diseases. Plants containing belladonna alkaloids are also ingested for their hallucinogenic properties. **Table 2** lists anticholinergic drugs from the 2019 Beers Criteria list in addition to compounds from other risk scales.

Table 2
Drugs with antimuscarinic properties

Class/Indication	Drugs	Other Receptors
Antiarrhythmic	Disopyramide	Sodium channel blocker
Anticholinergics	Atropine	—
Antidepressants	Paroxetine	Serotonin reuptake inhibitor
Antihistamines (first generation > second generation)	Bropheniramine, carbinoxamine, chlorpheniramine, clemastine, dexbropheniramine, dexchlorpheniramine, dimenhydrinate, diphenhydramine, doxylamine, hydroxyzine, homatropine, methscopolamine, propantheline, meclizine, promethazine, pyrilamine, triprolidine	Antihistamine
Antiparkinson	Benzatropine, trihexyphenidyl	Antihistamine, dopamine reuptake inhibition
Antipsychotics (first generation > second generation)	Fluphenazine, perphenazine, thoridazine, chlorpromazine, loxapine, methotrimeprazine, trifluoperazine Clozapine, olanzapine, quetiapine (mild)	Antidopaminergic
Muscle relaxants	Cyclobenzaprine, tizanidine, orphenadrine	Central α2-adrenergic agonism Similar to TCAs
Spasmolytic (GI)	Clidinium, dicyclomine, glycopyrrolate, hyoscyamine, propantheline, scopolamine	—
TCAs	Amitriptyline, doxepin >6 mg, desipramine Imipramine, nortriptyline, protriptyline, trimipramine	Sodium channel blocker Serotonin agonism, noradrenergic agonism, histamine antagonism, α1-adrenergic antagonism, GABA-A antagonism
Urinary incontinence	Oxybutynin, tolterodine, trospium, fesoterodine, flavoxate, solifenacin	—
Plants	*Mandragora* spp (mandrake, Devil's herb), *Burgmansia* spp (angel's trumpet), *Datura* spp (moonflower, jimsonweed, Devil's trumpet), *Solanum erinthum*, *Garrya* spp, *Campsis grandiflora*, *Lamprocapsnos spectabilis* (bleeding heart), *Ilex paraguariensis* (yerba mate)[7]	—

Abbreviation: GI, gastrointestinal.

Data from American Geriatrics Society Beers Criteria Update Expert Panel. American Geriatrics Society 2019 Updated AGS Beers Criteria® for Potentially Inappropriate Medication Use in Older Adults. *J Am Geriatr Soc.* 2019;67:674-694 and Rudolph J, Salow M, Angelini M. The Anticholinergic Risk Scale and Anticholinergic Adverse Effects in Older Persons. *J Am Med Assoc.* 2008;168(5):508-513.

Treatment

Treatment is mainly supportive, ensuring stabilization of airway, breathing, and circulation. Some patients benefit from therapy from physostigmine, an anticholinesterase inhibitor that penetrates the blood-brain barrier. Observationally, it is superior to benzodiazepines in the setting of moderate to severe agitation in promoting faster recovery and preventing intubations, but there are no randomized trials for safety and efficacy.[8] It is currently recommended for patients showing both peripheral and moderate to severe central anticholinergic toxicity, and should be administered with the guidance of a toxicologist or local poison control. Administration requires atropine at half dose and resuscitation equipment at bedside, because rapid infusion can cause bradycardia and asystole. It may also precipitate seizures if administered too rapidly. Relative contraindications are reactive airway disease, intestinal obstruction, epilepsy, and cardiac conduction abnormalities. It is not recommended in TCA poisoning because of wide QRS intervals and reports of asystole in TCA poisoning following physostigmine administration.[9] The half-life is approximately 15 minutes; smaller doses may be administered 20 to 30 minutes later if agitated delirium recurs. Symptoms generally resolve 6.5 hours after initial dose, but continuous infusions have been given for prolonged toxicity.[10,11] patients who do not have anticholinergic syndrome or in whom the dose of physostigmine is too high develop cholinergic toxicity, featuring salivation, lacrimation, vomiting, diarrhea, urinary incontinence, bradycardia, and bronchospasm.

Like TCAs, severe diphenhydramine overdose also creates sodium channel blockade, leading to intraventricular conduction delay. Wide QRS intervals should be treated with sodium bicarbonate. Intravenous (IV) lipid emulsion has been used in cases refractory to sodium bicarbonate.[6] Hyperthermia is managed with cooling. Benzodiazepines may be used for agitation and seizures. Activated charcoal is considered if exposure was less than 1 hour prior.

Sympathomimetic Syndrome

Sympathomimetics are substances that stimulate the sympathetic nervous system through increasing availability of the catecholamines norepinephrine, epinephrine, and dopamine, which leads to an overloading of the natural fight-or-flight response. Sympathomimetics are abused for their euphoric and addictive properties, producing toxic short-term and long-term effects.

Mechanism

Sympathomimetic drugs are classified as direct acting, indirect acting, or mixed acting. Direct sympathomimetic agents act on α and β adrenergic receptors. $\alpha 1$ Receptors control vasoconstriction and smooth muscle contractions on small blood vessels. $\alpha 2$ Receptors provide inhibitory feedback. $\beta 1$ Receptors increase heart rate and renin secretion. $\beta 2$ Receptors stimulate vasodilation and bronchodilation. Indirect-acting drugs increase the availability of catecholamines by displacing them from cytosolic vesicles, inhibiting reuptake into sympathetic neurons, or blocking the metabolizing enzymes monoamine oxidase and catechol-o-methyltransferase. Mixed-acting drugs act via both mechanisms.

Agonists with different α and β binding profiles are administered for hypotension, reactive airway disease, and heart failure. Most of these agents do not cross the blood-brain barrier. Drugs that do penetrate the CNS act indirectly through norepinephrine and dopamine that are synthesized in the brain. They often become drugs of abuse because of their euphoric effects and stimulation of the reward pathway. Dopamine plays a critical role in executive function, emotional behavior, and reward, resulting in addiction. Movement disorders and psychiatric features, such as paranoia, delusions, homicidal and suicidal ideation, and hallucinations, result from deranged dopaminergic neurotransmission.[12] Norepinephrine controls numerous brain functions, including body temperature, reproduction, and respiration, and may regulate the brain's overall state of activation.[13] It is an α and $\beta 1$ agonist, producing vasoconstriction through predominantly α-mediated effects. Serotonin mediates the euphoric effects and is discussed further later.

> **Clinics Care Points**
>
> - For management of refractory cocaine hypertensive emergency and myocardial ischemia, use phentolamine 1 to 2.5 mg IV administered every 5 to 15 minutes for alpha-mediated hypertension.
> - Alternative agents include nitroglycerin and nitroprusside.
> - Avoid pure beta-blockers in treatment of hypertension, as they may cause coronary vasospasm with unopposed alpha adrenergic stimulation, although this is controversial.
> - Mixed beta/alpha blockers such as labetalol have been used for cocaine toxicity without evidence of unopposed alpha effects.

Presentation

Cocaine is the prototypical drug associated with this toxidrome. **Table 3** outlines other drugs with variations of the typical sympathomimetic presentation.

Initial intoxication produces enhanced alertness, self-confidence, and euphoria, as well as an increase in heart rate and blood pressure. The experience is followed by a crash of depression with craving for more of the drug. At higher doses, the patient experiences euphoria, insomnia, and anorexia. Repeated dosing or high doses lead to anxiety, paranoia, seizures, as well as aggression. Other neurologic signs and symptoms may be tremor, ataxia, seizures, and coma. Hypertension, hyperthermia, tachycardia, tachypnea, mydriasis, and diaphoresis feature prominently. Severe overdose may present with hypotension and cardiac arrhythmias caused by sodium channel blockade, arrhythmia, or ischemia.

Because of the vasoconstrictive effects of catecholamines, vascular complications are seen, including stroke, reversible cerebral vasoconstriction syndrome, subarachnoid hemorrhage, intraparenchymal hemorrhage, cardiac arrest, and mesenteric ischemia. Rhabdomyolysis caused by agitation and hyperthermia with hyperkalemia and metabolic acidosis may result from psychomotor agitation and can be lethal. In severe adrenergic crisis, hepatorenal failure and disseminated intravascular coagulation (DIC) may also occur.[14]

Treatment

Benzodiazepines blunt the hyperadrenergic response and are first-line therapy. Severe agitation should be controlled with short-acting IV benzodiazepines such as midazolam or lorazepam.

For hyperthermia, ice packs may be used; in severe cases, with temperature greater than 41.1°C, paralysis with intubation and further cooling is necessary. Tylenol is ineffective because the hyperthermia is generated by muscular activity and not by a central set point. IV fluids should be given for rhabdomyolysis.[17] Succinylcholine is not recommended during intubation because it can worsen rhabdomyolysis; instead, rocuronium or vecuronium is recommended. Lactic acidosis and electrolyte abnormalities should be evaluated and corrected.

Cardiac ischemia is managed with nitroglycerin, and nitroprusside or calcium channel blockers can be used for hypertension and tachycardia. B-Blockers alone for hypertension and tachycardia should be avoided, because unopposed α stimulation may worsen hypertension. B-Blockers with combined α and β suppression, such as labetalol and carvedilol, have been used in practice.[18] An ECG should be checked to monitor the corrected QT interval. In cases of shock, resuscitation may require norepinephrine to prevent neurotransmitter depletion, alongside large fluid volumes.

Among the various dosing methods, ingestion through stuffing or packing needs to be considered and is detected by CT. Patients may require removal of retained packages endoscopically or through laparotomy to prevent mesenteric ischemia.[19]

Table 3
Drugs causing central nervous system sympathomimetic toxicity

Drug	Differentiating Symptoms
Amphetamine derivatives: amphetamine, dextroamphetamine	Agitation, tachycardia, psychosis
Ephedra (ma huang), ephedrine, pseudoephedrine	—
Methamphetamine	—
Methylphenidate	—
Cathinones (bath salts), khat (mephedrone, MDPV)	—
Cocaine	Agitation, hypertension, tachycardia, diaphoresis
PCP	Detachment, agitation, psychosis, nystagmus
Methylxanthines: Caffeine (>1 g), theophylline	Seizures, vomiting Lack of severe vital sign changes
MAOIs	Hypertensive emergency Serotonin syndrome
Ketamine	Sensory illusions, altered cognition, learning difficulty, persecutory ideas
MDMA (ecstasy) MDEA (Eve)	Hallucinations, anxiety Lack of severe vital sign changes

Abbreviations: MAOIs, monoamine oxidase inhibitors; MDEA, methyl diethanolamine; MDMA, 3,4-methylene-dioxymethamphetamine; MDPV, methylenedioxypyrovaleron; PCP, phenylcyclohexyl piperidine.
   Data from Refs.[14–16]

Serotonin Syndrome

Serotonin syndrome is caused by the overactivation of central and peripheral serotonin receptors. It features a core triad of altered mental status, neuromuscular excitement, and autonomic hyperactivity.

Mechanism

Serotonin is a neurotransmitter that modulates numerous brain functions, ranging from anxiety, mood, aggression, and sexual behavior, to sleep-wake cycle, nociception, motor activity, and hallucinations. Serotonergic neurons are major constituents of the raphe nuclei in brainstem. These neurons project to the forebrain and the spinal cord, and overall are widely distributed, with various subpopulations creating the effects listed earlier.[20] There are 7 families of 5-hydroxytryptamine receptors (5-HT), and, although 5-HT2A may play the largest role, multiple receptors contribute to the development of the syndrome. Various drug classes increase serotonin levels through the following: inhibition of serotonin uptake, decreased serotonin metabolism, increased serotonin synthesis, increased serotonin release, and activation of serotonergic receptors. Certain serotonergic drugs also increase CNS noradrenergic activity because of their activity on monoamine transporters.

Peripheral serotonin is produced by intestinal enterochromaffin cells and plays a role in metabolism, gastrointestinal (GI) motility, nausea, vasoconstriction, uterine contraction, and bronchoconstriction.

Presentation

Serotonin syndrome presents with a core triad of altered mental status (anxiety, agitation, disorientation, restlessness), neuromuscular excitement (hyperreflexia, myoclonus, ocular clonus, inducible clonus, peripheral hypertonicity), and autonomic hyperactivity (mydriasis, hypertension, tachycardia, tachypnea, hyperthermia, diaphoresis, hyperactive bowel).[21]

Mild serotonin syndrome features mydriasis, tremor, myoclonus, and hyperreflexia. Patients are afebrile, and have mild hypertension and tachycardia.

Moderate serotonin syndrome features hyperthermia to 40°C, with the symptoms listed earlier, but also with ocular clonus, agitation, hypervigilance, and pressured speech, along with hyperactive bowel sounds.

Severe serotonin syndrome features hyperthermia greater than 41.1°C, swings in heart rate, blood pressure, delirium, and rigidity, especially in the lower extremities. In extreme cases, seizures, rhabdomyolysis, respiratory failure, DIC, coma, and death may occur.

The Hunter Serotonin Toxicity Criteria are used to clinically diagnose the syndrome. To meet the criteria, patients with exposure to a serotonergic agent within the last 5 weeks must show one of the following:

1. Spontaneous clonus
2. Inducible clonus and agitation or diaphoresis
3. Ocular clonus and agitation or diaphoresis
4. Tremor and hyperreflexia
5. Hypertonia and temperature greater than 38°C and ocular clonus or inducible clonus

These criteria have a sensitivity of 84% and specificity of 97% compared with diagnosis by a clinical toxicologist.[22]

Neuromuscular excitement contributes most specifically to diagnosis of the syndrome. Diaphoresis and hyperactive bowel sounds can help differentiate this toxidrome from anticholinergic syndrome. Malignant hyperthermia, a reaction to inhalational anesthetics and succinylcholine in patients with ryanodine receptor mutations, also presents with hypertonicity. However, skin flushing and hyporeflexia can help differentiate this from serotonin syndrome.[23] Neuroleptic malignant syndrome is an idiopathic reaction to dopamine antagonists. In contrast with serotonin syndrome, it results in lead pipe rigidity and bradykinesia, rather than hyperkinesia in serotonin syndrome, and has a slower onset of development.[24]

Clinics Care Points

- Serotonin syndrome, Malignant Hyperthermia, and Neuroleptic Malignant Syndrome may present with similar findings including fever, elevated CK, and confusion. Key differentiating factors are listed below:

- Exposure history in NMS includes neuroleptic medications or with levodopa withdrawal in Parkinson's disease. NMS is accompanied by autonomic instability (blood pressure fluctuations, tachycardia, diaphoresis, sialorrhea, and incontinence). Tone is rigid, and evolution of symptoms occurs over days.

- Malignant hyperthermia is triggered by inhaled anesthetic or succinylcholine. Masseter rigidity is classically found. Hypercarbia is also seen on end tidal CO2 monitoring.

- Serotonin syndrome can be differentiated from these conditions by history of serotonergic medication exposure. There is rapid onset under 24 hours, and rapid offset with treatment. There is hyperreflexia, clonus, and tremor, in contrast to the rigidity of NMS and the sustained muscle contraction of MH.

Responsible Medications

Development of serotonin syndrome may be concentration dependent above a certain threshold, and can result from a single agent or drugs in combination from drugs listed in **Table 4**. Monoamine oxidase inhibitors (MAOIs) producing irreversible inhibition, when used in combination with selective serotonin reuptake inhibitors (SSRIs),

Table 4	
Drugs associated with serotonin syndrome	
Drug Class	**Medications**
SSRIs	Sertraline, fluoxetine, paroxetine, citalopram, fluvoxamine
SNRIs	Venlafaxine
MAOIs	Phenelzine, moclobemide, clorgiline, isocarboxazid, selegiline, Syrian rue, linezolid
TCAs	Clomipramine
Triazolopyridine derivatives	Trazodone, nefazodone
Cytochrome inhibitors (eg, CYP2D6 and CYP3A4)	Ritonavir, Ccprofloxacin, fluconazole
Anticonvulsants and antimigraine	Sumatriptan, valproic acid
Analgesics	Fentanyl, meperidine, tramadol, pentazocine, oxycodone
Antiemetics	Metaclopromide, ondansetron, granisetron
Bariatric medications	Sibutramine
Cough medication	Dextromethorphan
Hallucinogens	MDMA, LSD
Herbal supplements	St John's wort, ginseng, tryptophan

Abbreviations: LSD, lysergic acid diethylamide; SNRIs, serotonin norepinephrine reuptake inhibitors; SSRIs, selective serotonin reuptake inhibitors.

Data from Mitchell P. Drug interactions of clinical significance with selective serotonin reuptake inhibitors. *Drug Saf.* 1997;17(6):390-406.

meperidine, or dextromethorphan, are strongly associated with severe serotonin syndrome. Self-inhibition of metabolism also results in accumulation of certain drugs; this exacerbates the risk of SSRI buildup with an SSRI and tramadol.[25] SSRIs such as fluoxetine have prolonged half-lives and produce potentially dangerous overlap within 5 weeks of discontinuation.

Treatment

Offending agents should be discontinued, with the knowledge that the drugs may take days to weeks to clear. Supportive care is the mainstay of treatment.

For moderate and severe cases, cyproheptadine, a 5HT-2A antagonist, may be administered at a dose of 12 mg, with an additional 2 mg every 2 hours if symptoms persist. A maintenance dose of 8 mg should be used every 6 hours once the patient is stabilized.[26] There is evidence of symptomatic resolution, but it is unclear whether cyproheptadine improves patient outcomes. Chlorpromazine, a 5HT-2A agonist available through IV routes, is not preferred because of risk of hypotension, Neuroleptic Malignant Syndrome (NMS), and dystonic reactions.

Similar to the treatment of sympathomimetic syndrome, benzodiazepines blunt additional hyperadrenergic symptoms and control agitation. Chemical sedation is preferred to physical restraint because of muscle contractions producing lactic acidosis and hyperthermia. Overheating results from muscle activity and is not corrected using traditional antipyretics. Instead, cooling and sedation are administered, with intubation and paralysis at temperatures greater than 41°C. Succinylcholine should be avoided.

Short-acting agents that decrease blood pressure, such as esmolol or nitroprusside, are preferred to long-acting agents in order to avoid hypotension. Patients on propranolol and an MAOI can present with hypotension, and propranolol should be avoided.

Hallucinogens

Hallucinogens are psychoactive drugs that alter people's awareness and their experience of their environment, creating sensory misconceptions and false perceptions.

They have been historically incorporated into rituals and traditional medicines, and were used as an adjunct for psychotherapy until 1966.

Mechanism

Classic serotonergic hallucinogens are divided structurally into indolamines and phenylethylamines. Indolamines include lysergic acid diethylamide (LSD), psilocybin, and N,N-dimethyltryptamine (DMT). Phenylethylamines include mescaline, 2,5-dimethoxy-4-methylamphetamine, and other compounds.[27] Indolamines and phenylethylamines activate 5-HT2 receptors in the corticostriatothalamic circuitry, which could alter thalamocortical transmission and produce hallucinations. LSD has a dopamine-mediated effect that also produces ideas of reference or paranoid ideation.

Another class of hallucinogens are dissociative drugs, which include the N-methyl-D-aspartate (NMDA) antagonists phenylcyclohexyl piperidine (PCP), ketamine, and dextromethorphan. It has been proposed that NMDA antagonism in the corticostriatothalamic circuitry could disrupt thalamic filter functions and produce sensory overload of the cortical area,[28] producing effects in a common downstream pathway similar to the serotonergic hallucinogens.

A third class of compounds, termed enactogens, produce psychedelic effects of thought disorders and derealization without hallucinations, and are structurally similar to stimulant amphetamines. 3,4-Methylenedioxymethamphetamine (MDMA) is in this category, and has more direct dopamine and α2-adrenergic activity, creating sympathomimetic effects.[29]

Presentation

Hallucinogenic compounds produce many neuropsychiatric effects. Perceptual symptoms include altered shapes and colors (eg, geometric hallucinations, perceptions of movement, image trails, halos, macropsia, and micropsia), sharpened sense of hearing, and synesthesia. Psychic symptoms include alterations in mood, distortions in time, derealization and depersonalization, out-of-body experiences, difficulty communicating thoughts, and visual hallucinations. These psychic symptoms are unique and unlike any mental status alteration that occurs in sympathomimetic or anticholinergic toxicity. Somatic symptoms also occur, including tremors, nausea, blurred vision, dizziness, paresthesias, and weakness.[30]

Cognitively, patients develop attentional deficits and distractibility, lapses in working memory, and disruptions in ability to plan. Experiences may be positive, featuring sublime happiness or grandiosity. Negative effects include paranoia, panic, anxiety, frightening imagery, to the loss of control over thoughts and intentionality and psychosis, with many properties similar to schizophrenia.[28] Patients may incur severe injury or death by staring at the sun or jumping out of windows as a result of impaired judgment while intoxicated.[31]

Nausea and vomiting often precede psychedelic symptoms. Other systemic symptoms are not prominent. However, in extreme LSD overdose greater than 400 μg, life-threatening cardiovascular collapse and hyperthermia may occur. Use of dissociative hallucinogens and MDMA may produce tachycardia, hypertension, and hyperthermia. LSD, MDMA, and psilocybin (tryptamine) intoxication may also cause serotonin syndrome.

Duration of effects begins within minutes and can last for hours, depending on the substance and the route. Long-term effects of intoxication include persistent psychosis with visual disturbances, disorganized thinking, paranoia, and mood changes. Patients may also experience random flashbacks of visual perceptual distortions and sensations of derealization and depersonalization while not under the influence of the drug, termed hallucinogen persisting perception disorder.[32]

Responsible Medications
Many hallucinogenic compounds are found in nature. Psilocybin is derived from mushrooms; DMT is found in the Amazon, and is brewed into the tea ayahuasca. Mescaline is derived from a small cactus and made into peyote. There are numerous new synthetic derivatives, whose representative compounds are listed in **Table 5**.

Treatment
Treatment of acute hallucinogen intoxication begins with minimizing stimulation with a calm environment. Short-acting benzodiazepines such as midazolam, lorazepam, and diazepam are useful for agitation and dysphoria. Neuroleptics such as Haldol are useful adjuncts if psychotic symptoms persist. In severe overdoses, activated charcoal at 1 g/kg can be given, but only if ingestion was less than 1 hour before presentation. Urinary acidification followed by diuresis has a small effect on accelerating excretion of LSD and PCP but also enhances the risk of renal failure in patients with rhabdomyolysis, and is not recommended in most cases.[36]

γ-Aminobutyric Acid Agonist Withdrawal Syndromes

GABA agonists are often used as sedative agents because of their CNS-depressant effects. Withdrawal creates a state of extreme CNS hyperexcitation, which can be lethal. Alcohol withdrawal syndrome is the prototypical GABA agonist withdrawal syndrome, and should always be considered on the differential of acute-onset delirium.

Mechanism
GABAergic pathways regulate the firing of monoamine-containing neurons in the brain and spinal cord, inhibiting muscle hypertonia and seizure spreading.

The GABA-A receptor is the major inhibitory receptor in the CNS. Benzodiazepines, Z drugs, and barbiturates increase overall GABA-A channel opening. Alcohol works through multiple receptors, potentiating GABA-A effects and blocking NMDA excitatory effects. GABA-B receptors are also inhibitory, coupled to K^+ channels and ultimately decreasing Ca^{2+} channel conductance, mediating postsynaptic and presynaptic inhibition. Baclofen is the major agonist at this site.[37]

Long-term use of these substances (>2 weeks for benzodiazepines) causes the brain to decrease inhibitory transmission and enhance excitatory neurotransmission through increase of glutaminergic receptors. Absence of GABA potentiators in this new balance leads to hyperexcitation. Chronic alcohol use and cycles of withdrawal

Table 5 Hallucinogenic compounds		
Hallucinogen	**Sources**	**Sympathetic Activity**
Lysergic acid	LSD, morning glory, Hawaiian baby woodrose	Mild
Phenylethylamines	Mescaline, NBOMes (MDMA, amphetamines)	Moderate
Tryptamines	Psilocybin, AMT, DMT (ayahuasca), 5-Meo-DIPT	Mild
Salvinorin A	*Salvia* mint	Mild
Ketamine	Anesthetic	Prominent
Phencyclidine	PCP	Prominent
Dextromethorphan	Cough medicine	Prominent

Abbreviations: AMT, α-methyltryptamine; NBOMes, N-methoxybenzyl; 5-MeO-DIPT, 5-methoxydimethyltryptamine.
Data from Refs.[29,33–35]

permanently alter GABAergic function; withdrawal episodes may worsen over time with so-called neuronal kindling, resulting in excitotoxic damage.[38]

Common agents and their mechanisms of action are listed in **Table 6**.

Presentation

Alcohol withdrawal Mild withdrawal begins with tremors, anxiety, diaphoresis, palpitations, and GI upset. These symptoms develop 6 hours after the last drink. Alcoholic hallucinosis starts at between 12 and 24 hours of abstinence. Hallucinations may be visual, tactile, or auditory. Patients generally recognize that they are hallucinating, with intact mental status and normal vital signs.

Withdrawal seizures may occur within 12 to 48 hours of withdrawal in patients with chronic alcoholism, as well as in chronic benzodiazepine use. These seizures are usually generalized tonic-clonic and may cluster. Status epilepticus is less common and warrants further work-up.

In severe withdrawal, delirium tremens (DT) occurs from 48 hours to 96 hours since the last drink and lasts from 1 to 8 days. DT development is predicted by Clinical Institute Withdrawal Assessment for Alcohol Withdrawal Scale (CIWA-Ar) greater than 15, especially with systolic blood pressure greater than 150 mm Hg or pulse greater than 100 beats per minute, withdrawal seizures, older age, other medical problems, and prior withdrawal DT or seizures. The patient becomes disoriented, agitated, anxious, and begins hallucinating, with severe insomnia. Autonomic instability develops with hypertension, tachycardia, and diaphoresis. Death during this period may occur from arrhythmia; complicating illness such as pneumonia; or from another underlying comorbid disease such as pancreatitis, hepatitis, or CNS injury.[41]

Risk of DT increases with history of withdrawal seizures, DT, history of sustained drinking, and presence of withdrawal symptoms with an increased blood alcohol level.

Benzodiazepine withdrawal The presentation is similar to that of alcohol withdrawal, and worse with short-acting benzodiazepines. Immediately after withdrawal, there are 2 to 3 days of rebound anxiety and insomnia. Full-blown withdrawal can last 10 to 14 days and is characterized by insomnia, tension and anxiety, panic attacks, tremors, nausea, stiffness, headache, muscular pain, and perceptual changes. Seizures also occur, especially with chronic high dosing and abrupt discontinuation, and can present with intermittent subclinical seizures and status epilepticus.

Table 6
GABA agonists and their mechanisms of action

Drug	Mechanism
Alcohol	GABA-A and glycine potentiation, antagonizing NMDA and excitatory ion channels[39]
Benzodiazepines	Binds to allosteric benzodiazepine site on GABA-A receptor, increasing frequency of Cl− channel opening
Baclofen	GABA-B agonist in CNS and spinal cord; prevents calcium influx in presynaptic neurons, reduces presynaptic neurotransmitter release[40]
Barbiturates: phenobarbital	Bind to allosteric GABA-A receptor sites, enhance mean open time of Cl− channel
Z compounds: zaleplon, zolpidem, zopiclone, eszopiclone	Bind to GABA-A receptor benzodiazepine site
Carbamates: carisoprodol	GABA-A allosteric modulator and direct agonist, similar to barbiturates

Baclofen withdrawal Baclofen is administered by oral and intrathecal routes for spasticity. Withdrawal from oral agents from dose decreases in the setting of chronic use has been documented. Withdrawal from intrathecal agents can be dramatic, with onset within a few hours, lasting 1 to 2 weeks, and in some cases even lasting beyond 1 month with agitation, hypertonia, tachycardia, and hemodynamic instability,[42] usually in the setting of pump malfunction or replacement. The presentation may prominently feature delirium that is resistant to treatment with other medications. Symptoms range from increased spasticity and itching with delirium, changes to hyperthermia, seizures, DIC, and even death.

Treatment

Benzodiazepines are the staple of alcohol withdrawal treatment to prevent seizures, control autonomic symptoms, and suppress psychomotor agitation. Symptom-triggered approaches of dosing benzodiazepines include the CIWA-Ar, which rates severity based on subjective symptoms with thresholds to administer benzodiazepines. In a direct comparison of a symptom-triggered approach versus fixed scheduling using chlordiazepoxide, less medication was needed in the symptom-triggered group with a shorter treatment period, with similar clinical outcomes.[43] Short-acting benzodiazepines such as lorazepam are preferred in the setting of liver disease to avoid oversedation, although long-acting chlordiazepoxide tapers have also been used. Benzodiazepines also cause withdrawal, so, if high doses are administered, a benzodiazepine taper with 10% dose reduction per day is also recommended. For long-term benzodiazepine use, a taper over 10 weeks is preferable to prevent withdrawal and patient dropout.[44]

Clinics Care Points

- Some hospitals have transitioned towards using phenobarbital monotherapy first line for alcohol withdrawal.

- Multiple studies have shown a safety equivalent to benzodiazepines with similar rates of intubation, and success in treating withdrawal in sicker and more refractory patients, with shorter hospital stays.

- Widely accepted use has been limited by variations in protocol, and clinicians frequently underdose. Generally, a loading dose ranging from 6 to 15 mg/kg titrated to severity of symptoms and risk of respiratory compromise has been used, with maintenance dosing over 1 week to maintain steady drug levels followed by taper.[46]

Phenobarbital is used in benzodiazepine-resistant patients and has a long half-life with the benefit of self-taper. New evidence reveals that phenobarbital adjunctive or monotherapy may result in better outcomes with shorter hospital stays compared with symptom-triggered benzodiazepine schedules, and does not result in more frequent intubation from respiratory depression.[45,46]

Additional attention to nutritional deficiencies with vitamin supplementation, including thiamine and folate, should also be considered, and discussed further later.

Wernicke Encephalopathy

Wernicke encephalopathy is an acute confusional state precipitated by thiamine deficiency. It is characterized by the clinical triad of confusion, ophthalmoparesis with nystagmus, and ataxia. If treated early, the syndrome is reversible.

Mechanism

Thiamine acts as a cofactor for several enzymes in the Krebs cycle and the pentose phosphate pathway. Thiamine-dependent enzymes function as a connection between glycolytic and citric acid cycles. Deficiency leads to accumulation of lactate, pyruvate, and toxic intermediates, ultimately leading to neuronal cell death in the CNS and the peripheral nervous system.[47] Many areas metabolically injured in thiamine deficiency overlap with the memory formation centers, including the mammillary bodies and thalamus.

Thiamine is absorbed in the duodenum and crosses the blood-brain barrier through the bloodstream. Storage of thiamine lasts for about 18 days in the liver; thus, symptoms manifest approximately 2 weeks to 1 month after storage depletion. Demand for thiamine increases with higher carbohydrate load, which is why glucose administration without thiamine has been reported to precipitate acute Wernicke encephalopathy.[48] Various dietary sources contain thiamine, including meats, whole-grain cereals, nuts, and soybeans. The daily minimum requirement of thiamine on a 2000-kcal diet is 0.66 mg/d; the currently recommended intake is 1.1 mg for adult women and 1.2 mg for adult men.[49]

Clinics Care Points

- A dietary history may be critical to making a diagnosis of a nutritional deficiency, especially thiamine deficiency.
- Patients who eat predominantly processed junk foods high in carbohydrates have developed Wernicke's encephalopathy.
- The Paleo diet lacks fortified grains and may result in thiamine deficiency.

Causes
Thiamine deficiency is caused by any disease leading to malnutrition. It is most commonly associated with chronic alcohol use. Apart from the malnutrition associated with empty calorie consumption, alcohol itself can reduce thiamine absorption, impair storage in cirrhosis, and reduce thiamine phosphorylation. Other causes include GI surgical procedures, gastric or colon cancer, ulcerative colitis, peptic ulcer disease, intestinal obstruction, chronic diarrhea, pancreatitis, and hyperemesis. Malignancies such as leukemias and lymphomas, along with chemotherapeutics, also can cause thiamine deficiency. Systemic diseases occasionally cause thiamine deficiency, including acquired immunodeficiency syndrome, chronic infectious febrile illnesses, thyrotoxicosis, and renal disease with dialysis. Reduced intake occurs through starvation, as well as a diet of only polished white rice. Iatrogenic causes such as prolonged total parenteral nutrition (TPN) without thiamine administration, or lack of feeding followed by refeeding without thiamine supplementation, can also precipitate acute Wernicke encephalopathy.[48,50] Other thiamine deficiency syndromes include dry beriberi, a distal sensorimotor neuropathy with weakness and hyporeflexia, which can present concurrently with Wernicke, as well as wet beriberi, characterized by cardiac failure and fluid overload, which is more common in Asian people.[51]

Presentation
Wernicke encephalopathy classically presents with acute altered mental status, ophthalmoplegia and nystagmus, and ataxic gait, but the triad may only present in 16% to 20% of patients. The alteration in mental status may be as subtle as irritation, apathy, and inattention, with fatigue and loss of appetite, which progresses to disorientation, inability to calculate or comprehend abstraction, and lethargy. Hallucinations, agitation, and confabulation can also occur. At the extreme, coma and death can result. Ophthalmoplegia and cranial nerve deficits present with double vision, resulting from lesions in the pontine tegmentum or the abducens and oculomotor nuclei. Gait

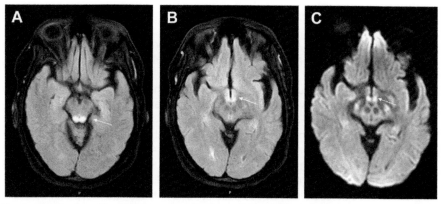

Fig. 1. MRI brain with classic imaging findings of thiamine deficiency. MRI brain without contrast showing fluid-attenuated inversion recovery (FLAIR) signal hyperintensity (*arrows*) involving the colliculi/midbrain tectum (*A*), mammillary bodies (*B*), and diffusion restriction in the mammillary bodies on diffusion-weighted imaging (*C*).

may vary from instability or wide-based gait to an inability to walk with severe ataxia. Autonomic instability with hypotension or hypothermia can also occur, along with seizures or progressive hearing loss (caused by midbrain tectal involvement).[51]

The syndrome overlaps with the same population at risk for alcohol intoxication and withdrawal. It is helpful in some cases to use radiographic and laboratory evidence to support the diagnosis. Thiamine levels are useful confirmatory tests, but levels may take 1 week to return. Empiric treatment should be initiated immediately.

Radiographically, cytotoxic and vasogenic edema appear as bilateral symmetric hyperintensities on T2 weighted magnetic resonance images in the periphery of the third ventricle, periaqueductal area, medial thalamus, mammillary bodies, and midbrain tectal plate (**Fig. 1**). Atypical locations include the caudate nucleus, cranial nerve nuclei, red nuclei, corpus callosum, dentate nuclei, cerebellum, and frontal/parietal cerebral cortices.[52] Sensitivity of MRI in revealing evidence of Wernicke encephalopathy is 53%, and specificity is 93% on T2 imaging without fluid-attenuated inversion recovery (FLAIR).[53]

Treatment

Wernicke encephalopathy is treated with 500 mg of IV thiamine 3 times daily for 3 days, followed by 250 mg IV daily for 3 to 5 days, followed by daily repletion with 100 mg orally. Acute Wernicke encephalopathy responds well to IV thiamine, with mental status improvement over several days. Symptoms of nystagmus or gait instability may last up to a few months. Traditionally, thiamine should be given with glucose in hypoglycemia because of the risk of precipitating Wernicke encephalopathy. Glucose should never be withheld for treatment of acute hypoglycemia, but thiamine should also be administered when available.[54] Any TPN should be administered with thiamine supplementation. Magnesium is required for conversion of thiamine into its active form, and should be checked and repleted as well.[55,56]

Korsakoff syndrome may result after a single acute episode of Wernicke encephalopathy, especially if untreated, and is characterized by impairment in anterograde and retrograde memory. This condition becomes evident after the initial encephalopathy resolves, and is an indication of more severe and permanent injury to the mammillothalamic tract.[57]

DISCLOSURE

A. Cai has nothing to disclose. X. Cai is an employee of Pfizer, Inc.

REFERENCES

1. Inouye S, van Dyck C, Alessi C, et al. Clarifying confusion: the confusion assessment method. A new method for detection of delirium. Ann Intern Med 1990; 113(12):941–8.
2. Montastruc J-L, Durrieu G, Sommet A, et al. Anticholinergics, antimuscarinics or atropinics? About the words in pharmacology: Letter to the Editors. Br J Clin Pharmacol 2010;69(5):561–2.
3. McGleenon BM, Dynan KB, Passmore AP. Acetylcholinesterase inhibitors in Alzheimer's disease. Br J Clin Pharmacol 1999;48(4):471–80.
4. Langmead CJ, Watson J, Reavill C. Muscarinic acetylcholine receptors as CNS drug targets. Pharmacol Ther 2008;117(2):232–43.
5. Abrams P, Andersson K-E, Buccafusco JJ, et al. Muscarinic receptors: their distribution and function in body systems, and the implications for treating overactive bladder. Br J Pharmacol 2006;148(5):565–78.
6. Abdi A, Rose E, Levine M. Diphenhydramine overdose with intraventricular conduction delay treated with hypertonic sodium bicarbonate and i.v. lipid emulsion. West J Emerg Med 2014;15(7):855–8.
7. Soulaidopoulos S, Sinakos E, Dimopoulou D, et al. Anticholinergic syndrome induced by toxic plants. World J Emerg Med 2017;8(4):297–301.
8. Burns MJ, Linden CH, Graudins A, et al. A comparison of physostigmine and benzodiazepines for the treatment of anticholinergic poisoning. Ann Emerg Med 2000;35(4):374–81.
9. Pentel P, Peterson CD. Asystole complicating physostigmine treatment of tricyclic antidepressant overdose. Ann Emerg Med 1980;9(11):588–90.
10. Rosenbaum C, Bird SB. Timing and Frequency of Physostigmine Redosing for Antimuscarinic Toxicity. J Med Toxicol 2010;6(4):386–92.
11. Phillips MA, Acquisto NM, Gorodetsky RM, et al. Use of a Physostigmine Continuous Infusion for the Treatment of Severe and Recurrent Antimuscarinic Toxicity in a Mixed Drug Overdose. J Med Toxicol 2014;10(2):205–9.
12. Zweben JE, Cohen JB, Christian D, et al. Psychiatric Symptoms in Methamphetamine Users. Am J Addict 2004;13(2):181–90.
13. Atzori M, Cuevas-Olguin R, Esquivel-Rendon E, et al. Locus Ceruleus Norepinephrine Release: A Central Regulator of CNS Spatio-Temporal Activation? Front Synaptic Neurosci 2016;8. https://doi.org/10.3389/fnsyn.2016.00025.
14. Gray S, Fatovich D, McCoubrie D, et al. Amphetamine-related presentations to an inner-city tertiary emergency department: a prospective evaluation. Med J Aust 2007;186(7):336–9.
15. Stavric B. Methylxanthines: Toxicity to humans. 2. Caffeine. Food Chem Toxicol 1988;26(7):645–62.
16. Williams RH, Erickson T, Broussard LA. Evaluating Sympathomimetic Intoxication in an Emergency Setting. Lab Med 2000;31(9):497–508.
17. Chan P, Chen J, Lee M, et al. Fatal and nonfatal methamphetamine intoxication in the intensive care unit. J Toxicol Clin Toxicol 1994;32(2):147–55.
18. Richards JR, Lange RA, Arnold TC, et al. Dual cocaine and methamphetamine cardiovascular toxicity: rapid resolution with labetalol. Am J Emerg Med 2017; 35(3):519.e1-4.
19. Maier L, Lionel T, Schmidt S, et al. Emergency department management of body packers and body stuffers. Swiss Med Wkly 2017;147(3738). https://doi.org/10.4414/smw.2017.14499.

20. Hornung J-P. The human raphe nuclei and the serotonergic system. J Chem Neuroanat 2003;26(4):331–43.

21. Mason P, Morris V, Balcezak T. Serotonin syndrome. Presentation of 2 cases and review of the literature. Medicine (Baltimore) 2000;79(4):201–9.

22. Dunkley EJC, Isbister GK, Sibbritt D, et al. The Hunter Serotonin Toxicity Criteria: simple and accurate diagnostic decision rules for serotonin toxicity. QJM 2003; 96(9):635–42.

23. Ali S, Taguchi A, Rosenberg H. Malignant hyperthermia - ScienceDirect. Best Pract Res Clin Anaesthesiol 2003;17(4):519–33.

24. Guze B, Baxter L. Neuroleptic Malignant Syndrome. N Engl J Med 1985;313: 163–6.

25. Mason B, Blackburn K. Possible serotonin syndrome associated with tramadol and sertraline coadministration. Ann Pharmacol 1997;31(2):175–7.

26. Graudins A, Stearman A, Chan B. Treatment of the serotonin syndrome with cyprohepatdine. The Journal of Emergency Medicine 1998;16(4):615-619. https:// doi.org/10.1016/S0736-4679(98)00057-2.

27. Halberstadt AL, Geyer MA. Multiple receptors contribute to the behavioral effects of indoleamine hallucinogens. Neuropharmacology 2011;61(3):364–81.

28. Vollenweider FX. Brain mechanisms of hallucinogens and entactogens. Dialogues Clin Neurosci 2001;3(4):265–79.

29. Kalant H. The pharmacology and toxicology of "ecstasy" (MDMA) and related drugs. Can Med Assoc J 2001;165(7):917–28.

30. Nichols DE. Hallucinogens. Pharmacol Ther 2004;101(2):131–81.

31. Tiscione NB, Miller MI. Psilocin identified in a DUID investigation. J Anal Toxicol 2006;30(5):342–5.

32. First M. DSM-5 handbook of differential diagnosis. 5th edition. Washington, DC: American Psychiatric Publishing; 2014. Available at: https://dsm. psychiatryonline.org/doi/full/10.5555/appi.books.9780890425596.Section1. Accessed December 9, 2019.

33. Williams RH, Erickson T. Evaluating Hallucinogenic or Psychedelic Drug Intoxication in an Emergency Setting. Lab Med 2000;31(7):394–401.

34. Bey T, Patel A. Phencyclidine Intoxication and Adverse Effects: A Clinical and Pharmacological Review of an Illicit Drug. Calif J Emerg Med 2007;8(1):9–14.

35. Roth BL, Baner K, Westkaemper R, et al. Salvinorin A: A potent naturally occurring nonnitrogenous opioid selective agonist. Proc Natl Acad Sci U S A 2002; 99(18):11934–9.

36. Barton CH, Sterling ML, Vaziri ND. Rhabdomyolysis and Acute Renal Failure Associated With Phencyclidine Intoxication. Arch Intern Med 1980;140(4):568–9.

37. Siegel G, Agranoff B, Albers RW, et al. Basic neurochemistry. 6th edition. Lippincott-Raven; 1999.

38. Becker HC. Kindling in Alcohol Withdrawal. Alcohol Health Res World 1998; 22(1):9.

39. Davies M. The role of GABAA receptors in mediating the effects of alcohol in the central nervous system. J Psychiatry Neurosci 2003;28(4):263–74.

40. Alvis BD, Sobey CM. Oral baclofen withdrawal resulting in progressive weakness and sedation requiring intensive care admission. Neurohospitalist 2017;7(1): 39–40.

41. Schuckit MA. Recognition and Management of Withdrawal Delirium (Delirium Tremens). N Engl J Med 2014;371(22):2109–13.

42. Hansen C, Gooch J, Such-Neibar T. Prolonged, Severe Intrathecal Baclofen Withdrawal Syndrome: A Case Report - Archives of Physical Medicine and Rehabilitation. Am Acad Phys Med Rehabil 2007;88(11):1468–71.

43. Saitz R, Mayo-Smith M, Roberts M, et al. Individualized Treatment for Alcohol Withdrawal: A Randomized Double-blind Controlled Trial. J Am Med Assoc 1994;272(7):519–23.

44. Denis C, Fatseas M, Lavie E, et al. Pharmacological interventions for benzodiazepine mono-dependence management in outpatient settings. Cochrane Database Syst Rev 2006;(3):CD005194.

45. Nisavic M, Nejad S, Isenberg B, et al. Use of phenobarbital in alcohol withdrawal management - a retrospective comparison study of phenobarbital and benzodiazepines for acute alcohol wit. Psychosomatics 2019;60(5):458–67.

46. Tidwell W, Thomas T, Pouliot J, et al. Treatment of Alcohol Withdrawal Syndrome: Phenobarbital vs CIWA-Ar Protocol. Am J Crit Care 2018;27(6):454–60.

47. Todd KG, Hazell A, Butterworth R. Alcohol-thiamine interactions: an update on the pathogenesis of Wernicke encephalopathy. Addict Biol 1999;4:261–72.

48. Drenick E, Joven C, Swendseid M. Occurrence of Acute Wernicke's Encephalopathy during Prolonged Starvation for the Treatment of Obesity. N Engl J Med 1966;274(17):937–9.

49. Ziporin ZZ, Nunes NT, Powell RC, et al. Thiamine requirement in the adult human as measured by urinary excretion of thiamine metabolites. J Nutr 1965;85(3):297–304.

50. Osiezagha K, Ali S, Freeman C, et al. Thiamine Deficiency and Delirium. Innov Clin Neurosci 2013;10(4):26–32.

51. Sechi G, Serra A. Wernicke's encephalopathy: new clinical settings and recent advances in diagnosis and management. Lancet Neurol 2007;6(5):442–55.

52. Zuccoli G, Pipitone N. Neuroimaging Findings in Acute Wernicke's Encephalopathy: Review of the Literature. Am J Roentgenol 2009;192(2):501–8.

53. Antunez E, Estruch R, Cardenal C, et al. Usefulness of CT and MR imaging in the diagnosis of acute Wernicke's encephalopathy. AJR Am J Roentgenol 1998;171(4):1131–7.

54. Donnino MW, Vega J, Miller J, et al. Myths and Misconceptions of Wernicke's Encephalopathy: What Every Emergency Physician Should Know. Ann Emerg Med 2007;50(6):715–21.

55. Zieve L. Influence of magnesium deficiency on the utilization of thiamine. Ann N Y Acad Sci 1969;162(2):732–43.

56. Dyckner T, Ek B, Nyhlin H, et al. Aggravation of thiamine deficiency by magnesium depletion. A case report. Acta Med Scand 1985;218(1):129–31.

57. Kopelman MD, Thomson AD, Guerrini I, et al. The Korsakoff Syndrome: Clinical Aspects, Psychology and Treatment. Alcohol Alcohol 2009;44(2):148–54.

Toxin-Induced Subacute Encephalopathy

David P. Lerner, MD[a],*, Aleksey Tadevosyan, MD[b], Joseph D. Burns, MD[a]

KEYWORDS

- Leukoencephalopathy • Antineoplastic drugs • Inorganic toxins • Antibiotics
- Antidepressants • Antipsychotic

KEY POINTS

- Inorganic toxins are ubiquitous but uncommonly result in toxicity. Both chronic exposure and more commonly single high-dose exposure can result in neurologic toxicity.
- Antibiotic-induced encephalopathy is likely an under-recognized entity because these patients commonly have additional metabolic, toxin, and infectious contributors to encephalopathy. There should be a low threshold for evaluation with concern for subclinical seizures as a significant concern.
- The encephalopathy associated with antineoplastic drugs is important to diagnose. The exclusion of malignancy within the central nervous system, paraneoplastic disorder, and ischemic or hemorrhagic stroke due to abnormal coagulopathy are important differential diagnoses that should be considered and excluded.
- Antidepressants and antipsychotic medications have activity on multiple neurotransmitter receptors with substantial overlap. Although serotonin syndrome and neuroleptic malignant syndrome are considered distinct entities, there likely is overlap and a spectrum of these diseases. Early consideration and recognition are important because these can be life-threatening diseases.

INTRODUCTION

Subacute toxic encephalopathies are challenging to identify due to their often insidious tempo of evolution, nonspecific manifestations, relative infrequency as individual entities, and frequent lack of specific diagnostic testing. Yet they are crucial to recognize—in aggregate, subacute toxic encephalopathies are a common problem that can lead to severe, irreversible harm if not diagnosed and treated efficiently. This article reviews the clinically relevant aspects of some of the more important subacute toxic

[a] Department of Neurology, Tufts University School of Medicine, Lahey Hospital and Medical Center, 41 Mall Road, Burlington, MA 01805, USA; [b] Department of Neurology, Lahey Hospital and Medical Center, 41 Mall Road, Burlington, MA 01805, USA
* Corresponding author.
E-mail address: david.lerner@lahey.org

Neurol Clin 38 (2020) 799–824
https://doi.org/10.1016/j.ncl.2020.07.006
0733-8619/20/© 2020 Elsevier Inc. All rights reserved.

encephalopathy syndromes caused by inorganic toxins, carbon monoxide (CO), antibiotics, antineoplastic agents, and psychiatric medications.

DISCUSSION
Inorganic Toxins

Bismuth
Multiple industries continue to use bismuth to date, including cosmetics, industrial/manufacturing, and pharmaceuticals (**Table 1**). The most common exposure to bismuth and means of toxicity is ingestion of bismuth salts, namely bismuth subsalicylate, used to treat diarrhea and other gastrointestinal (GI) upset symptoms (eg, Pepto-Bismol). Historically, bismuth was used in treatment of syphilis and amebiasis and resulted in numerous cases of toxicity, including an episode of 70 deaths in a 7-year period in France.[1] Since the advent of additional antibiotic therapy, use of bismuth salt for treatment of infections and consequently rates of overdose have dramatically declined. Although bismuth toxicity now is rare, it remains important to recognize its physical examination, laboratory, and radiographic manifestations.

As with many heavy metals, there is a risk of systemic and neurologic toxicity associated with bismuth. Bismuth has markedly lower toxicity than other heavy metals.[2] Intoxication can occur from chronic exposure, high-dose single administration, or a combination of both.[3–5] Chronic toxicity has been associated with serum concentrations of 50 µg/L to 1600 µg/L, and those presenting with encephalopathy typically have a serum range from 680 µg/L to 700 µg/L.[6] Bismuth levels can also be checked in the urine (commonly 150–1250 µg/L) and cerebrospinal fluid.[3–5]

Findings of intoxication include increased salivation, bluish/brownish gingival lining, and black spots on mucosal membranes, which are uncommon but can assist with the diagnosis of chronic ingestion. Gingival and mucosal changes rarely are seen in acute intoxication. The encephalopathy associated with either acute or chronic intoxication follows a common pattern: prodromal phase with slow progression over weeks to a month followed by a rapid deterioration.[7,8] The encephalopathy is associated with myoclonus, ataxia, dysarthria, parkinsonism, and rarely seizures and focal neurologic deficits.[2–4,8] Neuropsychiatric symptoms, including auditory and visual hallucinations, also can occur.[3]

Bismuth deposition within the brain results in the neurologic manifestations of intoxication, discussed previously. The metal is radio-opaque and on computerized tomography (CT) can demonstrate hyperdensity within the dorsomedial thalamus, cerebral cortex, and cerebellum.[9,10]

Treatment of overdose is symptomatic and supportive. If the ingestion occurred within hours, a single dose of activated charcoal may be useful in preventing absorption. Renal dysfunction can slow clearance, so ensuring adequate hydration is essential. Although chelation has demonstrated an increased rate of excretion, there are no data addressing its effect on patient outcome.[8] In the setting of combined renal failure and bismuth toxicity, hemodialysis could be considered because it can clear the heavy metal.[11] Typically, chronic ingestion encephalopathy can improve with removal of the offending agent/medication and supportive care, but this can take weeks to months and may not be fully reversible.[8]

Lithium
Lithium is a widely prescribed medication for use in bipolar disorder, suicide prevention in depression, and maintenance therapy for these diseases. Despite its wide use, toxicity is common due to its narrow therapeutic window.[12] Approximately 75% of patients taking lithium have side effects from the medication, most of which are mild.[12]

Table 1
Inorganic toxins

Inorganic Toxin	Common Laboratory Value	Systemic Symptoms	Neurologic Symptoms	Treatment
Bismuth	Serum Chronic toxicity, 50–1600 µg/L Neurologic toxicity, 680–700 µg/L Urine Chronic toxicity, 150–1250 µg/L	Salivation, bluing of gingival lining, black spots on mucosa	Rapidly progressive encephalopathy, myoclonus, ataxia, dysarthria, parkinsonism	Supportive care consideration for hemodialysis
Lithium	Serum Acute/chronic toxicity, >1.5 mEq/L	ECG changes, nausea/vomiting/diarrhea, polyuria	Action tremor, dysarthria, lethargy, ataxia, fasciculations, myoclonus	Sodium polystyrene sulfonate Consideration for hemodialysis
Aluminum	Serum Acute/chronic toxicity, 20–1000 µg/L	Myalgia, bone pain, proximal weakness, hypercalcemia	Lethargy and progression to coma, commonly seizures, dysarthria, myoclonus, hallucinations	Deferoxamine administration with hemodialysis
CO	Serum Carboxyhemoglobin Nonsmoker, <3% Chronic smoker, <10%–12%	Nausea, cherry red lips, nose, ears	Headache, dizziness, confusion with progression to coma	High-flow oxygen, nonrebreather oxygen supplementation Consideration for hyperbaric oxygen treatment

For example, in the United States in 2014, there were 6840 cases of lithium toxicity, 160 of these with severe symptoms and 7 deaths.[13] Because lithium, sodium, and volume status all are closely intertwined, changes to a person's water and salt intake can change the serum lithium level greatly even when on chronic, stable dosing.

Toxicity from lithium overdose—acute, acute-on-chronic, or chronic—can be seen at serum concentrations of 1.5 mEq/L to 2.5 mEq/L (therapeutic level 0.6–1.2 mEq/L).[14,15] Although there is correlation between the serum lithium level and severity of symptoms, a single serum lithium level may not correlate with clinical signs of toxicity because central nervous system concentration lags serum levels.[14,15] In acute ingestion, the serum concentration may be elevated without substantial neurologic symptoms, whereas chronic ingestion may demonstrate near-normal drug levels with marked neurologic symptoms.[14] Toxicity associated with chronic use of lithium presents in a more protracted fashion but with the same neurologic symptoms as acute intoxication. Those patients older than age 50, with comorbid hyperthyroidism or chronic kidney disease, are at higher risk.[16]

Initial symptoms include fine action tremor, dysarthria, and mild lethargy. As central nervous system concentrations increase, the tremor becomes present at rest and the amplitude can increase.[14] The tremor typically precedes ataxia and neuromuscular excitability, including fasciculations and spontaneous myoclonus.[14,15] Encephalopathy and confusion result from greater CNS concentration, and, if the intoxication is severe, seizures and status epilepticus can occur.[12] Although the symptoms typically are reversible, the syndrome of irreversible lithium-effectuated neurotoxicity (SILENT) can occur, with chronic cerebellar ataxia, extrapyramidal symptoms, and dementia.[17]

Common systemic findings include cardiovascular changes—T-wave flattening, QT prolongation, and rarely sinus node dysfunction or ventricular arrhythmias.[18] Additional signs and symptoms include GI disturbances with nausea, vomiting, and diarrhea, and renal manifestations, chiefly polyuria, with associated hyponatremia and dehydration.[19]

In the setting of acute intoxication, even with early recognition, activated charcoal is not recommended because it does not prevent absorption.[20] Sodium polystyrene sulfonate whole-bowel irrigation has been used with success at preventing absorption.[21] Typically, a diagnosis is not made in the hyperacute setting and, rather than prevention of absorption, rapid removal is the cornerstone of management. Lithium is removed easily by hemodialysis.[16,22,23] There are not firmly established guidelines for initiation of hemodialysis, but considerations include[16,22,23]

- Serum lithium levels greater than 5 mEq/L
- Serum lithium level greater than 4 mEq/L and a serum creatinine greater than 2 mg/dL
- Any level with depressed level of consciousness, seizures, or other life-threatening manifestations

Aluminum

Aluminum exposure occurs commonly, yet toxicity is rare. Large exposure and toxicity are encountered predominantly in patients with chronic kidney disease stage IV or stage V on aluminum-containing phosphate binders and those on hemodialysis.[24–26] In 2003, the reported aluminum toxicity rate for those on hemodialysis was 0.5% t0 0.8%.[27] Because hemodialysis requires exposure to a large volume of water, even slight changes in the aluminum concentration of municipal water supply can result in toxicity and commonly results in localized outbreaks of exposure and toxicity.[25,26] Recent reports of acute intoxication have been the result of changes to municipal water supply.[25,26] Aluminum exposure also can occur due to medications, including iron-containing and calcium-containing drugs, calcitriol, vitamin B complex supplements, acetylsalicylic acid, and clonidine, although normal renal function typically allows for excretion of excessive aluminum.[28]

Those patients with aluminum toxicity may present with acute or chronic intoxication syndromes. Acute intoxication occurs during dialysis that involves exposure to very high concentrations of aluminum in dialysate. Manifestations include encephalopathy that may progress to coma, frequently accompanied by seizures.[29] Acute, high levels of serum aluminum may occur (normal serum concentration <20 μg/L) and reported levels of 400 μg/L to 1000 μg/L are associated with increased mortality.[29]

More commonly, chronic exposure to aluminum results in toxicity. This can occur from aluminum-containing phosphate binder ingestion, which no longer is recommended because there is no known safe dosing amount.[28] Chronic exposure results in aluminum deposition in multiple tissues, including bone and muscle, resulting in diffuse bone pain and myalgias, proximal muscle weakness, hypercalcemia, microcytic anemia, and progressive dementia. The dementing illness first presents with language disorders.[30] The initial changes are subtle with dysarthria, stuttering, and changes in periodicity.[30] The language changes can progress with worsening dysarthria, myoclonus, hallucinations, and seizures.[29]

In the late 1970s, the description, "dialysis dementia," was coined and linked to aluminum deposition within the cerebral cortex.[31] The dementing illness presented initially with lack of concentration and retrograde amnesia. This illness was followed by time disorientation and memory impairment.[31] Mood changes are a major component of the described syndrome and include variable features, such as irritability, hostility, euphoria, violence, depression, and apathy as well as psychotic features of paranoia, delusions, and mixed auditory and visual hallucinations.[31]

A diagnosis of aluminum toxicity can be made with serum concentration testing at the end of hemodialysis sessions. Any level greater than 20 μg/L is considered abnormal.[32] For those with symptoms of aluminum toxicity but levels below the abnormal threshold, a deferoxamine stimulation test can be completed. An increase in serum levels by greater than 50 μg/L is considered positive and consistent with excessive stores of aluminum. Additional testing can include bone biopsy—which rarely is done—with demonstration of aluminum staining.[31] Care must be taken when considering deferoxamine stimulation testing because the body stores of aluminum release and may result in worsening neurotoxicity.[33] Electroencephalography (EEG) can show a characteristic pattern of diffuse background slowing with superimposed frontal intermittent rhythmic delta and bursts of frontocentral sharp waves.[30,34]

The Kidney Disease Outcomes Quality Initiative recommends annual serum aluminum level checks for those undergoing hemodialysis and quarterly for those taking aluminum-containing phosphate binders.[35] Treatment duration varies based on the aluminum level and severity of symptoms, but the removal of whole-body stores of aluminum with deferoxamine administration during hemodialysis weekly is central.[36]

Carbon monoxide

CO is an odorless, colorless gas produced from incomplete hydrocarbon combustion. Although CO is present in the atmosphere at low levels, in closed environments concentrations it easily can reach toxic levels that result in impaired oxygen transportation and oxidative phosphorylation. Frequency of CO intoxication cases typically varies by season, with more cases during colder months as a result of increased heating requirements. In the United States, CO poisoning results in 50,000 emergency department visits and approximately 1200 deaths per year.[37–39] The mortality rate is estimated at 1% to 3%.[38,39] Potential sources of CO include poorly functioning heating systems, improperly vented fuel burning systems, hookah use, and exposure to methylene chloride (used as a paint stripper, degreasing agent, or extraction solvent), which is metabolized to CO.[37,40–43]

CO binds to the heme ring in erythrocytes with a greater than 200-times affinity compared with oxygen.[8] The binding results in allosteric changes to the heme ring, which preclude additional oxygen molecule binding and prevent offloading of oxygen in tissues resulting in hypoxic tissue injury.[8] CO that is distributed into tissues further exacerbates the effects of tissue hypoxia by causing inactivation of cytochrome oxidase and causes anaerobic oxidation.[44] Finally, ischemic-reperfusion injury occurs during the treatment phase of CO poisoning.[37,44,45] This results in lipid peroxidation and generation of excitotoxicity, depolarization, and nitrative stress.[45]

To make a diagnosis of CO poisoning, a high index of suspicion in the appropriate setting leading to demonstration of a risk factor for exposure by clinical history are paramount.[37] Common symptoms include headache (80%), nausea (50%), dizziness (55%), and mild confusion (30%).[46] As the carboxyhemoglobin level increases, the severity of symptoms worsens and may result in coma (up to 30% of acute toxicity presentations).[37] The commonly described cherry red lips and skin are insensitive and present in only approximately 30% of cases.[37] Common systemic toxicity includes cardiac toxicity and is present in one-third of patients, and those presenting with acute toxicity should undergo electrocardiogram (ECG) and cardiac biomarker assessment.[47] It is crucial to recall that standard pulse oximetry demonstrates normal oxygen saturation despite the fact that tissue is hypoxic.

Among patients with CO exposure, 40% have delayed neurologic sequelae.[48] These can include cognitive deficits, personality changes, depression, anxiety, and movement disorders that may persist for years after exposure, with imaging findings commonly demonstrating bilateral hippocampus and globus pallidus destruction[37,49,50] (**Fig. 1**). Although there is not a correlation with exact carboxyhemoglobin

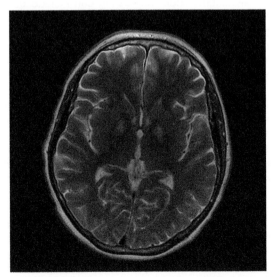

Fig. 1. T2-weighted MRI. There is bilateral T2 signal hyperintensity in the globus pallidus. (*Courtesy* of Dr. Juan Small, Lahey Hospital and Medical Center, Burlington, MA.)

level, depressed level of consciousness at the time of presentation is associated with greater risk of delayed neurologic symptoms.[37,44] Age greater than 36 and exposure greater than 24 hours increase the risk of long-term disability.[51] The long-term relative risk of dementia is 1.6 (relative risk 1.11–2.04).[50]

Acute management of CO toxicity includes removing the patient from the exposure source and ensuring at the time of discharge that exposure does not reoccur. High-flow oxygen via face mask, including potential nonrebreather use, should be initiated immediately because this dramatically decreases the elimination time of CO, from 300 minutes to 90 minutes.[37] Hyperbaric oxygen at 2 or more atmospheres of pressure can decrease this time even further, to 30 minutes.[52,53] Recommendations for use of hyperbaric oxygen include[52,53]

- Patients with carboxyhemoglobin level greater than 25% (or 20% in pregnancy)
- Depressed level of consciousness
- Severe acidosis, with pH less than 7.1
- Other signs of end-organ ischemia

Antibiotics

Antibiotics are one of the most frequently prescribed classes of medication in both inpatient and outpatient settings and, like all medications, are not without risk (**Table 2**). Central nervous system toxicity is likely an under-recognized consequence because it easily can be clouded by other causes of encephalopathy.[54] Serous central nervous system side effects commonly have been reported at a frequency of approximately 1%, but newer antibiotics have reported CNS toxicity rates of 15%.[54–56] A high degree of suspicion for antibiotic-associated CNS toxicity is essential.

Many factors are associated with increased susceptibility for neurotoxicity, including age (older age with higher risk), nutritional status, integrity of the blood-brain barrier, rate and route of medication delivery, activation and elimination of the drug and metabolites, and comedication administration.[57] Retrospective reviews report neurologic toxicity with at least 12 different classes of antibiotics and 54 specific antibiotics.[57,58] Different classes of antibiotics have different clinical neurotoxic syndromes due to differing pathophysiologic mechanisms of.[58]

The clinical features of neurotoxicity vary with the antibiotic administered but there is overlap.[58] The most common symptoms include psychosis with delusions or hallucinations (47% of reported cases), myoclonus (15%), convulsive and nonconvulsive seizures (14%), and cerebellar symptoms with ataxia or dysmetria (5%).[58] Neurologic symptoms can occur from the first dose of antibiotic or emerge months after treatment, but the median time of onset to symptoms is 5 days.[58] The time to resolution of encephalopathy after antibiotic discontinuation or change also is approximately5 days.[58] Common diagnostic evaluation completed for neurotoxicity in the setting of antibiotic use includes magnetic resonance imaging (MRI), CT, and EEG. MRI typically is normal, with the exception of metronidazole-associated neurotoxicity (discussed later), but EEG is abnormal in 70% of cases, with the most common abnormalities nonspecific slowing and generalized periodic discharges.[58]

The potentially serious but commonly reversible neurologic toxicity noted with antibiotics likely is an underdiagnosed condition.[58,59] Dose reduction in those patients at high risk of neurotoxicity may decrease the risk, but close neurologic monitoring is the mainstay of diagnostic evaluation. Treatment consists of discontinuation of the offending agent, use of antiepileptic medications for seizure and/or status epilepticus,

Table 2
Antibiotic classes and neurologic toxicity

Antibiotic Class	Neurotoxic Effects	Mechanism of Neurotoxicity	Risk Factors
Penicillins Penicillin G Piperacillin Ampicillin Oxacillin	Seizures Tremor Encepha- lopathy Psychosis	Inhibition of GABA$_A$ receptors	Renal failure/ dysfunction Older age Abnormal CNS penetration
Cephalosporins Cefepime Ceftazidime Cefazolin Cephalexin Ceftriaxone	Seizures Myoclonus Asterixis	Inhibition of GABA$_A$ release Increase glutamate	Renal failure/ dysfunction Older age Abnormal CNS penetration
Carbapenems Imipenem Meropenem Ertapenem Doripenem	Encepha- lopathy Seizures Myoclonus	Inhibition of GABA$_A$ receptors Binding of glutamate receptors	Renal failure/ dysfunction Older age Abnormal CNS penetration
Aminoglycosides Gentamicin	Encepha- lopathy Mesence- phalic glial death	NMDA receptor activation	Abnormal CNS penetration
Quinolones Ciprofloxacin Ofloxacin Norfloxacin	Encepha- lopathy Psychosis Seizure Myoclonus Tourette-like syndrome	Inhibition of GABA$_A$ receptor NMDA receptor activation Possible dopamine receptor activation	Abnormal CNS penetration Extremes of age
Tetracyclines	Intracranial hypertension Encephalopathy		
Metronidazole	Ataxia Dysarthria	Neuronal death within cerebellar dentate nuclei, brainstem, and corpus callosum	

antipsychotic medications for psychosis, and supportive care. Hemodialysis can be considered in select cases.[57]

Penicillins

Penicillins were the first antibiotic class to cause neurotoxicity. Penicillin G procaine resulted in anxiety and somatization in patients due to procaine's cocaine-like effect of dopamine release.[57,59] Penicillins exert inhibition on GABA transmission due to similar structure of β-lactam rings and γ-aminobutyric acid (GABA) neurotransmitters.[60] If the lactam ring is cleaved, the epileptogenic potential is lost.[61] The array of symptoms associated with penicillin-induced neurotoxicity includes psychological manifestations, such as anxiety and confusion, myoclonus, and subclinical and focal seizures.[57] Those with abnormal renal function, prior CNS disease, or at the extremes of age are at increased risk.[57]

Cephalosporins

Cephalosporin-induced neurotoxicity is associated with all generations of the drugs. Its manifestations include encephalopathy (with increased or decreased level of arousal), myoclonus, truncal asterixis, chorea, convulsive seizures, nonconvulsive status epilepticus, and coma.[57,59,62] The primary risk factors for CNS toxicity include renal dysfunction and prior CNS disease.[63,64] Neurologic symptoms can include

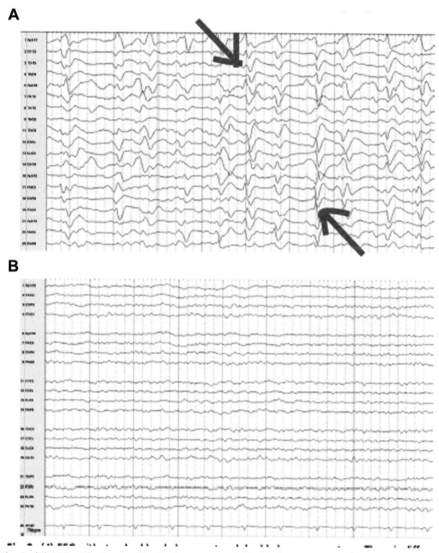

Fig. 2. (A) EEG with standard lead placement and double banana montage. There is diffuse severe generalized slowing and approximately 1-Hz generalized periodic discharges with triphasic morphology (arrow). There is ongoing cefepime administration at the time of the EEG. (B) Repeat EEG 5 days after cessation of cefepime with standard lead placement and double banana montage. There is resolution of the generalized periodic discharges with emergence of mild diffuse posterior dominate rhythm slowing.

lethargy, confusion, agitation, and chorea that progresses over days.[59] Nonconvuslive seizures and status epilepticus has been in as many as 15% of patients treated with cefepime and these patients often require anticonvulsants[59] (**Fig. 2**). CNS toxicity is due to decreased GABA release, increase excitatory amino acid release, and high affinity for and antagonism of $GABA_A$ receptors.[58,59] Typical onset of symptoms is 1 day to 10 days from medication onset.[65]

Carbapenems

Carbapenems are associated with seizures, with an estimated incidence of 3%.[59] Again the pathophysiology of increased seizure risk, shared with the other β-lactam ring containing penicillins and cephalosporins, is related to GABA receptor blockade and possibly enhancement of glutamate binding to the N-methyl-D-aspartate (NMDA) receptor.[59,66] The complexity of the side chain decreases the neurotoxicity[67] (**Fig. 3**). More common neurologic symptoms include headache and disorientation.[57] As with the other β-lactam medications, older age, prior CNS disease, and renal dysfunction are risk factors for neurologic toxicity.

Aminoglycosides

Aminoglycosides can affect most of the neuraxis: neuromuscular junction, peripheral nerve, cranial nerves, and brain/brainstem (namely, cochlear dysfunction and ototoxicity). Encephalopathy and other manifestations of CNS neurotoxicity, however, are rare. One case report noted pontine and mesencephalic axon, astrocyte, and oligodendroglia loss after intrathecal gentamicin administration.[57] The pathophysiology of CNS toxicity is thought to occur through the NMDA receptor as coadministration

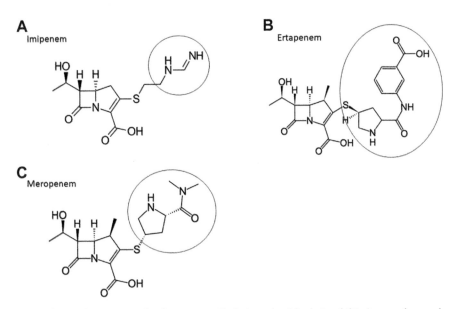

Fig. 3. Chemical structures of carbapenems. Circled are the side chains. (A) Imipenem has a relatively less complex side chain and is associated with increased neurologic toxicity. The more complex side changes ([B] ertapenem and [C] meropenem) result in decreased neurologic toxicity. Images adapted from Fvasconcellos public domain. (National Center for Biotechnology Information. "PubChem Compound Summary for CID 11145493, Ertapenem monosodium" PubChem, https://pubchem.ncbi.nlm.nih.gov/compound/Ertapenem-monosodium. Accessed 3 August, 2020.)

of NMDA antagonists diminish the toxicity.[68] The major risk factor for CNS toxicity associated with aminoglycosides is abnormal CNS permeability.[69]

Quinolones

Quinolones have multiple neurotoxic effects, including seizures, encephalopathy, myoclonus, and psychosis.[57] CNS toxicity is reported with an incidence of 0.89%.[70] The pathophysiology is uncertain but thought to include inhibition of $GABA_A$ receptors and activation of NMDA receptors.[71] There are reports of a Tourette-like syndrome with orofacial and limb automatisms and echolalia that raises the possible dopaminergic component of neurotoxicity.[72] Risk factors for toxicity include prior CNS injury and extremes of age.[73]

Tetracyclines

Tetracycline can cause intracranial hypertension and associated encephalopathy.[74]

Sulfa

Sulfamethoxazole has been associated with encephalopathy and psychosis. Extremes of age and immunocompromised patients are at greater risk for neurotoxicity.[75] The pathophysiology is unknown but it is known that sulfamethoxazole has excellent CNS penetration.

Metronidazole

Metronidazole is of special consideration because the typical neurologic manifestation is a cerebellar syndrome of ataxia and dysarthria.[58] Onset of neurologic symptoms typically occurs weeks after medication administration.[58,76] MRI abnormalities are frequent and consist most commonly of T2 hyperintensity within the cerebellar dentate nuclei, brainstem, and corpus callosum.[58,77] The MRI changes and neurologic symptoms commonly are reversible.[77]

Chemotherapy

Antineoplastic treatments can result in a wide range of peripheral and central nervous system disorders (**Table 3**). Although the most common neurologic complication of

Table 3 Chemotherapy and neurologic toxicity	
Chemotherapy Class	**Acute Neurotoxic Effects**
Methotrexate	Common: fatigue, confusion, headache, stroke-like syndromes Rare: seizure
Cytarabine	Common: aseptic meningitis, headache, seizure, myelopathy Rare: cerebellar dysfunction
5-FU	Common: encephalopathy Rare: cerebellar dysfunction, extrapyramidal movement disorder, seizures
Cyclophosphamide/ ifosfamide	Common: encephalopathy, blurry vision Rare: cerebellar dysfunction, extrapyramidal movement disorder, seizures, hallucinations
Kinase inhibitors	Common: dizziness, gait disturbance, tremor, cognitive disorder
Nitrosourea	Uncommon: encephalopathy and seizure
Asparaginase	Common: fatigue and confusion Rare: cerebral venous thrombosis and acute ischemic stroke
Platinum compound	Uncommon: headache, encephalopathy, cortical blindness

antineoplastic treatment is peripheral neuropathy, central nervous system dysfunction is an important complication.[78,79] Discerning chemotherapeutic neurologic toxicity from potential metastatic disease or paraneoplastic syndromes is paramount. CNS toxicity may result from direct toxic effects of the antineoplastic drug, cerebrovascular dysfunction, or autoimmune disorders. Although outside the scope of this article, chronic changes in cognitive function after chemotherapeutic treatment is not uncommon.

As seen with other medication classes, toxic effects are related to premorbid patient conditions and the medication, dose, route of administration, and concomitant medication administration. Premorbid blood-brain barrier integrity also is an important risk factor and commonly is affected adversely in patients with cancer by brain radiation.[80] Early identification of central neurotoxic effects is important because early dose reduction and possible drug change are essential components of management.[80]

Methotrexate

Methotrexate is an antimetabolite chemotherapeutic that can be administered inttathecal for treatment of leptomeningeal spread of malignancy.[80] Both the total dose and route of administration are risk factors for CNS toxicity. Acute toxicity typically is encountered 2 to 4 hours after high dose administration and lasts for 12 hours to 72 hours.[80] The most common symptoms include fatigue, confusion, and headache. Seizures are rare but may occur. Symptoms typically resolve and retreatment with methotrexate generally is considered appropriate.[81] Aseptic meningitis can occur in the acute setting in high-dose, frequent administration.[82] Intrathecal administration is associated with increased risk for aseptic meningitis as well as myelopathy.[80]

More subacute presentations include stroke-like syndromes, such as hemiparesis, ataxia, aphasia, and confusion that typically occur 2 days to 14 days after administration and can last up to 72 hours.[81,83,84] MRI commonly demonstrates T2-weighted hyperintensities and related diffusion restriction that is localized to white matter.[83,84] Children receiving moderate to high doses of methotrexate for acute lymphocytic lymphoma are the most common cohort to present with the stroke-like syndrome, but it is reported in nearly all age groups.[85] The pediatric cohort demonstrated seizures in 60% of cases, diffusion restriction in 40% of cases, ataxia in 5%.[85]

Chronic CNS complications of methotrexate administration are of greatest concern due to their irreversibility and progressive nature.[80] The progressive leukoencephalopathy associated with methotrexate, the risk of which is increased with whole-brain radiation, results in progressive development of white matter T2/fluid-attenuated inversion recovery (FLAIR) signal hyperintense lesions.[86,87] Associated neurologic symptoms include progressive cognitive impairment, gait disturbance, and aphasia.[88,89] It appears to occur in approximately 25% of adult and pediatric patients treated with high-dose methotrexate.[88-90] Folinic acid commonly is administered with methotrexate to treat GI and bone marrow toxicity but it does not prevent or reverse neurologic toxicity.[80]

Cytarabine

Cytarabine is a pyrimidine analog that inhibits DNA synthesis and is used to treat leukemias, lymphomas, and leptomeningeal spread of malignancies.[91] Intrathecal administration can result in aseptic meningitis, headache, seizure, and myelopathy, similar to the effects of intrathecal methotrexate.[78,92,93] Intravenous administration rarely can cause encephalopathy, which occurs 2 days to 5 days after initiation of treatment and typically is followed by cerebellar dysfunction.[80,91] Cerebellar dysfunction can occur at low doses but typically occurs with the total dose is greater than 30 g/m^2.[80] Older age (greater than 40 years), abnormal liver and renal function, and premorbid neurologic dysfunction increase the risk of cerebellar toxicity, which manifests as dysarthria, nystagmus, and gait ataxia.[80] MRI in these patients demonstrates cerebellar atrophy and reversible white matter T2/FLAIR hyperintensities.[80]

Fluorouracil
Fluorouracil (5-FU) inhibits DNA synthesis by inhibiting pyrimidine synthesis and is used to treat GI, head and neck, and breast tumors.[80,94,95] Rarely, 5-FU can result in CNS toxicity, but those with dihydropyridine dehydrogenase deficiency are at greater risk for encephalopathy.[96] Additional rare CNS toxicity includes cerebellar dysfunction (ataxia, dysmetria, dysarthria, and nystagmus), extrapyramidal movement disorders, and seizures.[94,95,97] Hyperammonemia without other evidence of liver dysfunction can occur and result in CNS toxicity. It should be considered in patients with movement disorders following administration.[98]

Cyclophosphamide and ifosfamide
Both cyclophosphamide and ifosfamide are alkylating agents that require activation in the liver to form active metabolites. Cyclophosphamide and its active metabolites rarely cross the blood-brain barrier, resulting in rare CNS side effects, including confusion and blurred vision.[99] Ifosfamide, on the other hand, can cross the blood-brain barrier more readily and causes encephalopathy in 10% to 30% of patients.[100,101] Risk factors include renal dysfunction, hypoalbuminemia, concurrent antiemetic use, and prior cisplatin administration.[100] Additional symptoms can include cerebellar dysfunction, extrapyramidal symptoms, hallucinations, and seizures.[102] Symptoms typically begin within several hours to a day after administration and resolve in 3 days to 4 days.[80] There are few data, but thiamine and methylene blue may prevent the encephalopathy associated with ifosfamide.[103,104]

Kinase inhibitors
Kinase inhibitors are a ubiquitous chemotherapeutic class that have rare neurologic toxicity. Imatinib, a tyrosine kinase inhibitor, has resulted in posterior reversible encephalopathy syndrome.[78] Larotrectinib, a neurotropic tropomyosin receptor kinase, commonly is associated with mild neurologic deficits including dizziness, gait disturbance, tremor, and memory impairment in up to 53% of those treated, but, of those cases, symptoms are moderate or severe in only 7%.[105] Lorlatinib is an ROS1 tyrosine kinase inhibitor with common but generally mild neuropsychiatric side effects, including cognitive dysfunction (18%), mood disturbance including emotional lability and irritability (18%), and hallucinations (5%).[106]

Nitrosoureas
Carmustine and lomustine cross the blood-brain barrier easily but typically do not result in neurotoxicity. Encephalopathy and seizures have occurred in patients with prior brain injury, including CNS malignancy.[107] The CNS toxicity typically occurs weeks to months after administration.[78]

Asparaginase
Asparaginase is used to treat leukemia and lymphomas. There is an associated coagulopathy effect that includes both thrombosis and hemorrhage. Although rare, cerebral venous sinus thrombosis and acute ischemic stroke due to arterial thrombosis are potentially life-threatening complications.[108] Neurologic symptoms of fatigue and disorientation are reported in the acute phase in up to 10% of patients.[108]

Platinum compounds

Platinum-containing chemotherapy includes cisplatin, carboplatin, and oxaliplatin. These medications uncommonly cause CNS adverse effects due to minimal diffusion across the blood-brain barrier. Common neurologic side effects include headache, encephalopathy, ischemic stroke, seizure, and cortical blindness.[109] Carboplatin can reach the highest CSF concentrations.[109] The mechanism for CNS toxicity is unknown, but the associated encephalopathy may be due, at least in part, to the electrolyte disorders associated with use (ie, hyponatremia and hypocalcemia).

Antidepressants and Antipsychotics

Antidepressant and antipsychotic drug use is common and increasing.[110-116] (**Table 4**). Not surprisingly, the prevalence of adverse effects associated with them

Table 4
Summary of medications/drugs causing serotonin syndrome and hypothesized mechanisms of action

Mechanism of Action	Drug/Medication
Promotion of synthesis of serotonin in the serotonergic presynaptic cells	L-tryptophan
Inhibition of serotonin degradation in the presynaptic cells (inhibition of monoamine oxidase)	MAOIs Methylene blue Linezolid
Stimulation of serotonin release from vesicles in the presynaptic cells	Amphetamines Mirtazapine Dextromethorphan MDMA Opioids (oxycodone, meperidine) Tramadol
Inhibition of serotonin reuptake transporter on the presynaptic cells (leading to increase of serotonin in synaptic cleft)	SSRI/SNRI TCA Opiates (meperidine, methadone) Tramadol Trazodone Bupropion MDMA Cocaine/amphetamines St. John's wort
Direct serotonin agonism (activation of postsynaptic 5-HT$_{1A}$ receptor)	Buspirone LSD Triptan class of medications Ergot class of medication Fentanyl Lithium Metoclopramide
Indirect serotonin agonism	Cytochrome P450 modulators • Altered drug metabolism and clearance Opioids (morphine) • Activation of GABA and glutamate receptors, and indirect stimulation or proserotonergic cells

Abbreviations: LSD, Lysergic acid diethylamide; SSRI/SNRI, selective serotonin reuptake inhibitor/serotonin and norepinephrine reuptake inhibitor; TCA, Tricyclic antidepressants.
   Data from Refs.[123,124,160]

is increasing as well.[117–120] For example, In the most recent (2017) annual report from the American Association of Poison Control Center, the selective serotonin reuptake inhibitor (SSRI)/serotonin and norepinephrine reuptake inhibitor (SNRI) group of medications was responsible for approximately 3.8% (n = 122) of mortalities as well as 29,522 incidences of single exposure.[120] Serotonin syndrome and neuroleptic malignant syndrome (NMS) are the most important causes of encephalopathy associated with these medications because they are very treatable yet can be fatal when not recognized and treated efficiently. Although closely related in terms of pharmacology, clinical manifestations, and treatment, these largely are distinct entities with important differences in management.

Serotonin syndrome

Serotonin syndrome is a sudden-onset, severe toxic syndrome caused by a sudden pathologic increase in CNS serotonergic neurotransmission. Serotonin in the CNS is involved in cognition, learning, memory, reward, and other complex processes. Peripherally, it modulates vasoconstriction, uterine contraction, and GI motility and also is released by platelets and functions in platelet aggregation.[121] In the CNS, serotonin acts on 7 groups of serotonin receptor families (5-HT_1–5-HT_7), many of which have multiple receptor subtypes with a total of 14 different serotonin receptors.[122] It is hypothesized that many CNS processes influenced by serotonin, including the manifestations of serotonin syndrome, occur largely via activation of the postsynaptic 5-HT_{1A} receptor system.[123,124]

Most cases of serotonin syndrome occur in patients taking multiple serotonergic medications or large doses of a single drug. In a meta-analysis of 299 cases published between 2004 and 2014, the most common cause of serotonin syndrome was a combination of antidepressants and opiates use (16.1% of cases), closely followed by single-agent overdose at 15.4%, with the latter responsible for most intensive care unit (ICU) admissions.[125] Nonetheless, serotonin syndrome can occur in patients taking normal doses of single serotonergic antidepressants.[126,127] A wide variety of drugs have been associated with serotonin syndrome (see **Table 4**). SSRIs and SNRIs probably are the most common contributors to serotonin syndrome due to the frequency of their use and direct effect on serotonergic neurotransmission. A variety of medications not typically recognized as having proserotonergic effects have been associated, including other antidepressants (bupropion, monoamine oxidase inhibitors [MAOIs], tricyclic antidepressants, and St. John's wort), analgesics (tramadol, meperidine, and fentanyl), antiemetics (metoclopramide), antiepileptics (valproate and carbamazepine), antibiotics (linezolid), antitussives (dextromethorphan), and muscle relaxants (cyclobenzaprine), among many others. Multiple illicit drugs have been associated with serotonin syndrome, including amphetamines, cocaine, and 3,4-methyl enedioxy methamphetamine (MDMA). Somewhat counterintuitively, abrupt withdrawal of serotonin antagonists, notably the atypical antipsychotic clozapine, also can cause serotonin syndrome.[128–130]

The onset of serotonin syndrome typically is rapid, usually taking place less than 13 hours after starting a new or overdosing on a serotonergic drug, or changing the dose of a chronically taken serotonergic drug.[131,132] Delayed presentation, however, often over days, may occur, especially in patients taking a mixture of serotonergic (eg, SSRI and SNRI) and antiserotonergic medications (eg, antipsychotics).[133] The typical syndrome is the triad of altered mental status, neuromuscular excitability, and autonomic hyperactivity. Encephalopathy may exist in many forms—frank agitation, hallucination, anxiety, and, when severe, depressed level of consciousness including coma.[123] Motor signs include rigidity, tremor, hyper-reflexia, and clonus (spontaneous and inducible), with a predilection for the lower extremities.[134] Presence of spontaneous lower extremity clonus as well as ocular clonus is fairly specific and especially helpful in narrowing the diagnosis to serotonin syndrome.[135] Dysautonomic signs and symptoms include diaphoresis, hyperthermia, diarrhea, and hemodynamic instability. Without treatment, serotonin syndrome can progress to seizures and coma with multiple systemic complications, including respiratory failure, acute renal failure, cardiac dysrhythmias, and disseminated intravascular coagulation.[123,136]

There are several different diagnostic criteria used to assess for the presence of serotonin syndrome[135] (**Table 5**). There is no combination, however, of tests or clinical syndrome that identifies serotonin syndrome with high specificity. Therefore, using history, laboratory testing, imaging, and a reasonable index of suspicion for this condition, serotonin syndrome must be differentiated from other conditions with a similar clinical presentation, including NMS; malignant hyperthermia; anticholinergic or sympathomimetic drug toxicity; neurotoxicity related to cephalosporins or calcineurin inhibitors; withdrawal from sedatives including ethanol, benzodiazepines, baclofen (especially intrathecal), and barbiturates; CNS infections; septic encephalopathy from a non-CNS infection; thyrotoxicosis; and rarely severe intracranial hypertension.

Treatment of patients with serotonin syndrome begins with management of acute, severe non-neurologic organ system dysfunction, including tracheal intubation and mechanical ventilation for respiratory failure; treatment of cardiac dysrhythmias and hemodynamic instability; and appropriate fluid resuscitation for hypotension, renal dysfunction, and electrolyte abnormalities. All potentially proserotonergic drugs immediately must be discontinued completely and care should be taken to not inadvertently introduce new proserotonergic agents (starting fentanyl in the ICU a common mistake). Benzodiazepines are an essential component of management, effective for decreasing the severity of agitated encephalopathy, seizures, neuromuscular hyperactivity, and cardiovascular instability. Antiadrenergic agents should be avoided for treatment of dysautonomic tachycardia or hypertension because of the potential for unpredictable exaggerated or paradoxic effects. If increasing doses of

Table 5 Clinical criteria used to evaluate serotonin syndrome		
	Sternbach Criteria	**Hunter Criteria**
Medication	• Recent addition or increase in known serotonergic medication • No recent addition of or increase in known neuroleptic medication	• The presence of a known serotonergic medication
Exclusion	• Absence of other possible causes	

Clinical findings	• Any 3 of the following:
	  ○ Altered mental status
	  ○ Myoclonus
	  ○ Hyperreflexia
	  ○ Diaphoresis
	  ○ Shivering
	  ○ Tremor
	  ○ Diarrhea
	  ○ Incoordination
	  ○ Fever
		• One of the following:
		  ○ Spontaneous clonus
		  ○ Inducible clonus OR ocular clonus WITH either
		    ■ Diaphoresis OR agitation
		    ■ Fever AND hypertonicity
		• Tremor AND hyperreflexia

Data from Dunkley EJ, Isbister GK, Sibbritt D, Dawson AH, Whyte IM. The Hunter Serotonin Toxicity Criteria: simple and accurate diagnostic decision rules for serotonin toxicity. QJM. 2003;96(9):635-42.

benzodiazepines do not accurately control these problems, small doses of IV morphine can be used. For hypertension, conservative titration of the ultra–short-acting calcium channel antagonist clevidipine is reasonable; longer-acting vasodilators should be avoided due to the potential for exaggerated effects with consequent hypotension. Cyproheptadine, due to its antagonism 5-HT$_{1A}$ and 5-HT$_{2A}$ receptors, is a fairly specific antidote for serotonin syndrome. It should be added in patients with severe serotonin syndrome who do not respond to the previously described treatment. Proserotonergic agents should be avoided for the duration of the acute phase of the illness, and a careful risk:benefit analysis should occur before restarting such drugs in the future.

Neuroleptic malignant syndrome

NMS is the most severe adverse reaction associated with antipsychotic medications. Although the incidence of NMS is relatively low, occurring in 0.02% to 3% in patients taking antipsychotic medications,[137–139] the importance of NMS derives from the high population prevalence of antipsychotic drug use[110–113] combined with impressive in-hospital mortality of 3% to 20% and significant associated morbidity, including respiratory failure, venous thromboembolism, acute renal failure, and systemic infections.[140–144] The exact pathophysiology of NMS is not known, but it is clear that decreased activity at central dopamine D2 receptors, with resultant severe sympathetic and neuromuscular hyperactivity, is key.

NMS most commonly presents as the tetrad of encephalopathy, rigidity, fever, and dysautonomia. In most cases, encephalopathy is the first symptom of NMS and can have multiple phenotypes, including agitation, psychosis, catatonia, and, when severe, coma.[145] Fever can be severe and take the form of dangerous hyperthermia. Dysautonomia is problematic, most frequently consisting of tachycardia and labile hypertension, but dysrhythmias can occur. Rigidity is a prominent feature, causing elevation of serum creatine kinase, present in approximately 75% of cases, and rhabdomyolysis in approximately one-third of patients.[146] Pneumonia and acute respiratory failure requiring intubation complicates NMS in 12% to 19% of patients.[138,147] Respiratory failure was determined to be the strongest independent predictor of mortality in a recent larger study using the US Healthcare Cost and Utilization Project nationwide inpatient sample database.[144] Other independent predictors of mortality from this study include acute kidney injury, acute liver failure, acute myocardial infarction, and sepsis.

When caused by first generation antipsychotics, NMS typically evolves over several days.[148] Cases caused by atypical antipsychotics or antidopaminergic antiemetics, however, can have a more insidious onset. Combined with a less typical clinical syndrome, often with absence of hyperpyrexia and rigidity, diagnosis of NMS associated with these drugs can be especially challenging.[139,149,150] In one of the largest studies, the mortality from NMS in patients taking atypical antipsychotics was almost 2-times lower than those taking typical antipsychotics, although not reaching statistical significance (3.3% vs 7.6%, respectively).[147] Of the atypical antipsychotics, rigidity and tremor were thought to occur less frequently from clozapine-induced NMS.[151] One interpretation of these data is that the toxic syndrome associated with atypical antipsychotics is not NMS but an overlap syndrome involving features of NMS and serotonin syndrome, caused by more complex abnormalities in monoaminergic neurotransmission related to their more complex, broader spectrum of monoamine receptor modulation.

There are multiple diagnostic mimickers of NMS that should be considered when NMS is suspected. The most common and diagnostically challenging is serotonin syndrome. Importantly, clonus, whether inducible or spontaneous, as well as hyper-reflexia is absent in NMS and one of the main features of serotonin syndrome. Malignant catatonia can be difficult to distinguish from NMS, a problem compounded by the fact that risk factors for the conditions essentially are identical. A days-long to weeks-long prodrome of behavioral changes, lack of extremely severe rigidity or dysautonomia, and lack of improvement with benzodiazepines and removal of dopamine antagonists should prompt consideration of malignant catatonia.[152] Parkinson-hyperpyrexia syndrome essentially is identical to NMS and occurs in patients with Parkinson disease in whom dopamine agonists are decreased or discontinued abruptly and/or a new dopamine antagonist is started.[153,154] Other conditions in the differential diagnosis for NMS include malignant hyperthermia; anticholinergic or sympathomimetic drug toxicity; severe withdrawal from sedatives, including ethanol and benzodiazepines, baclofen (especially intrathecal), and barbiturates; CNS infections; thyrotoxicosis; and, rarely, severe intracranial hypertension.

Treatment of NMS is similar to that of serotonin syndrome, as described previously. After stopping the inciting agents, care must be taken to treat end-organ dysfunction. Benzodiazepines and bromocriptine are the mainstays of therapy to treat agitation, hyperpyrexia, and muscle rigidity and spasm. Dopaminergic agents other than bromocriptine, such as amantadine and levodopa, have been used as adjuncts.[155] Dantrolene, which acts only to relax skeletal muscle and, therefore, does not treat all elements of NMS, is used in severe cases that do not respond to these treatments or when the rigidity and hyperthermia are immediately life-threatening. Dexmedetomidine has been used to treat the agitation and hemodynamic instability (tachypnea and tachycardia).[156] ECT and perhaps systemic corticosteroids can be useful in severe cases recalcitrant to other therapy.[157,158] In most cases, atypical antipsychotics can be restarted safely in patients who have had NMS 4 weeks after complete resolution; however, this must be done cautiously and with close follow-up because approximately 10% to 20% of patients experience a recurrence.[159]

CLINICS CARE POINTS

- Inorganic toxins are ubiquitous and, although toxicity is rare, can present insidiously. Metal intoxication (bismuth, lithium, and aluminum) toxidromes commonly have additional neurologic findings on examination, including tremors, ataxia, and seizures. The removal of the offending agent is the mainstay of treatment and, in appropriate clinical context, hemodialysis should be considered.
- Although most antibiotic classes have associated neurologic toxicity, penicillin, cephalosporins, and carbapenems are associated most commonly with encephalopathy. Those patients with advanced age and renal dysfunction are at increased risk for such toxicity. When there is an incongruent change in mental status while there is systemic improvement from infection, concern for neurotoxicity due to antibiotic therapy should strongly be considered.
- Antineoplastic medications can present with myriad neurologic toxicity syndromes affecting the whole neuraxis. For those patients presenting with subacute neurologic symptoms, it is imperative to exclude central or peripheral nervous system disease due to the oncologic process. The differential diagnosis is broad, but consideration for metastatic disease and ischemic or hemorrhagic stroke must be excluded.
- There is substantial overlap between NMS and serotonin syndrome. It is common that intentional or unintentional overdose of these medications is polysubstance. The mainstay treatment is removal of the offending agent and

supportive care. Early benzodiazepine administration treats the hyperactivity, but close monitoring of vital signs requires additional vigilance.

DISCLOSURE

Dr D.P. Lerner receives royalty payments from McGraw-Hill for editorial services. Dr A. Tadevosyan and Dr J.D. Burns have nothing to disclose.

REFERENCES

1. Martin-Bouyer G, Foulon G, Guerbois H, et al. Epidemological study of encephalopathies following bismuth administration per os. Characteristics of intoxicated subjects: comparison with a control group. Clin Toxicol 1981;18:1277–83.
2. Weast R. CRC, Handbook of chemistryand physics. Boca Raton (FL): Chemical Rubber Company Publishing; 1984.
3. Sampognaro P, Vo KT, Richie M, et al. Bismuth subgallate toxicity in the age of online supplement use. Neurologist 2017;22:237–40.
4. Hogan DB, Bharbride C, Duncan A. Bismuth toxicity presenting as declining mobility and falls. Can Geriatr J 2018;21:307–9.
5. Le Quesne PM. Toxic substances and the nervous system: the role of clinical observation. J Neurol Neurosurg Psychiatry 1981;44:1–8.
6. Hillemand P, Palliere M, Laquais B, et al. Bismuth treatment and blood mismuth levels. Sem Hop 1977;53:1663–9.
7. Jungreis AC, Schaumburg HH. Encephalopathy from abuse of bismuth subsalicylate (Pepto-Bismol). Neurol 1993;43:1265.
8. Reynold PT, Abalos KC, Hopp J, et al. Bismuth toxicity: a rare cause of neurological dysfunction. Int J Clin Med 2012;3:46–8.
9. Siram R, Botta R, Kashikunte C, et al. Chronic encephalopathy with ataxia, myoclonus, and auditory neuropathy. A case of bismuth poisoning. Neurol India 2017;65:186–7.
10. Buge A, Supino-Viterbo V, Rancurel G, et al. Epileptic phenomena in bismuth toxic encephalopathy. J Neurol Neurosurg Psychiatry 1981;44:62–7.
11. Stevens PE, Moore DF, House IM, et al. Significant elimination of bismuth by haemodilaysis with a new heavy metal chelating agent. Nephrol Dial Transplant 1995;10:696–8.
12. Strobusch AD, Jefferson JW. The checkered history of lithium in medicine. Pharm Hist 1980;22:72.
13. Mowry JM, Sypker DA, Brooks DE, et al. Annual report of the american association of poison control centers national poison data system (NPDS): 32nd annual report. Clin Toxicol 2015;53:962–1147.
14. Speirs J, Hirsch SR. "Severe lithium toxicity with "normal serum concentrations. Br Med J 1978;1:815.
15. Venkatarathnamma PN, Patil AR, Nanjudaiah N. Fatal lithium toxicity with therapeutic levels-a case report. Int J Clin Pharmacol Ther 2011;49:336.
16. Lavonas EJ, Buchanan J. Hemodialysis for lithium poisoning. Cochrane Database Syst Rev 2015;(9):CD007951.
17. Adityanjee, Munshi KR, Thampy A. The syndrome of irreversible-lithium effectuated neurotoxicity. Clin Neuropharmacol 2005;28:38.
18. Tilkian AG, Schroeder JS, Kao JJ, et al. The cardiovascular effects of lithium in man. A review of the literature. Am J Med 1976;61:665–70.
19. Kelley S, Gibson CAM. Lithium toxicity: The illusion of PTSD. Ann Psychiatry Ment Health 2017;5:1109–12.

20. Smith SW, Ling LJ, Halstenson CE. Whole bowel irrigation as a treatment for acute lithium overdose. Ann Emerg Med 1991;20:536.
21. Belanger Dr, Tierney MG, Dickinson G. Effect of sodium polystyrene sulfonate on lithium bioavailability. Ann Emerg Med 1992;21:1312.
22. Hauger RL, O'Connor KA, Yudofsky S, et al. Lithium toxicity: when is hemodialysis necessary? Acta Psychiatr Scand 1990;81:515.
23. Vodovar D, El Balkhi S, Curis E, et al. Lithium poisoning in the intensive care unit: predictive factors of severity and indications for extracorporeal toxin removal to improve outcome. Clin Toxicol (Phila) 2016;54:615.
24. Pierides AM, Edwards WG Jr, Cullum UX Jr, et al. Hemodialysis encephalopathy with osteomalacic fractures and muscle weakness. Kidney Int 1980;18:115.
25. Caramelo CA, Cannata JB, Rodeles MR, et al. Mechanisms of aluminum-induced microcytosis: lessons from accidental aluminum intoxication. Kidney Int 1995;47:164.
26. Burwen DR, Olsen SM, Bland LA, et al. Epidemic aluminum intoxication in hemodialysis patients tracted to use of an aluminum pump. Kidney Int 1995;47:164.
27. Schifman RB, Luevano DR. Aluminum Toxicity: Evaluation of 16-Year Trend Among 14,919 Patients and 45,480 Results. Arch Pathol Lab Med 2018;142:742.
28. Bohrer D, Bertagnolli DC, de Oliveria SM, et al. Drugs as a hidden source of aluminum for chronic renal patients. Nephrol Dial Transplant 2007;22:605.
29. Bansal VK, Bansal S. Nervous system disorders in dialysis patients. Handb Clin Neurol 2014;119:395.
30. Chen Y, Tian X, Wang X. Advances in dialysis encepahlopathy research: a review. Neurol Sci 2018;39:1151–9.
31. Alfrey AC, LeGendre GR, Kaehny WD. The dialysis encephalopathy syndrome - possible aluminum intoxication. N Engl J Med 1976;294:184.
32. Salusky IB, Foley J, Nelson P, et al. Aluminum accuulation during treatment with aluminum hydroxide and dialysis in children and young adults with chronic renal disease. N Engl J Med 1991;324:527.
33. Ellenberg R, King AL, Sica DA, et al. Cerebrospinal fluid aluminum levels following deferoxamine. Am J Kidney Dis 1990;16:157.
34. Modelli Andrade LG, Garcia FD, Silva VS, et al. Dialysis encephalopathy secondary to aluminum toxicity diagnosed by bone biopsy. Nephrol Dial Transplant 2005;20:2581–2.
35. National Kiney Foundation. K/DOQI clinical practice guidelines for bone metabolism and disease in chronic kidney disease. Am J Kidney Dis 2003;42:S1.
36. Ackrill P, Ralston AJ, Day JP, et al. Successful removal of aluminum form patients with dialysis encephalopathy. Lancet 1980;2:692.
37. Ernst A, Zibrak JD. Carbon monoxide poisoning. N Engl J Med 1998;339:1603.
38. Hampson NB. US mortality due to carbon monoxide poisoning, 1999-2014. accidental and intentional deaths. Ann Am Thorac Soc 2016;13:1768.
39. Rose JJ, Wang L, Xu Q, et al. Carbon monoxide poisoning: pathogenesis, management and future directions of therapy. Am J Respir Crit Care Med 2017;195:596.
40. Thomassen O, Brattebo G, Rostrum M. Carbon monoxide poisoning while using a small cooking stove in a tent. Am J Emerg Med 2004;22:204.
41. Centers for Disease Control and Prevention (CDC). Carbon monoxide poisoning attributed to underground utility cable fifers–New York. January 20000-June 2004. MMWR Morb Mortal Wkly Rep 2004;53:920.

42. Hampson NP, Dunn SL. Carbon monoxide poisoning from portable electrical generators. J Emerg Med 2015;49:125.

43. Retzky SS. Carbon monoxide poisoning from hookah smoking: an emerging public health problem. J Med Toxicol 2017;13:193.

44. Hardy KR, Thom SR. Pathophysiology and treatment of carbon monoxide poisoning. J Toxicol Clin Toxicol 1994;32:613.

45. Doyle KP, Simon RP, Stenzel-Poore MP. Mechanisms of ischemic brain damage. Neuropharmacology 2008;55:310–8.

46. Pages B, Planton M, Buys S, et al. Neuropsychological outcome after carbon monoxide exposure following a storm: a case-control study. BMC Neurol 2014;14:153.

47. Satran D, Henry CR, Adkinson C, et al. Cardiovascular injury and long-term mortality following moderate to severe carbon monoxide poisoning. JAMA 2006; 295:398.

48. Nakano T, Hasegawa T, Suzuki D, et al. Amantadine improves delayed neuropsychiatric sequelae of carbon monoxide poisoning: a case report. Brain Sci 2019;9:292.

49. Hampson NP, Piantadosi CA, Thom SR, et al. Practice recommendations in the diagnosis, management and prevention of carbon monoxide poisoning. Am J Respir Crit Care Med 2012;186:1095–101.

50. Lia CY, Huang YW, Tseng CH, et al. Patients with Carbon monoxide poisoning and subsequent dementia: a population-based cohort study. Medicine (Baltimore) 2016;95:e2418.

51. Weaver LK, Valentin KJ, Hopkins RO. Carbon monoxide poisoning: risk factors for cognitive sequelae and the role of hyperbaric oxygen. Am J Respir Crit Care Med 2007;176:491–7.

52. Hyperbaric recommendations: Undersea Hyperbaric Medical Society. Hyperbaric Oxygen Committee. Hyperbaric Oxygen Therapy Indications: The Hyperbaric Oxygen Therapy Committee Report. 2008.

53. Hampson NB, Little CE. Hyperbaric treatment of patients with carbon monoxide poisoning in the United States. Undersea Hyperb Med 2005;32:21.

54. Fugate JE, Kalimullah EA, Hocker SE, et al. Cefepime neurotoxicity in the intensive care unit: a cause of severe, underappreciated encephalopathy. Crit Care 2013;17:R264.

55. Owens RC, Ambrose PG. Antimicrobial safety: focus on fluoroquinolones. Clin Infect Dis 2005;41(suppl 2):S144–57.

56. Mattappalil A, Mergenhagen KA. Neurotoxicity with antimicrobials in the elderly: a review. Clin Ther 2014;36:1489–511.

57. Grill MF, Maganti RK. Neurotoxic effects associated with antibiotic use: management considerations. Br J Clin Pharmacol 2011;72:381–93.

58. Bhattacharyya S, Darby RR, Raibagkar P, et al. Antibiotic-associated encephalopathy. Neurology 2016;86:963–71.

59. Grill MF, Maganti R. Cephalosporin-induced neurotoxicity: clinical manifestations, potential pathogenic mechanisms, and the role of electroencephalographic monitoring. Ann Pharmacother 2008;42:1843–50.

60. Schliamser SE, Cars O, Norrby SR. Neurotoxicity of beta-lactam antibiotics: predisposing factors and pathogenesis. J Antimicrob Chemother 1991;27:405–25.

61. Gutnick MJ, Prince DA. Penicillinase and the convulsant action of penicillin. Neurology 1971;21:759–64.

62. Martin TCS, Chow S, Johns TS, et al. Ceftaroline-associated encephalopathy in patient with severe renal impairment. Clin Infect Dis 2019. https://doi.org/10.1093/cid/ciz857. ciz857.

63. Roncon-Albuquerque R Jr, Pires I, Martins R, et al. Ceftriaxone-induced acute reversible encephalopathy in a patient treated for a urinary tract infection. Neth J Med 2009;67:72–5.

64. Calandra G, Lydick E, Carrigan J, et al. Factors predisposing to seizures in seriously ill infected patients receiving antibiotics: experience with imipenem/cilastatin. Am J Med 1988;84:911–8.

65. Dakdouki GK, Al-Awar GN. Cefepime-induced encephalopathy. Int J Infect Dis 2004;8:59–61.

66. Koppel BS, Hauswer WA, Politis C, et al. Seizures in the critically ill: the role of imipenem. Epilepsia 2001;42:1590–3.

67. Sunagawa M, Matsumura H, Sumita Y, et al. Structural features resulting in convulsive activity of carbapenem compounds: effect of C-2 side chain. J Antibiot 1995;48:408–16.

68. Darlington CL, Smith PF. Vestibulotoxicity following aminoglycoside antibiotics and its prevention. Curr Opin Investig Drugs 2003;4:841–7.

69. Segal JA, Harris BD, Kustova Y, et al. Aminoglycoside neurotoxicity involves NMDA receptor activation. Brain Res 1999;815:270–7.

70. Jungst G, Mohr R. Side effects of ofloxacin in clinical trials and in postmarketing surveillance. Drugs 1987;34:S144–9.

71. Akahane K, Tsutomi Y, Kimura Y, et al. Levofloxacin, an optical isomer of ofloxacin, has attenudated epileptogenic activity in mice and inhibitory potency in GABA receptor binding. Chemotherapy 1994;40:412–7.

72. Thomas RJ, Reagan DR. Association of a Tourette-like syndrome with ofloxacin. Ann Pharmocother 1996;30:138–41.

73. Lee CH, Cheung RT, Chan TM. Ciprofloxacin-induced oral-facial dyskinesia in a patient with normal liver and renal function. Hosp Med 2000;61:142–3.

74. Snavely SR, Hodges GR. The neurotoxicity of antibacterial agents. Ann Intern Med 1984;101:92–104.

75. Saidinejad M, Ewald MB, Shannon MW. Transient psychosis in an immunecompetent patient after oral trimethoprim-sulfamethoxazole administration. Pediatrics 2005;115:e739–41.

76. Patel K, Green-Hopkins I, Lu S, et al. Cerebellar ataxia following prolonged use of metronidazole: case report and literature review. Int J Infect Dis 2008;12:e111–4.

77. Kuriyama A, Jackson JL, Doi A, et al. Metronidazole-induced central nervous system toxicity: a systematic review. Clin Neuropharmacol 2011;34:241–7.

78. DeAngelis LM, Posner JB. Side effects of chemotherapy. In: Deangelis LM, Posner JB, editors. Neurologic complications of cancer. 2nd edition. New York: Oxford University Press; 2009. p. 447–510.

79. Dietrich J, Wen PY. Neurologic complications of chemotherapy. In: Schiff D, Kesari S, Wen PY, editors. Cancer neurology in clinical practice. 2nd edition. Totowa (NJ): Humana Press; 2008. p. 287–326.

80. Verstappen CC, Heimans JJ, Hoekman K, et al. Neurotoxic complications of chemotherapy in patients with cancer: clinical signs and optimal management. Drugs 2003;63:1549–63.

81. Walker RW, Allen JC, Rosen G, et al. Transient cerebral dysfunction secondary to high-dose methotrexate. J Clin Oncol 1986;4:1845.

82. Mott MG, Stevenon P, Wood CB. Methotrexate meningitis. Lancet 1972;2:656.

83. Inaba H, Khan RB, Laningham FH, et al. Clinical and radiological characteristcs of methotrexate-induced acute encephalopathy in pediatric patients with cancer. Ann Oncol 2008;19:178.

84. Borgna-Pignatti C, Battisti L, Marradi P, et al. Transient neurologic disturbances in a child treated with moderate-dose methotrexate. Br J Haematol 1992;81:448.

85. Bhojwani D, Sabin ND, Pei D, et al. Methotrexate-induced neurotoxicity and leukocenphalopathy in childhood acute lymphoblastic leukemia. J Clin Oncol 2014; 32:949.

86. Rubinstein LJ, Herman MM, Long TF, et al. Disseminated necrotizing leukoencephalopathy: a complication of treated central nervous system leukemia and lymphoma. Cancer 1975;35:291.

87. Pizzo PA, Poplack DG, Bleyer WA. Neurotoxicities of current leukemia therapy. Am J Pediatr Hematol Oncol 1979;1:127.

88. Oka M, Terae S, Kobayashi R, et al. MRI in methotrexate-related leukoencephalopathy: Disseminated necrotising leukoencephalopathy in comparison with mild leukoencephalopathy. Neuroradiology 2003;45:493.

89. Robain O, Dulac O, Dommergues JP, et al. Necrotisin leukoencephalopathy complicating treatment of childhood leukaemia. J Neurol Neurosurg Psychiatry 1984;47:65.

90. Blay JY, Conroy T, Chevreau C, et al. High-dose methotrexate for the treatment of primary cerebral lymphoma: analysis of survival and late neurologic toxicity in a retrospective series. J Clin Oncol 1998;16:864–71.

91. Smith GA, Damon LE, Rugo HS, et al. High-dose cytarabine dose modification reduces the incidence of neurotoxicity in patients with renal insufficiency. J Clin Oncol 1997;15:833.

92. Ven den Berg H, van der Flier M, van de Wetering MD. Cytarabine-induced aseptic meningitis. Leukemia 2001;15:697–9.

93. Dunton SF, Nitschke R, Spruce WE, et al. Progressive ascending paralysis following administration of intrathecal and intravenous cytosine arabinoside: a Pediatric Oncology Group Study. Cancer 1986;57:1083.

94. Riehl JL, Brown WJ. Acute cerebellar syndrome secondary to 5-fluorouracil therapy. Neurology 1964;14:961.

95. Gottlieb JA, Luce JK. Cerebellar ataxia with weekly 5-fluorouracil administration. Lancet 1971;1:138.

96. Takimoto CH, Lu ZH, Ahang R, et al. Severe neurotoxicity following 5-fluorouracil based chemotherapy in a patient with dihydropyrimidine dehydrogenase deficiency. Clin Cancer Res 1996;2:477–81.

97. Howell SB, Pfeifle CE, Wung WE. Effect of allopurinol on the toxicity of high-dose 5-fluorouracil administered by intermittent bolus injection. Cancer 1983;51: 220–5.

98. Liaw CC, Wang HM, Wang CH, et al. Risk of transient hyperammonemic encephalopathy in cancers patients who received continuous infusion of 5-fluorouracil with the complication of dehydration and infection. Anticancer Drugs 1999;10:275.

99. Kende G, Sirkin SR, Thomas PR, et al. Blurring of vision: a previously undescribed complication of cyclophosphamide therapy. Cancer 1979;44:69–71.

100. David KA, Picus J. Evaluating risk factors for the development of ifosfamide encepahlopathy. Am J Clin Oncol 2005;28:277.

101. Rieger C, Fiegl M, Ischer J, et al. Incidence and severeity of ifosfamide-induced encephalopathy. Anitcancer Drugs 2004;15:347.

102. DiMaggio JR, Brown R, Baile WF, et al. Hallucinations and ifosfamide-induced neurotoxicity. Cancer 1994;73:1509–14.
103. Pelgrims J, DeVos F, Vanden Brande J, et al. Methylene blue in the treatment and prevention of ifosfamide-induced encephalopathy: report of 12 cases and a review of the literature. Br J Cancer 2000;82:291.
104. Buesa JM, Carcia-Teijido P, Losa R, et al. Treatment of ifosfamide encephalopathy with intravenous thiamine. Clin Cancer Res 2003;9:4636.
105. Drilon A, Laetsch TW, Kummar S, et al. Efficacy of larotrectinib in TRK fusion-positive cancers in adults and children. N Engl J Med 2018;378:731.
106. Solomon BJ, Besse B, Bauer TM, et al. Lorlatinib in patients with ALK-positive non-small cell lung cancer: results from a global phase 2 study. Lancet Oncol 2018;19:1654–67.
107. Shingleton BJ, Bienfang DC, Albert DM, et al. Ocular toxicity associated with high-dose carmustine. Arch Ophthalmol 1982;100:1766–72.
108. Muller H. Use of L-asparaginase in childhood ALL. Crit Rev Oncol Hematol 1998;28:97–113.
109. Vieillot S, Pouessel D, de Champfleur NM, et al. Reversible posterior leukoencephalopathy syndrome after carboplatin therapy. Ann Oncol 2007;18:608.
110. Oteri A, Mazzaglia G, Pecchioli S, et al. Prescribing pattern of antipsychotic drugs during the years 1996–2010: a population based database study in Europe with a focus on torsadogenic drugs. Br J Clin Pharmacol 2016;82:487–97.
111. Sultan RS, Correll CU, Schoenbaum M, et al. National patterns of commonly prescribed psychotropic medications to young people. J Child Adolesc Psychopharmacol 2018;28(3):158–65.
112. Alexander GC, Gallagher SA, Mascola A, et al. Increasing off-label use of antipsychotic medications in the United State, 1995-2008. Pharmacoepidemiol Drug Saf 2011;20(2):177–84.
113. Van Brunt DL, Gibson PJ, Ramsey JL, et al. Outpatient use of major antipsychotic drugs in ambulatory care settings in the United States, 1997-2000. Medscape Gen Med 2003;5(3):16.
114. Pratt LA, Brody DJ, Gu Q. Antidepressant use in persons aged 12 and over: United States, 2005-2008. NCHS Data Brief 2011;76:1–8.
115. Pratt LA, Brody DJ, Gu Q. Antidepressant use among persons aged 12 and over: United States, 2011–2014. NCHS data brief, no 283. Hyattsville (MD): National Center for Health Statistics; 2017.
116. OECD. Health at a glance 2015: OECD indicators OECD indicators. Paris: OECD Publishing; 2015. p. 217.
117. Read J, Williams J. Adverse effects of antidepressants reported by a large international cohort: emotional blunting, suicidality, and withdrawal effects. Curr Drug Saf 2018;13(3):176–86.
118. Tamblyn R, Bates DW, Buckeridge DL, et al. Multinational comparison of new antidepressant use in older adults: a cohort study. BMJ Open 2019;9:e027663.
119. Murray-Thomas T, Jones ME, Patel D, et al. Risk of mortality (including sudden cardiac death) and major cardiovascular events in atypical and typical antipsychotic users: a study with the general practice research database. Cardiovasc Psychiatry Neurol 2013;2013:247486.
120. Gummin DD, Mowry JB, Spyker DA, et al. Clinical toxicology. 2017 annual report of the American Association of Poison Control Centers' National Poison Data System (NPDS): 35th annual report. Clin Toxicol (Phila) 2018;56(12):1213–415.
121. Berger M, Gray JA, Roth BL. The expanded biology of serotonin. Annu Rev Med 2009;60:355–66.

122. Barnes NM, Sharp T. A review of central 5-HT receptors and their function. Neuropharmacology 1999;38(8):1083–152.
123. Boyer EW, Shannon M. The serotonin syndrome. N Engl J Med 2005;352(11): 1112–20.
124. Francescangeli J, Karamchandani K, Powell M, et al. The serotonin syndrome: from molecular mechanisms to clinical practice. Int J Mol Sci 2019;20(9):2288.
125. Werneke U, Jamshidi F, Taylor DM, et al. Conundrums in neurology: diagnosing serotonin syndrome – a meta-analysis of cases. BMC Neurol 2016;16:97.
126. Liu Y, Yang H, He F, et al. An atypical case of serotonin syndrome with normal dose of selective serotonin inhibitors. Medicine 2019;98:19.
127. Arora B, Kannikeswaran N. The serotonin syndrome-the need for physician's awareness. Int J Emerg Med 2010;3:373–7.
128. Stevenson E, Schembri F, Green DM, et al. Serotonin syndrome associated with clozapine withdrawal. JAMA Neurol 2013;70(8):1054–5.
129. Zerjav-Lacombe S, Dewan V. Possible serotonin syndrome associated with clomipramine after withdrawal of clozapine. Ann Pharmacother 2001;35(2):180–2.
130. Zesiewicz TA, Borra S, Hauser RA. Clozapine withdrawal symptoms in a Parkinson's disease patient. Mov Disord 2002;17(6):1365–7.
131. Nelson LS, Erdman AR, Booze LL, et al. Selective serotonin reuptake inhibitor poisoning: An evidence-based consensus guideline for out-of-hospital management. Clin Toxicol 2007;45(4):315–32.
132. Birmes P, Coppin D, Schmitt L, et al. Serotonin syndrome: a brief review. Can Med Assoc J 2003;168(11):1439–42.
133. Little K, Lin CM, Reynolds PM. Delayed serotonin syndrome in the setting of a mixed fluoxetine and serotonin antagonist overdose. Am J Case Rep 2018;19: 604–7.
134. Ener RA, Meglathery SB, Van Decker WA, et al. Serotonin syndrome and other serotonergic disorders. Pain Med 2003;4(1):63–74.
135. Dunkley EJ, Isbister GK, Sibbritt D, et al. The Hunter Serotonin Toxicity Criteria: simple and accurate diagnostic decision rules for serotonin toxicity. QJM 2003; 96(9):635–42.
136. Jones D, Story DA. Serotonin syndrome and the anaesthetist. Anaesth Intensive Care 2005;33(2):181–7.
137. Velamoor VR. Neuroleptic malignant syndrome. Recognition, prevention and management. Drug Saf 1998;1:73–82.
138. Levenson JL. Neuroleptic malignant syndrome. Am J Psychiatry 1985;142(10): 1137–45.
139. Caroff SN, Mann SC. Neuroleptic malignant syndrome. Med Clin North Am 1993;77(1):185–202.
140. Caroff SN. The neuroleptic malignant syndrome. J Clin Psychiatry 1980;41(3): 79–83.
141. Shalev A, Hermesh H, Munitz H. Mortality from neuroleptic malignant syndrome. J Clin Psychiatry 1989;50(1):18–25.
142. Taniguchi N, Tanii H, Nishikawa T, et al. Classification system of complications in neuroleptic malignant syndrome. Methods Find Exp Clin Pharmacol 1997;19(3): 193–9.
143. Addonizio G, Susman VL, Roth SD. Neuroleptic malignant syndrome: review and analysis of 115 cases. Biol Psychiatry 1987;22(8):1004–20.
144. Modi S, Dharaiya D, Schultz L, et al. Neuroleptic malignant syndrome: complications, outcomes, and mortality. Neurocrit Care 2016;24(1):97–103.

145. Rosebush PI, Anglin RE, Richards C, et al. Neuroleptic malignant syndrome and the acute phase response. J Clin Psychopharmacol 2008;28(4):459–61.

146. Lang FU1, Lang S, Becker T, et al. Neuroleptic malignant syndrome or catatonia? Trying to solve the catatonic dilemma. Psychopharmacology 2015; 232(1):1–5.

147. Nakamura M, Yasunaga H, Miyata H, et al. Mortality of neuroleptic malignant syndrome induced by typical and atypical antipsychotic drugs: a propensity-matched analysis from the Japanese Diagnosis Procedure Combination database. J Clin Psychiatry 2012;73(4):427–30.

148. Seitz DP, Gill SS. Neuroleptic malignant syndrome complicating antipsychotic treatment of delirium or agitation in medical and surgical patients: case reports and a review of the literature. Psychosomatics 2009;50(1):8–15.

149. Caroff SN, Mann SC. Neuroleptic malignant syndrome and malignant hyperthermia. Anaesth Intensive Care 1993;21(4):477–8.

150. Kogoj A, Velikonja I. Olanzapine induced neuroleptic malignant syndrome–a case review. Hum Psychopharmacol 2003;18(4):301–9.

151. Belvederi Murri M, Guaglianone A, Bugliani M, et al. Second-generation antipsychotics and neuroleptic malignant syndrome: systematic review and case report analysis. Drugs in R&D 2015;15(1):45–62.

152. Dessens FM, van Paassen J, van Westerloo DJ, et al. Electroconvulsive therapy in the intensive care unit for the treatment of catatonia: a case series and review of the literature. Gen Hosp Psychiatry 2016;38:37–41.

153. Friedman JH, Feinberg SS, Feldman RG. A neuroleptic malignant like syndrome due to levodopa therapy withdrawal. JAMA 1985;254(19):2792–5.

154. Serrano-Dueñas M. Neuroleptic malignant syndrome-like, or–dopaminergic malignant syndrome–due to levodopa therapy withdrawal. Clinical features in 11 patients. Parkinsonism Relat Disord 2003;9(3):175–8.

155. Carbone JR. The neuroleptic malignant and serotonin syndromes. Emerg Med Clin North Am 2000;18(2):317–25.

156. Tsaousi GG, Lamperti M, Bilotta F. Role of dexmedetomidine for sedation in neurocritical care patients: a qualitative systematic review and meta-analysis of current evidence. Clin Neuropharmacol 2016;39(3):144–51.

157. Fornaro M. Catatonia: a narrative review. Cent Nerv Syst Agents Med Chem 2011;11(1):73–9.

158. Sato Y, Asoh T, Metoki N, et al. Efficacy of methylprednisolone pulse therapy on neuroleptic malignant syndrome in Parkinson's disease. J Neurol Neurosurg Psychiatry 2003;74(5):574–6.

159. Ananth J1, Parameswaran S, Gunatilake S, et al. Neuroleptic malignant syndrome and atypical antipsychotic drugs. J Clin Psychiatry 2004;65(4):464–70.

160. Volpi-Abadie J, Kaye AM, Kaye AD. Serotonin syndrome. Ochsner J 2013;13(4): 533–40.

Toxin-Induced Coma and Central Nervous System Depression

Monica Krause, MD[a],*, Sara Hocker, MD[b]

KEYWORDS

- Neurotoxicity • Anesthetic • Sedative hypnotic • Cocaine washout syndrome
- Brain-death mimickers

KEY POINTS

- Intravenous and inhaled anesthetics intentionally depress consciousness but, in doing so, may lead to movement disorders, long-term cognitive impairment, and seizures.
- Sedative hypnotics are a broad category of medications with severe central nervous system (CNS) depression and complicated interactions with the nervous system in addition to their impact on consciousness.
- Abrupt discontinuation of cocaine may cause a profound comatose state that, with supportive care alone, resolves within 24 to 48 hours.
- High clinical suspicion is required to diagnose acute and chronic carbon monoxide poisoning given the nonspecific presentation.
- Prescription and environmental toxins may produce CNS effects that mimic brain death.

INTRODUCTION

Induction of coma and central nervous system (CNS) depression is at times a desired part of patient care. Such actions are particularly important in operating rooms and intensive care units (ICUs) to keep patients safe and comfortable. Despite the necessity of coma and CNS depression, undesired toxic effects may occur. In addition, certain medications and toxins may alter consciousness in an undesired manner. This article discusses medications and toxins that intentionally and unintentionally lead to depressed level of consciousness and the additional neurotoxicities that may result. It is not intended to be exhaustive but to provide key concepts for

[a] Department of Neurology, Mayo Clinic College of Medicine, 200 First Street Southwest, Rochester, MN 55905, USA; [b] Division of Neurocritical Care and Hospital Neurology, Department of Neurology, Mayo Clinic College of Medicine, 200 First Street Southwest, Rochester, MN 55905, USA
* Corresponding author.
E-mail address: Krause.Monica@mayo.edu

Neurol Clin 38 (2020) 825–841
https://doi.org/10.1016/j.ncl.2020.07.002   **neurologic.theclinics.com**
0733-8619/20/© 2020 Elsevier Inc. All rights reserved.

representative anesthetics, pain medications, sedative hypnotics, stimulant washout syndromes, carbon monoxide (CO) poisoning, and toxin-induced brain-death mimickers.

ANESTHETIC EFFECT ON THE BRAIN

Anesthetic medications are most frequently used for their sedative ability during surgical procedures or in the ICU. For most patients, these medications are well tolerated. However, with both the inhaled and intravenous forms, there are well-recognized and uncommon neurologic adverse manifestations. Given the vast number of anesthetic agents, this the focus here is on those most commonly used, including propofol, ketamine, nitrous oxide, isoflurane, and sevoflurane. **Table 1** summarizes the key points about these representative analgesics.

Intravenous Anesthetics

Propofol
Propofol induces sedation by binding to central alpha-2 receptors.[1] Given its highly lipophilic nature, patients can have a delayed emergence after cessation, particularly after a prolonged course. Movement disorders have also been attributed to this medication, including tremors, dystonias, multifocal myoclonus, and opisthotonus. [1–7] Although at times the movements appear seizurelike, no epileptogenic activity is appreciated when an electroencephalogram (EEG) is obtained.[3,6,8] Several mechanisms have been suggested for the cause of these movement disorders:

- Excess neuroexcitation via desensitization of the gamma-aminobutyric acid (GABA)–A receptor resulting in abnormalities of membrane currents and interneuron asynchrony.[4,9,10]
- Antagonism of the glycine receptors, particularly in the spinal cord where they have an important inhibitory effect.[1,4,8]
- Toxic metabolite buildup leading to abnormal movements.[9,10]

Ketamine
Ketamine is a promising sedating and analgesic medication that acts as a noncompetitive antagonist of N-methyl-D-aspartate (NMDA) receptors. In addition, ketamine interacts with opioid receptors and the monoamine, cholinergic, and adrenoreceptor systems. Its use is associated with profound emergence reactions/dreams and hallucinations as well as potential addiction.[11] When used long term or abused, it is associated with memory impairment. In addition, given its mechanism of action, repeated exposure may result in upregulation of the NMDA receptor sensitizing the neuron to glutamate. This process enhances calcium influx, ultimately causing apoptosis.[12] The exact clinical outcome of this effect is unknown at this time but this does raise the question of the ability to use ketamine in the developing brain.

Inhaled Anesthetics

One potential neurotoxic effect of all inhaled anesthetics (except nitrous oxide) is malignant hyperthermia, which manifests as tachycardia, hyperthermia, increase in end-tidal carbon dioxide level, and generalized rigidity. Typically, this occurs within an hour of administration.[1] If not promptly recognized, severe respiratory and metabolic acidosis develops, leading to life-threatening hyperkalemia and rhabdomyolysis within hours.[13] Malignant hyperthermia occurs in genetically predisposed patients (ryanodine receptor-1 positivity) exposed to the inhaled anesthetics or to extreme

Table 1
Summary of intravenous and inhaled anesthetics, their mechanism of action, and special considerations

Drug	Mechanism	Special Considerations for Depressant Effects	Other Nervous System Adverse Effects
Propofol	Alpha-2 agonist	• Delayed emergence	Movement disorders • Tremors • Dystonias • Multifocal myoclonus • Opisthotonus • Seizurelike phenomenon
Ketamine	Noncompetitive antagonist of NMDA receptors • Also interacts with opioid receptors and monoamine, cholinergic, and adrenoreceptor systems	• Profound emergence reactions/dreams • May be apoptotic through upregulation of NMDA receptors	• Memory impairment • Hallucinations • Potential for addiction
Nitrous oxide	Not well understood • May stabilize axon membranes to partially inhibit action potentials • May partially interact with opioid receptors	—	• Subacute combined degeneration
Isoflurane	Not well understood • May alter sensitivity of multiple ion channels	• Associated with malignant hyperthermia • May be apoptotic	• Leads to increase in enzymes that produce amyloid-β • Neurotoxicity in highly metabolic brain tissue
Sevoflurane		• Associated with malignant hyperthermia	• Potentially epileptogenic

Abbreviation: NMDA, N-methyl-D-aspartate.

environmental temperature/stress.[13] The treatment of choice is dantrolene, which reduces the activity of the ryanodine receptor.[1,13]

Nitrous oxide

Nitrous oxide's mechanism of sedation is not well understood. It may stabilize axon membranes to partially inhibit action potentials and it may produce a degree of analgesia from partial interaction with opioid receptors.[14] When abused in the medical or recreational setting, it is associated with subacute combined degeneration. This disorder manifests as paresthesias and unsteady gait caused by the degeneration of the sensory nerve fibers.[15]

Isoflurane

The exact mechanism for all inhaled anesthetics is not well understood. It is proposed that these medications work through alterations in the sensitivities of ion channels via neurotransmitter interactions with multiple receptors, including GABA-A, glycine, nicotinic acetylcholine, serotonin, and glutamate receptors.[16] Neurotoxicity of isoflurane is also poorly understood, with most research being conducted in animal and cellular studies. These studies have shown altered glucose metabolism, induction of cellular markers of apoptosis, and upregulation of enzymes responsible for β-amyloid protein production.[17,18] The results raise concerns for neurodegeneration and worsening Alzheimer disorder caused by isoflurane. A case report of 2 patients treated with a prolonged course of high-dose isoflurane for severe refractory status epilepticus showed T2-hyperintensity changes in thalamus, cerebellum, and medulla on MRI.[19] Although the clinical implications, if any, of these findings are unknown, this raises concern for isoflurane neurotoxicity, particularly in highly metabolic areas of the brain.

Sevoflurane

Other than sedation, one of the major neurologic effects of sevoflurane is potential perioperative convulsions.[20] However, determining the exact epileptogenic nature of sevoflurane is difficult because there are mixed studies outside of case reports.[19,21,22] In high-risk patients, it is reasonable to consider use of adjuvant anesthetic medication (opioids, benzodiazepines, nitrous oxide) to limit the risk of a possible epileptogenic state with sevoflurane.[22]

PAIN MEDICATIONS

Pain management provides significant challenges but is important for patient comfort and quality of life. However, pain medications have side effects, particularly on the nervous system. Countless options for pain management exist, but 2 of the most frequently used prescription pain medications are highlighted here: opioids and gabapentinoids. Other neuropathic pain medications (baclofen and tricyclic antidepressants) are discussed later given their other neurologic manifestations.

Opioids

Opioids, mu-receptor agonists, are frequent first-line medications for acute severe pain in the hospital and have common reversible nervous system effects, as listed in **Box 1**.[1] One notable effect of opioids is an increase in intracranial pressure (ICP). In 1 case report, an intensive care patient treated with morphine and fentanyl experienced severe increases in ICP that only resolved after discontinuation of the 2 medications.[23] At present, 1 proposed mechanism for ICP increase is the vasodilatory effects of opioid medication. However, the exact mechanism is still undetermined.

Box 1
Reversible adverse central nervous system effects of opioids

- Miosis
- Depressed level of consciousness
- Depressed respiratory drive
- Seizures (particularly with tramadol)
- Myoclonus (drug and dose specific)
- Increased intracranial pressure (ICP)

Fentanyl

Fentanyl is an ideal opioid used in the ICU given its analgesic/anesthetic properties and intravenous route of administration. However, when used in combination with other serotonin agents, fentanyl can lead to serotonin syndrome because of its inherent serotonergic activity.[1] Serotonin syndrome is characterized by altered mental status, neuromuscular irritability, and autonomic instability from excessive activation of postsynaptic serotonin receptor activation. Delayed recognition of this disease can be fatal. Treatment generally includes removal of the offending agent and supportive measures, although benzodiazepines have also been used.[24] Note that, although fentanyl has the highest serotonergic effect of the opiates, tramadol, meperidine, and methadone also have serotonin activity and could lead to serotonin syndrome.[24]

Gabapentinoids

Gabapentin and its cousin pregabalin, originally designed as anticonvulsants, are effective against neuropathic pain via a mechanism not yet fully understood. They commonly cause sedation, imbalance, and ataxia, particularly when initiating the medication.[1] These toxicities are much more common in patients with renal disease given their renal metabolism. Patients with renal disease have been reported to develop severe, disabling myoclonus. In the case reports, removal of the gabapentin or pregabalin and dialysis (if the patient is dialysis dependent) may reverse the severe myoclonus.[25–28]

SEDATIVE HYPNOTICS

Sedative hypnotics, as their name suggests, lead to altered levels of consciousness that allow surgical procedures or enhance sleep in patients with insomnia. **Table 2** highlights key details of the medications described here.

Benzodiazepines

Benzodiazepines increase the frequency of opening of postsynaptic chloride channels, thereby slowing action potential propagation. This slowed propagation depresses the electrical activity of the brain, allowing sedation as well as prevention of epileptic activity.[29] Neurotoxicities associated with benzodiazepines are associated with slowed electrical activity and include decreased respiratory drive and delayed emergence.[1] They may also be associated with increased ICP.[1] In addition, a small proportion of the population experiences a paradoxic reaction to benzodiazepines with severe agitation, hostility, or disinhibition and hyperactivity.[30–32] It is hypothesized that the paradoxic reaction is caused by loss of cortical restraint through the inhibitory actions of benzodiazepines. When the paradoxic reaction occurs, flumazenil may

Table 2
Summary of sedative hypnotics, their mechanism of action, and special considerations

Drug	Mechanism of Action	Special Consideration for Depressant Effects	Other Nervous System Adverse Effects
Benzodiazepines	Increase frequency of postsynaptic chloride channel opening	• Delayed emergence • Paradoxic reaction possible	• Decreased respiratory drive • Increased ICP
Barbiturates	Increase duration of postsynaptic chloride channel opening	• Prolonged use can lead to severe systemic complications	• Cognitive slowing • Movement disorders • Hyperactivity in children
Alcohols			
Ethanol	Facilitation of GABA receptors and inhibition of excitatory glutamate receptors	Acute intoxication • Black-out phenomenon Chronic intoxication • Withdrawal (seizures and delirium tremens) • Wernicke-Korsakoff syndrome • Hepatic encephalopathy	—
Ethylene glycol	—	• Somnolence and coma associated with cerebral edema	• Slurred speech • Ataxia • Nausea/vomiting

Methanol	—	• Coma complicated by severe lactic acidosis	• Long-term effects
			  ○ Optic neuropathy
			  ○ Tremor
			• Bilateral putaminal necrosis on MRI

Baclofen	Central GABA derivative	• Encephalopathy with triphasic waves • Theoretic attenuation with repeated exposures	• Myoclonus
Clonidine	Central and peripheral α2-adrenoreceptor agonist	• May induce coma	• Decreased sympathetic output • Severe systemic hypertension that may lead to SAH

GHB	GABA-like compound	• Transient amnesia and comma	• Convulsions • Hypotonia • Vertigo • Abuse potential
Zolpidem	GABA-receptor agonist	• Amnesia • Driving parasomnias	• Depression • Visual hallucinations • Nightmares • Dizziness • Addiction potential

Abbreviations: GHB, gamma-hydroxybutyrate; SAH, subarachnoid hemorrhage.

abort this reaction. Otherwise, treatment includes withdrawal of the medication and supportive care to ensure that patients do not hurt themselves or others.[30]

Barbiturates

Barbiturates, similarly to benzodiazepines, work on the postsynaptic chloride channel. However, they increase the duration of the chloride channel opening to alter action potential propagation.[33] Members of this class of medication can be used for both surgical sedation and second-line or third-line agents for seizure management.[29] Barbiturates, including thiopental and methohexital, are associated with movement disorders such as tremor and dystonia during continuous infusion and anesthetic induction.[7,34] In contrast, phenobarbital is overall well tolerated from a neurologic standpoint, with the most common neurotoxic effects being sedation, behavior (primarily hyperactivity in children), and cognitive slowing.[33] Other more well-known effects from phenobarbital are systemic, with increased risk of liver disease and connective tissue disease.[33]

Alcohols

Alcohols, particularly ethanol, are commonly abused substances readily accessible to patients of all ages. Nontraditional but highly toxic alcohols include ethylene glycol and methanol, which may be ingested in an accidental manner by animals or children. However, in other instances, ethylene glycol and methanol consumption may be intentional in the setting of suicide attempts. Neurotoxic effects of ethanol, methylene glycol, and methanol are discussed below.

Ethanol

The mechanism of action of ethanol most likely involves facilitation of GABA receptors and inhibition of excitatory glutamate receptors.[35] Toxic effects from ethanol are caused by complex interplay between direct neurologic effects, nutritional deficiencies, neurotransmitter alterations, and enhancement of neuroinflammatory processes.[36] The neurotoxic presentation varies based on the acuity of intoxication and chronicity of use.

- Acute intoxication
  - Black-out phenomenon: patients have minimal recollection of events, possibly caused by ethanol's effect on the hippocampus.[35,36]
- Chronic intoxication:
  - Confusion during the withdrawal period:
    - Complicated by seizures and delirium tremens[35,36]
  - Hepatic encephalopathy caused by alcoholic cirrhosis[36]
  - Wernicke-Korsakoff syndrome caused by thiamine deficiency
    - Wernicke encephalopathy: patients present with altered mental status (impaired memory, disorientation, and diminished spontaneous speech output), gait ataxia, and ophthalmoplegia, although not all 3 must be present[35,36]
    - Korsakoff syndrome: syndrome may later develop and is characterized by confabulation with anterograde and retrograde amnesia[36]
    - Treatment with high-dose thiamine is important to treat Wernicke encephalopathy with the goal of preventing Korsakoff syndrome[35]

Ethylene glycol

Ethylene glycol is an odorless, colorless, sweet-tasting liquid found in many household products.[37] Ethylene glycol itself is not toxic but its metabolites (glycolic acid and oxalate) lead to toxicity. The neurotoxicity occurs in the first phase of the toxidrome with slurred speech, ataxia, nausea, and vomiting. Profound somnolence and coma associated with cerebral edema may then occur.[38] These neurologic side effects are compounded by the development of a profound metabolic acidosis, which can lead to further decrease in the level of consciousness.[37] Ultimately ethylene glycol toxicity produces cardiopulmonary collapse and profound renal injury.[37,38] Early recognition is imperative. Treatment focuses on correcting the severe acidosis and administration of fomepizole/ethanol to prevent further metabolism of ethylene glycol.[37,38]

Methanol

Methanol is a colorless toxic liquid found in industrial solvents, such as windshield-washer fluid. Like ethylene glycol, methanol itself is not toxic but is metabolized by the liver to toxic metabolites, formaldehyde and formic acid, that produce a severe lactic acidosis.[39] The severe lactic acidosis can result in depressed level of consciousness and coma.[39] Before the profound alteration in sensorium, nonspecific neurologic findings include headache, nausea, vomiting, and dizziness.[40] Following the acute insult, lasting neurologic effects can include tremor and visual disturbance from optic neuropathy.[39] Characteristic MRI findings in methanol toxicity include bilateral putaminal necrosis with or without hemorrhage.[39,40] Treatment involves correction of metabolic acidosis and dialysis to remove the methanol and its metabolites.[39]

Baclofen

Baclofen, a centrally acting GABA derivative, is frequently used for its muscle relaxant properties in spastic patients, treatment of neuropathic pain, and more recently in chronic alcohol withdrawal.[41–43] The most common neurotoxic effect involves a mild encephalopathy that may be associated with myoclonus. More severe encephalopathy may develop, with significant EEG findings including mild to severe generalized slowing and triphasic waves.[43] A case report of baclofen toxicity showed a severe burst-suppression pattern associated with encephalopathy.[42] An overdose study of rats yielded early-onset and prolonged marked encephalopathy confirmed with EEG. The encephalopathy could be attenuated by prior repeated exposure to baclofen, suggesting tolerance that may play a role in future understanding of baclofen toxicity.[41]

Clonidine

Clonidine is a central and peripheral alpha2-adrenoreceptor agonist with multiple clinical indications, including anesthetic adjuvant and intrathecal analgesia.[44,45] It also decreases sympathetic output and is a potent antihypertensive.[46] When clonidine levels become toxic, seizures, confusion, and depressed level of consciousness, including coma, can ensue.[45,47] Agitation is also common in the pediatric population.[48] High doses of clonidine in the immediate phase can cause hypertensive emergency and vasospasm caused by the peripheral adrenoreceptor response, which in turn can lead to subarachnoid hemorrhage and hypertensive emergency.[45,47,48] Treatment of overdoses is typically supportive, with control of blood pressure, bradycardia, and respiratory depression being key. Some investigators have trialed naloxone to reverse the natural opioid release that clonidine can trigger.[49]

Gamma-Hydroxybutyrate

Gamma-hydroxybutyrate (GHB) is a GABA-like compound found naturally in the CNS and as a byproduct of intrinsic GABA metabolism.[50,51] Biochemically, it shows analgesic properties with the ability to increase brain opioids, enhance dopaminergic activity, increase serotonin levels, and promote endorphin release.[50,51] Although clinically it is used as an anesthetic induction agent and in the treatment of narcolepsy and alcohol withdrawal, it has more recently been recognized as a substance of abuse.[50,51] GHB can produce a high, enhance the ability to increase muscle bulk in bodybuilders, and cause a profound sedation that has been implicated in sexual assults.[50–52] The profound sedation has been described as transient amnesia or even coma.[50,51] Additional neurotoxic effects of GHB include convulsions, confusion, combative/self-injurious behavior, drowsiness, hypotonia, and vertigo.[50–52] Treatment is supportive, with intubation being required in patients who are unable to protect their airways.[50] After removal of GHB, patients typically recover within hours.[50]

Zolpidem and Related Nonbenzodiazepine Insomnia Medications

Zolpidem is a GABA-receptor agonist commonly used for insomnia treatment when life-style modification is inadequate.[53] Other medications within this group include zaleplon, eszopiclone, and zopiclone. The most common neurologic adverse effects from zolpidem include confusion, depression, visual hallucinations, nightmares, dizziness, and amnesia. These effects are both time and dose dependent.[53–55] Zaleplon and zopiclone have similar side effects to zolpidem. Eszopiclone has the additional side effects of neuralgia and dysgeusia.[54] Less common but more severe neurotoxic effects, particularly reported with zolpidem, involve complex parasomnias such as sleep driving that can result in significant bodily harm to the patient and others.[53–55] Concurrent ethanol use increases the risk for development of the complex parasomnias.[54] In addition, there is a theoretic risk for addiction and abuse.[54]

COCAINE WASHOUT SYNDROME

Cocaine is an illicit stimulant that produces local anesthetic and potent vasoconstriction.[56,57] Typically, it causes a euphoric experience, although patients may also have agitation, anxiety, panic, and psychosis.[56] Cocaine can cause a comatoselike state when abused long-term and then abruptly discontinued. This state is known as cocaine washout syndrome and is summarized in **Box 2**.[58] There may be hyporeflexia and lack of response to stimuli (including noxious stimuli) or the remainder of the neurologic examination may be normal.[58,59] Patients frequently are intubated for airway protection and can have a mild degree of hypotension or bradycardia.[58] However, in at least 1 reported instance, a patient had refractory hypotension was nonresponsive to 3 vasopressors.[60] Recovery spontaneously occurs after 24 to 48 hours of drug removal.[58,60] The exact pathophysiology of cocaine washout syndrome is not fully understood. It is thought to be related to chronic overstimulation of the CNS and neurotransmitter depletion.[59]

Box 2
Cocaine washout syndrome presentation

- Depressed level of consciousness to point of coma
- Hyporeflexia
- Hypotension
- Bradycardia
- Reduced respiratory drive

CARBON MONOXIDE POISONING

CO is a tasteless, odorless, highly toxic gas that more readily binds to hemoglobin than oxygen and decreases the oxygen carrying capacity of hemoglobin. CO further reduces the amount of oxygen released into peripheral tissues through a left shift in the oxygen dissociation curve. Ultimately, this leads to tissue hypoxia and acute and chronic neurologic sequelae.[61] The acute symptoms present in the immediate time following exposure. Chronic CO neurotoxicity occurs days to weeks after the initial exposure and severity may depend on degree of consciousness during the acute insult.[62] Between acute and chronic symptoms, patients are typically close to or completely back to their preexposure baseline. Acute and chronic symptoms are outlined in **Box 3**. Treatment in acute and chronic CO toxicity is supportive. There are mixed studies showing some utility of hyperbaric oxygen therapy in the acute poisoning phase for patients who present in a comatose state.[61–64]

In both acute and chronic CO toxicity, characteristic but not specific MRI changes occur and can help confirm the diagnosis of CO poisoning, as described in **Box 4**.

TOXIN-INDUCED BRAIN-DEATH MIMICKERS

Many substances may mimic coma. The selection discussed here is not meant to be exhaustive but highlights 4 frequent and potentially fatal toxin-induced mimickers of coma that must be recognized to prevent morbidity and fatality.

Tricyclic Antidepressants

Tricyclic antidepressants (TCAs) were originally designed as treatment of depression but have recently found more favor in their treatment of headache and chronic pain. Their mechanism of action has 4 main actions: inhibition of norepinephrine uptake, alpha-adrenergic blockade, myocardial membrane stabilization, and anticholinergic effects.[65] When taken in excess, these pharmacologic properties can produce severe neurologic toxicity, as outlined in **Box 5**.[65,66]

In addition to significant neurotoxicity, TCA overdose can result in a profound cardiac toxicity with prolongation of the PR, QRS, and QT intervals.[65] Treatment of TCA toxicity is supportive, with intubation for respiratory compromise, pressor support for severe hypotension, and administration of sodium bicarbonate for acidosis correction.[65,66]

Box 3
Presentation of carbon monoxide toxicity

Acute toxicity
- Mild symptoms
  - Weakness, nausea, confusion, shortness of breath
- Severe symptoms
  - Visual changes, chest pain, loss of consciousness
    - Loss of consciousness is thought to arise from increased ICP and cerebral edema from the hypoxia induced by CO poisoning.

Chronic toxicity
- Memory and cognitive defects
- Apathy
- Mutism
- Urinary incontinence
- Gait disturbance

Box 4
MRI brain findings in carbon monoxide toxicity

Acute poisoning
- Most common
  - T2 hyperintensity within the globus pallidus
- Less common
  - T2 hyperintensities within the cerebral cortex, cerebellum, and hippocampi

Chronic poisoning
- Confluent T2 hyperintensity in the white matter sparing the cortex

---

Organophosphate Poisoning

Organophosphates are commonly found in insecticides and pesticides and are absorbed through inhalation, ingestion, or dermal contact.[67] The toxins bind to and inactivate acetylcholinesterase, resulting in excessive cholinergic activity, which leads to bronchospasm, fasciculations, hypertension, salivation, emesis, diaphoresis, and seizures.[67,68] Flaccid paralysis may develop, which is life threatening and may result in respiratory arrest.[67,68] Treatment involves airway support, ensuring further exposure does not occur by thorough skin cleansing, and administration of atropine and pralidoxime.[68] Even with these measures, mortality remains high.[68]

Cefepime Neurotoxicity

Cefepime is a fourth-generation cephalosporin used to treat neutropenic fever and health care–associated infections. Although cefepime is an important antibiotic, given its pseudomonal coverage, neurotoxic effects are becoming more apparent, particularly in the setting of ICU delirium and depressed level of consciousness. Neurotoxic effects are thought to be related to inhibition of GABA-A receptors or release of GABA.[69] Cefepime-associated neurotoxic effects include:

- Diminished level of consciousness, even to the point of coma[69–71]
  - Triphasic waves may be present on EEG[69]
- Delirium or agitation[69]
- Myoclonus[69–71]
- Nonconvulsive status epilepticus (rare)[69,71]
- Aphasia[69]

Symptom onset is typically 4 to 5 days after cefepime initiation.[69,70] Risk factors for cefepime neurotoxicity include renal impairment. Even when the dose is adjusted for decreased renal clearance, toxicity may still be seen.[69,71] Treatment involves discontinuation of cefepime and supportive care.[69,71]

Box 5
Neurotoxicity in tricyclic antidepressant overdose

Anticholinergic symptoms (generally first neurologic manifestations)
- Dry mouth, blurred vision, mydriasis, urinary retention, and constipation

CNS symptoms (can rapidly develop)
- Somnolence, delirium, hallucinations, and eventual coma with severe respiratory depression
- Generalized tonic-clonic seizures

> **Box 6**
> **Botulism presentation**
>
> - Symmetric cranial nerve palsies
> - Descending flaccid paralysis
> - Autonomic symptoms: anhidrosis, severe dry mouth, orthostatic hypotension, constipation
> - Progressive loss of deep tendon reflexes
> - Respiratory compromise
> - Preserved cognition

Botulism

Botulism is a rare disease with a characteristic toxidrome resulting from toxins produced by *Clostridium botulinum*, as summarized in **Box 6**.[72,73]

Symptoms result from blockade of presynaptic acetylcholine transmission in the motor neuron.[72,74] *C botulinum* can be found naturally in soils and its spores can survive standard cooking and food-processing measures. When these spores are consumed by infants, infantile botulism can develop because of the infants' underdeveloped gastrointestinal flora.[72,73] Botulism can also result from germination of *C botulinum* within wounds (characteristically the wounds of injection drug users).[72]

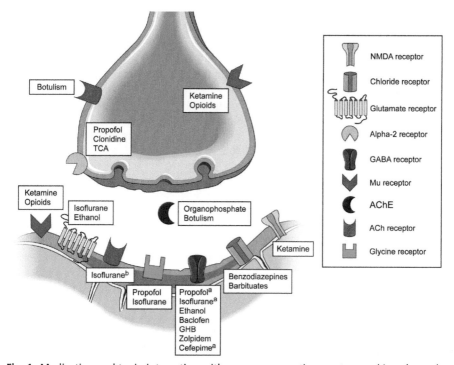

Fig. 1. Medication and toxin interaction with common synaptic receptors and ion channels. [a] GABA-A receptor interaction predominantly. [b] Nicotinic acetylcholine receptor interaction. Ach, acetylecholine; AChE, acetylcholinesterase.

Treatment involves quick recognition and supportive care in an ICU with intubation if respiratory compromise occurs. Once hemodynamic stability is achieved, antitoxin administration early in the course can decrease the duration of paralysis and dependence on mechanical ventilation.[72,73]

SUMMARY

Several medications and toxins can lead to CNS depression and additional neurotoxicity as described in this article. **Fig. 1** summarizes the main synaptic receptors affected by these medications and toxins. Much more research needs to be done to further clarify the mechanisms, risk factors, and treatments for these neurotoxic effects so that in the future they may be avoided or quickly reversed. In the meantime, clinicians must have high suspicion for these effects in order to accurately identify and subsequently care for patients who experience these toxicities.

DISCLOSURE

The authors have nothing to disclose.

REFERENCES

1. Dawson ET, Hocker SE. Neurologic Complications of Commonly Used Drugs in the Hospital Setting. Curr Neurol Neurosci Rep 2016;16(4):35.
2. Kumar N, Hu WT. Extrapyramidal reaction to ondansetron and propofol. Mov Disord 2009;24(2):312–3.
3. Saravanakumar K, Venkatesh P, Bromley P. Delayed onset refractory dystonic movements following propofol anesthesia. Paediatr Anaesth 2005;15(7):597–601.
4. Carvalho DZ, Townley RA, Burkle CM, et al. Propofol Frenzy: Clinical Spectrum in 3 Patients. Mayo Clin Proc 2017;92(11):1682–7.
5. Reynolds LM, Koh JL. Prolonged spontaneous movement following emergence from propofol/nitrous oxide anesthesia. Anesth Analg 1993;76(1):192–3.
6. Saunders PR, Harris MN. Opisthotonus and other unusual neurological sequelae after outpatient anaesthesia. Anaesthesia 1990;45(7):552–7.
7. Reddy RV, Moorthy SS, Dierdorf SF, et al. Excitatory effects and electroencephalographic correlation of etomidate, thiopental, methohexital, and propofol. Anesth Analg 1993;77(5):1008–11.
8. Fernando SM, Fitzpatrick T, Hurdle H, et al. Recurrent non-epileptiform seizure-like phenomena secondary to propofol administration. Can J Anaesth 2017; 64(7):783–5.
9. Tam MK, Irwin MG, Tse ML, et al. Prolonged myoclonus after a single bolus dose of propofol. Anaesthesia 2009;64(11):1254–7.
10. Islander G, Vinge E. Severe neuroexcitatory symptoms after anaesthesia–with focus on propofol anaesthesia. Acta Anaesthesiol Scand 2000;44(2):144–9.
11. Kurdi MS, Theerth KA, Deva RS. Ketamine: Current applications in anesthesia, pain, and critical care. Anesth Essays Res 2014;8(3):283–90.
12. Biddle C, Ford V. The Neurotoxicity of General Anesthetic Drugs: Emphasis on the Extremes of Age. Annu Rev Nurs Res 2017;35(1):201–19.
13. Rosenberg H, Pollock N, Schiemann A, et al. Malignant hyperthermia: a review. Orphanet J Rare Dis 2015;10:93.
14. Nitrous Oxide. Lexicomp Online Database. Wolters Kluwer Clinical Drug Information. Accessed 8 November 2019.

15. Oussalah A, Julien M, Levy J, et al. Global Burden Related to Nitrous Oxide Exposure in Medical and Recreational Settings: A Systematic Review and Individual Patient Data Meta-Analysis. J Clin Med 2019;8(4):551.

16. Stachnik J. Inhaled anesthetic agents. Am J Health Syst Pharm 2006;63(7): 623–34.

17. Ori C, Dam M, Pizzolato G, et al. Effects of isoflurane anesthesia on local cerebral glucose utilization in the rat. Anesthesiology 1986;65(2):152–6.

18. Xie Z, Dong Y, Maeda U, et al. The inhalation anesthetic isoflurane induces a vicious cycle of apoptosis and amyloid beta-protein accumulation. J Neurosci 2007;27(6):1247–54.

19. Fugate JE, Burns JD, Wijdicks EF, et al. Prolonged high-dose isoflurane for refractory status epilepticus: is it safe? Anesth Analg 2010;111(6):1520–4.

20. Terasako K, Ishii S. Postoperative seizure-like activity following sevoflurane anesthesia. Acta Anaesthesiol Scand 1996;40(8 Pt 1):953–4.

21. Modica PA, Tempelhoff R, White PF. Pro- and anticonvulsant effects of anesthetics (Part I). Anesth Analg 1990;70(3):303–15.

22. Voss LJ, Sleigh JW, Barnard JP, et al. The howling cortex: seizures and general anesthetic drugs. Anesth Analg 2008;107(5):1689–703.

23. Hocker SE, Fogelson J, Rabinstein AA. Refractory intracranial hypertension due to fentanyl administration following closed head injury. Front Neurol 2013;4:3.

24. Pedavally S, Fugate JE, Rabinstein AA. Serotonin syndrome in the intensive care unit: clinical presentations and precipitating medications. Neurocrit Care 2014; 21(1):108–13.

25. Clark S, Rabinstein AA, Hocker SE. Disabling Asterixis Induced by Gabapentin. J Med Cases 2015;6(7):285–6.

26. Kaufman KR, Parikh A, Chan L, et al. Myoclonus in renal failure: Two cases of gabapentin toxicity. Epilepsy Behav Case Rep 2014;2:8–10.

27. Healy DG, Ingle GT, Brown P. Pregabalin- and gabapentin-associated myoclonus in a patient with chronic renal failure. Mov Disord 2009;24(13):2028–9.

28. Bookwalter T, Gitlin M. Gabapentin-induced neurologic toxicities. Pharmacotherapy 2005;25(12):1817–9.

29. Hocker SE. Status Epilepticus. Continuum (Minneap Minn) 2015;21(5 Neurocritical Care):1362–83.

30. McKenzie WS, Rosenberg M. Paradoxical reaction following administration of a benzodiazepine. J Oral Maxillofac Surg 2010;68(12):3034–6.

31. Tae CH, Kang KJ, Min BH, et al. Paradoxical reaction to midazolam in patients undergoing endoscopy under sedation: Incidence, risk factors and the effect of flumazenil. Dig Liver Dis 2014;46(8):710–5.

32. Kohli N, Bordeaux JS. Involuntary movements during periocular reconstruction secondary to lorazepam. Dermatol Surg 2015;41(3):432–3.

33. Kwan P, Brodie MJ. Phenobarbital for the treatment of epilepsy in the 21st century: a critical review. Epilepsia 2004;45(9):1141–9.

34. Nair PP, Wadwekar V, Murgai A, et al. Refractory status epilepticus complicated by drug-induced involuntary movements. BMJ Case Rep 2014;2014.

35. Noble JM, Weimer LH. Neurologic complications of alcoholism. Continuum (Minneap Minn) 2014;20(3 Neurology of Systemic Disease):624–41.

36. Hammoud N, Jimenez-Shahed J. Chronic Neurologic Effects of Alcohol. Clin Liver Dis 2019;23(1):141–55.

37. Singh R, Arain E, Buth A, et al. Ethylene Glycol Poisoning: An Unusual Cause of Altered Mental Status and the Lessons Learned from Management of the Disease in the Acute Setting. Case Rep Crit Care 2016;2016:9157393.

38. McQuade DJ, Dargan PI, Wood DM. Challenges in the diagnosis of ethylene glycol poisoning. Ann Clin Biochem 2014;51(Pt 2):167–78.
39. Nazir S, Melnick S, Ansari S, et al. Mind the gap: a case of severe methanol intoxication. BMJ Case Rep 2016;2016.
40. Jain N, Himanshu D, Verma SP, et al. Methanol poisoning: characteristic MRI findings. Ann Saudi Med 2013;33(1):68–9.
41. Chartier M, Malissin I, Tannous S, et al. Baclofen-induced encephalopathy in overdose - Modeling of the electroencephalographic effect/concentration relationships and contribution of tolerance in the rat. Prog Neuropsychopharmacol Biol Psychiatry 2018;86:131–9.
42. Kumar G, Sahaya K, Goyal MK, et al. Electroencephalographic abnormalities in baclofen-induced encephalopathy. J Clin Neurosci 2010;17(12):1594–6.
43. Triplett JD, Lawn ND, Dunne JW. Baclofen Neurotoxicity: A Metabolic Encephalopathy Susceptible to Exacerbation by Benzodiazepine Therapy. J Clin Neurophysiol 2019;36(3):209–12.
44. Maze M, Tranquilli W. Alpha-2 adrenoceptor agonists: defining the role in clinical anesthesia. Anesthesiology 1991;74(3):581–605.
45. Pomerleau AC, Gooden CE, Fantz CR, et al. Dermal exposure to a compounded pain cream resulting in severely elevated clonidine concentration. J Med Toxicol 2014;10(1):61–4.
46. Scholz J, Tonner PH. α2-Adrenoceptor agonists in anaesthesia: a new paradigm. Curr Opin Anesthesiol 2000;13(4):437–42.
47. Frye CB, Vance MA. Hypertensive crisis and myocardial infarction following massive clonidine overdose. Ann Pharmacother 2000;34(5):611–5.
48. Farooqi M, Seifert S, Kunkel S, et al. Toxicity from a clonidine suspension. J Med Toxicol 2009;5(3):130–3.
49. Manzon L, Nappe TM, Maguire NJ. Clonidine Toxicity. In: StatPearls. Treasure Island (FL): StatPearls Publishing LLC; 2019.
50. Dupont P, Thornton J. Near-fatal gamma-butyrolactone intoxication–first report in the UK. Hum Exp Toxicol 2001;20(1):19–22.
51. Friedman J, Westlake R, Furman M. Grievous bodily harm:" gamma hydroxybutyrate abuse leading to a Wernicke-Korsakoff syndrome. Neurology 1996;46(2):469–71.
52. Zvosec DL, Smith SW. Agitation is common in gamma-hydroxybutyrate toxicity. Am J Emerg Med 2005;23(3):316–20.
53. Ben-Hamou M, Marshall NS, Grunstein RR, et al. Spontaneous adverse event reports associated with zolpidem in Australia 2001-2008. J Sleep Res 2011;20(4):559–68.
54. Zammit G. Comparative tolerability of newer agents for insomnia. Drug Saf 2009;32(9):735–48.
55. Wong CK, Marshall NS, Grunstein RR, et al. Spontaneous Adverse Event Reports Associated with Zolpidem in the United States 2003-2012. J Clin Sleep Med 2017;13(2):223–34.
56. Glauser J, Queen JR. An overview of non-cardiac cocaine toxicity. J Emerg Med 2007;32(2):181–6.
57. Mendelson JH, Mello NK. Management of cocaine abuse and dependence. N Engl J Med 1996;334(15):965–72.
58. Roberts JR, Greenberg MI. Cocaine washout syndrome. Ann Intern Med 2000;132(8):679–80.
59. Sporer KA, Lesser SH. Cocaine washed-out syndrome. Ann Emerg Med 1992;21(1):112.

60. Rhee JH, Yadavalli VS, Mekaroonkamol P, et al. Cocaine Washout Syndrome: A Rare Case Presentation With Refractory Shock. Chest 2012;142(4):344A.
61. Prockop LD, Chichkova RI. Carbon monoxide intoxication: an updated review. J Neurol Sci 2007;262(1–2):122–30.
62. Tormoehlen LM. Toxic leukoencephalopathies. Neurol Clin 2011;29(3):591–605.
63. Kumar N. Industrial and environmental toxins. Continuum: Lifelong Learning in Neurology 2008;14(5):102–37.
64. Sykes OT, Walker E. The neurotoxicology of carbon monoxide - Historical perspective and review. Cortex 2016;74:440–8.
65. Kerr GW, McGuffie AC, Wilkie S. Tricyclic antidepressant overdose: a review. Emerg Med J 2001;18(4):236–41.
66. Frommer DA, Kulig KW, Marx JA, et al. Tricyclic Antidepressant Overdose: A Review. JAMA 1987;257(4):521–6.
67. Robb EL, Baker MB. Organophosphate toxicity. In: Abai B, et al, editors. StatPearls. Treasure Island (FL): StatPearls Publishing LLC.; 2019.
68. Naughton SX, Terry AV Jr. Neurotoxicity in acute and repeated organophosphate exposure. Toxicology 2018;408:101–12.
69. Appa AA, Jain R, Rakita RM, et al. Characterizing Cefepime Neurotoxicity: A Systematic Review. Open Forum Infect Dis 2017;4(4):ofx170.
70. Subedi A, Songmen S, Manchala V, et al. Cefepime-Induced Neurotoxicity: An Underappreciated Cause of Encephalopathy. Am J Ther 2019;26(4):e547–8.
71. Fugate JE, Kalimullah EA, Hocker SE, et al. Cefepime neurotoxicity in the intensive care unit: a cause of severe, underappreciated encephalopathy. Crit Care 2013;17(6):R264.
72. Sobel J. Botulism. Clin Infect Dis 2005;41(8):1167–73.
73. Carrillo-Marquez MA. Botulism. Pediatr Rev 2016;37(5):183–92.
74. Dressler D, Saberi FA, Barbosa ER. Botulinum toxin: mechanisms of action. Arq Neuropsiquiatr 2005;63(1):180–5.

Toxin-Induced Cerebellar Disorders

Katelyn Dolbec, MD[a], Michael R. Dobbs, MD, MHCM[b],
Mam Ibraheem, MD, MPH, CPH, ABPN Diplomate[c,d],*

KEYWORDS

- Cerebellum • Neurotoxicity • Ataxia • Nystagmus • Anticonvulsants • Ethanol
- Industrial exposure • Toxicology

KEY POINTS

- The cerebellum plays an important role in both motor and nonmotor symptoms, and is particularly sensitive to certain neurotoxins.
- Toluene and mercury are encountered often in industrial settings as an accidental exposure with subsequent cerebellar disorder. Toluene is additionally used as an agent of abuse with neurotoxic complications.
- Anticonvulsants, primarily phenytoin and carbamazepine, are associated with cerebellar toxicity, with both acute and chronic neurologic manifestations.
- Acute and chronic ethanol use have distinct neurologic presentations, but both can cause white matter and cerebellar disorders.
- Recognition of an agent causing the particular disorder is important so that the route of exposure and subsequent treatment options can be identified.

INTRODUCTION

In general, the central nervous system is sensitive to toxic exposures for numerous reasons related to the way the central nervous system is formed and repaired. The nervous system is formed in a stepwise process with each stage in development essential to the proper formation. Each step, including migration, differentiation, and synaptic pruning, is essential to the normal functioning of the nervous system.[1] Beyond the initial formation of the central nervous system, mature neurons are postmitotic cells without the ability to be repaired from surrounding cells.[1] Neurons have a high

[a] Department of Neurology, Beth Israel Deaconess Medical Center, 330 Brookline Avenue, Boston, MA 0225, USA; [b] Department of Neurology, University of Texas Rio Grande Valley School of Medicine, 2102 Treasure Hills, Harlingen, TX 78550, USA; [c] Department of Neurology, University of Kentucky, 740 South Limestone, KY Clinic, J401, Lexington, KY 40536, USA; [d] US Department of Veterans Affairs, Lexington VA Medical Center-Troy Bowling Campus, 1101 Veterans Drive, Room A303a, Mail Code: 127-CD, Lexington, KY, USA
* Corresponding author.
E-mail address: Mam.Ibraheem@uky.edu

Neurol Clin 38 (2020) 843–852
https://doi.org/10.1016/j.ncl.2020.07.003
0733-8619/20/© 2020 Elsevier Inc. All rights reserved.

metabolic demand and are therefore sensitivity to metabolic derangements and subsequent damage.[1]

Although the entire peripheral and central nervous systems are susceptible to the effects of toxins, the cerebellum, in particular the cerebellar cortex and Purkinje cells, is preferentially damaged.[2] Coordination, motor control, and eye movements are reliant on the normal physiology and can all be impaired if there is injury to the cerebellum.[3]

The cerebellum plays an important role in motor systems and, to a lesser extent, nonmotor systems, with damage resulting in clinical manifestations including weakness, ataxia, incoordination, dysarthria, and nystagmus. With the interference of any step in the formation of the brain or derangements in normal physiology with toxin exposure, clinical manifestations of cerebellar injury may be present (**Table 1**).

TOLUENE

Toluene is commonly found as a component of industrial solvents and, given its widespread use, it can result in acute and chronic exposures, and accidental overdose, and it has found use as a drug of abuse.[4] Toluene is used as an additive to numerous industrial solvents and is commonly found in gasoline, paints, and rubber manufacturing.[5] A potential source of toluene involved in both accidental exposure and as a source of abuse is as a component of glue. Outside of the industrial setting, in the community there is the possibility of exposure through paints, adhesives, nail polish, and cigarettes.[5] The most common route of exposure is through inhalation; however, given the widespread use of toluene in the industrial setting, dermal exposure is also possible.[5]

Toluene has been found to be present in highly lipid-rich areas of the brain, and the high lipid content of myelin explains why white matter structures seem to be preferentially affected.[6] Animal studies have shown similar results, with toluene seeming to preferentially damage highly lipid-prevalent areas with relative sparing of regions with reduced myelination.[6] However, the exact mechanism by which damage occurs remains under investigation.

Clinical Manifestations

Although typically the exposure has primarily neurologic complications, it has been found to be irritable to the eyes and respiratory tract, with secondary effects in the liver and renal system.[5] However, the central nervous system manifestations, which are graded based on the degree of exposure to toluene, are the most prominent effects as a result of exposure. Globally, alterations in level of consciousness are observed in addition to lightheadedness, dizziness, incoordination, and ataxia.[5]

Chronic exposure can result in hematologic abnormalities and psychomotor disturbances, and has been associated with teratogenicity in pregnant women.[5] The damage to the cerebellum in toluene toxicity results in the incoordination, ataxia, and dizziness sensations that can be observed as a result of acute or chronic exposure. In addition, given the apparent predilection of toluene for white matter, leukoencephalopathy with a clinical presentation similar to dementia has been observed.[6]

Although there is known teratogenicity to the fetus from exposure to toluene, the presentation can be variable in children with various disorders, including microcephaly, hyperactivity, developmental delay, craniofacial, and limb abnormalities.[5]

Diagnosis

Exposure to toluene may be detected via direct toluene levels; however, bioassays for hippuric acid, o-cresol levels, and benzylmercapturic acid in urine studies may aid in

Table 1 Toxin-induced cerebellar disorders: summary learning points	
Toluene solvent abuse syndrome	Sources: Toluene-containing paint thinner, paint stripper, and glue. Route of exposure: Inhalational: huffing (inhaling soaked rags) or bagging (inhaling from bags containing solvent) Systemic signs: Abdominal pain, anorexia, weight loss, gastritis, possible renal tubular acidosis (hypokalemia and acidosis), rhabdomyolysis, hepatitis, solvent odor on breath Neurologic manifestations: Tremor of the head and extremities, ataxia, staggering gait, cognitive deficits, personality changes, optic nerve atrophy, hearing loss, loss of smell, spasticity, and hyperreflexia Diagnosis: 1. Laboratory: increased serum toluene levels and urine hippuric acid levels confirm exposure, but are not always detected 2. Imaging: MRI of the brain often shows cerebellar and cerebral atrophy. Evidence of white matter disease can be seen with increased signal intensity on T2-weighted images in the periventricular, internal capsular, and brainstem pyramidal regions 3. Electrophysiologic studies: brainstem auditory evoked response testing may show sparing of early components and loss or decrement of the late components (waves III and IV). Abnormal pattern visual evoked cortical potentials and prolonged P100 peak latency may occur in patients with toxic optic neuropathy caused by toluene abuse Treatment: Supportive care and addiction rehabilitation
Mercury poisoning	Poisoning with elemental mercury vapor or organic mercury (along with other symptoms of peripheral nervous system) can result in cerebellar symptoms, including ataxia and tremor, with pathologic neuronal damage seen in visual cortex, cerebellar vermis and hemispheres, and postcentral cortex
Anticonvulsant drugs	Anticonvulsant drugs, including phenobarbital, phenytoin, and carbamazepine, in increased concentration or acute overdose, manifest toxicity with predominantly ataxia, nystagmus, and central nervous system depression. Chronic use of phenytoin may also result in cerebellar atrophy
Ethanol	Both acute intoxication and chronic abuse of ethanol can result in ataxia, tremor, and altered mental status. Wernicke encephalopathy should be considered when any patient with chronic alcoholism has changes in mental status and ataxia not related to acute intoxication

Data from Tormoehlen LM, Rusyniak DE. Chapter 59 – Neurotoxicology. In: Biller J, editor. Practical Neurology, 5th Ed. Wolters Kluwer, 2017: 763-780.

detection of toluene.[7] There are endogenous sources of hippuric acid, which may result in a false-positive when trying to assess for toxicity related to toluene exposure.[7] However, there is no single confirmatory finding on imaging. Given that the findings are not pathognomonic, clinical history obtained from the patient about potential sources or exposure is essential to the diagnosis of toluene toxicity.

Treatment

There is no currently available reversal agent for toluene, so the treatment is primarily supportive. Management is aimed at specific manifestations of toluene toxicity, including renal or respiratory injury, with ongoing education about cessation of illicit substances with addiction counseling resources.[8] A high index of suspicion based on the clinical presentation for toluene toxicity can result in early detection and subsequent treatment.

MERCURY POISONING

In the past, before the recognition of the potential for neurotoxicity, mercury was used universally in the production of both medical and commercial items. Previously mercury was a component in medical products, with use in thermometers, blood pressure cuffs, batteries, light bulbs, and electrodes.[9] Given the improved understanding of the potential toxicity of mercury, the main ways in which humans are exposed to mercury currently is via consumption of contaminated seafood and dental mixtures.[9]

The route of exposure determines the clinical presentation as well as the appropriate treatment. The main routes of exposure are vapor from liquid mercury, and consumption of methyl mercury via seafood ingestion.[9] Elemental mercury exposure typically results from inhalation of the vapors.[10] Inorganic mercury results primarily in disorders outside of the central nervous system, with primarily gastrointestinal and renal complications.[10]

In addition, organic mercury exposures are responsible for most of the neurologic complications commonly associated with toxicity.[10]

Clinical Manifestations

Numerous systemic signs can be observed in both acute and chronic exposure to the various forms of mercury. Pulmonary manifestation include irritation to the bronchi and lung parenchyma, whereas gastrointestinal manifestations range from metallic taste to stomatitis and gastroenteritis.[9] Renal symptoms include tubular necrosis with resultant proteinuria.[9] In the peripheral nervous system, the common presentation is paresthesias caused by underlying neuropathy.[9]

Methyl mercury in contaminated fish was first identified in Minimata, Japan, with the subsequent constellation of systems related to methyl mercury positioning referred to as Minimata disease.[11]

Typical central nervous system symptoms as a result of acute poisoning include vision and hearing impairments, changes in sense of smell and taste, and somatosensory and psychiatric disturbances.[11] The cerebellum seems to be predominately affected in acute toxicity, with evidence of dysmetria, dysdiadochokinesia, dysarthria, and writing and gait abnormalities with notable ataxia.[11] Further tremor, other movement disorders, and memory disturbances are on the spectrum of mercury poisoning based on the time of exposures and the concentration of mercury.[10]

Notably, in utero exposure has been found with patients presenting with variable symptoms ranging from intellectual disability, epilepsy, and difficulty with coordinated movements to the most severe forms with akinetic mutism.[11] At the cellular level, there has been notable cerebellar atrophy, with loss of granule cells within the cerebellum found at autopsy.[11]

Diagnosis

In assessing for mercury exposure or toxicity, there are 2 main modalities in which exposure can be assessed. The first is by testing 24-hour urine collection; however, in addition to urine collection, whole-blood mercury levels must also be drawn, because organic mercury is not primarily excreted via the urinary system.[10] Therefore, it is essential that both urine and serum levels are obtained because, if the toxicity was only as a result of organic mercury exposure, it may be missed in urine studies.

In terms of imaging, there are certain modalities with particular findings that can be supportive of a diagnosis of mercury exposure. A study evaluating regional cerebral blood flow with single-photon computed tomography found that there was no difference in cortical regional cerebral blood flow in patients with exposure to mercury; however, there was also a notable decrease in regional blood flow within the cerebellum.[12] Cerebellar atrophy assessed on MRI was present in 27% of patients with methylmercury exposure compared with zero patients in the comparison group.[12] In addition, in terms of electrophysiology contribution to diagnosis, there have been notable abnormalities with somatosensory evoked potentials after mercury toxicity. In short latency somatosensory evoked potential in patients with mercury exposure, the N20 component was found to be absent.[11]

Treatment

In relation to the multisystem involvement of mercury toxicity, initial treatment is to ensure patient stability with a focus on supportive care. If the exposure is from inorganic mercury or elemental mercury, treatment with a chelator is recommended, primarily with intramuscular dimercaprol followed by oral succimer.[10] In toxicity related to organic mercury, typically related to seafood ingestion, oral succimer is used as monotherapy.[10]

ANTICONVULSANT DRUGS
Phenobarbital

Phenobarbital belongs to the barbiturate class of drugs, a class of medications that act on GABA-A receptors.[13] GABA is the primary inhibitory neurotransmitter within the central nervous system.[13] The way in which phenobarbital functions as an anticonvulsant is by binding the GABA-A receptor, with resultant prolonged opening of the chloride channel, and subsequent intracellular influx of chloride ions, thus decreasing cellular excitability.[14] Phenobarbital has a particularly long half-life, in part because of slow absorption and redistribution within the body.

The main source of exposure is from prescriptions, because barbiturates were previously commonly used for treatment of seizure disorders. When used for seizure management, the medication can be administered orally, intravenously, or via intramuscular injection.

Clinical manifestations

Most commonly there are limited systemic signs associated with phenobarbital toxicity, but folate deficiencies, osteomalacia, hepatotoxicity, aggravation of porphyria, and teratogenicity have been reported.[15] The neurologic manifestations are variable, and typically present in a dose-dependent fashion with the most severe being related to central nervous system depression.[16] Phenobarbital toxicity has additionally been found to present clinically with nystagmus, tremor, and ataxia as a result of cerebellar involvement.[17]

Treatment
Whether toxicity is a result of intentional or accidental use, the treatment remains primarily supportive. In the setting of overdose related to phenobarbital use, there should be a special focus on the respiratory depression and cardiac complications of bradycardia and hypotension.[14]

Phenytoin

Phenytoin has long been used as an anticonvulsant in the treatment of primarily focal epilepsies. Phenytoin is metabolized via the cytochrome P450 system, which has overlap in the overall breakdown of numerous drugs. Given the overlap in metabolism, the level of phenytoin within the serum can vary based on the specific drug-drug interaction. The drug levels are also sensitive to interactions with other changes in physiology, such as hypoalbuminemia, malnutrition, and liver or kidney injury.[18]

Clinical manifestations

In terms of systemic manifestations, chronic phenytoin is associated with phenytoin-induced gingival enlargement and drug reaction with eosinophilia and systemic symptoms, which can have multi–organ system involvement, including liver and kidney injury.[18] In addition, there are known skin reactions as a result of phenytoin use, which include Stevens-Johnson syndrome, toxic epidermal necrolysis , and purple glove syndrome, with discoloration, edema, and ischemia of the skin as a result of intravenous phenytoin use.[18] There is concern for abnormalities with bone mineral density with resultant osteoporosis with long-term use.[19] During administration of the medication, cardiovascular toxicity is a significant concern with intravenous infusions with the potential of hypotension, arrhythmias, and bradycardia.[18] In laboratory studies, phenytoin has been found to damage Purkinje cells; however, the mechanism that leads to cerebellar degeneration and subsequent clinical presentation remains unclear.[19]

Clinical manifestations of toxicity include cerebellar findings such as nystagmoid eye movements, ataxia, dysarthria, tremor, seizures, and depressed level of consciousness.[18,20] Phenytoin is known to be neurotoxic; the clinical presentation correlates with the unbound plasma concentration, and typically occurs in a dose-dependent manner.[18]

Notably, the time of exposure to phenytoin seems to be strongly correlated with the cerebellar atrophy.[21] Phenytoin use has been associated, independent of underlying generalized seizures or brain damage, with cerebellar atrophy. In retrospective analysis of patients on chronic phenytoin therapy, 40% had cerebellar ataxia, with many having reduced cerebellar volume, with an apparent predilection for vermis degeneration.[19]

Treatment

Management of acute toxicity is primarily supportive, because there is no reversal agent for use in the setting of toxicity.[22] The identification of phenytoin-induced acute or chronic toxicity is important given that withdrawal of the medication promptly can result in reversal of acute cerebellar symptoms. Discontinuation of chronic phenytoin use in patients with evidence of toxicity is important to reduce progression of symptoms.

Carbamazepine

Carbamazepine is a sodium channel blocker with additional anticholinergic properties.[23] Its main use is for the treatment of focal epilepsy, although carbamazepine can also be used for other conditions, including trigeminal neuralgia and neuropathic pain, and as a mood stabilizer.[23] Toxicity from the use of carbamazepine can result from coadministration of other medications that are metabolized via the same cytochrome P450 system.[23]

Clinical manifestations

Clinical manifestations of toxicity related to carbamazepine are variable, including headache, nystagmus, dizziness or dysequilibrium, ataxia, seizures, and alterations in level of consciousness.[23,24] The exact mechanism by which carbamazepine is a neurotoxic agent remains unclear. There is evidence that patients with epilepsy with cerebellar atrophy are at increased risk for the potential of adverse side effects from carbamazepine.[25]

Treatment
Management is focused on reducing absorption or further metabolism with activated charcoal to reduce absorption and, if necessary, hemodialysis, plasmapheresis, or continuous venovenous hemofiltration.[23]

Ethanol

There are nearly 14 million individuals in the United States that meet diagnostic criteria for alcoholism, and, given the high prevalence of abuse and the known neurotoxic effects of alcohol, there is high potential for associated morbidity.[26]

Pathophysiology
Studies from autopsy have revealed that certain areas of the brain seem to be more susceptible to ethanol use, particularly the frontal lobes and the cerebellum.[26] Typical changes at the cellular level include decrease in myelinated fibers with resultant increase in white matter disease compared with gray matter.[26] There is a noted susceptibility of cholinergic nuclei, locus coeruleus, and the raphe nucleus to ethanol use.[26] Further, astrocytes, oligodendrocytes, and synaptic terminals seem to be affected preferentially.[27] Although the cerebellum is globally injured, the vermis is most commonly and significantly affected by ethanol use.[27]

The cerebellum seems to be preferentially targeted by ethanol use, with a potential mechanism of derangement in GABA-A receptor–dependent neurotransmission, because GABA-A release is altered within Purkinje cells, interneurons, and granule cells.[28] Although there are numerous propositions as to the pathophysiology, the exact mechanism resulting in cerebellar injury from ethanol use remains unclear.

Clinical manifestations
The clinical manifestations of ethanol use are variable, with the most severe resulting from chronic use. With prolonged exposure to ethanol, Wernicke-Korsakoff syndrome can occur. Wernicke-Korsakoff presents with confusion, ataxia, visual changes, and amnesia.[26] Early recognition is important, because treatment with high-dose thiamine and alcohol cessation can be useful in reversal of some of the severity of the clinical manifestations.[26]

Despite the evidence of prominent neurotoxicity with chronic alcohol use, systemic manifestations, particularly within the liver, can also result in secondary neurologic presentations. With liver disorder, and subsequent dysfunction, hepatic encephalopathy can result. Hepatic encephalopathy is characterized by confusion, alterations in level of consciousness, asterixis, dysarthria, and ataxia.[27] Acute hepatic encephalopathy is typically a result of increased ammonia levels. At autopsy, hepatic encephalopathy disorder is characterized by prominence of Alzheimer type II astrocytes within the cortex and deep gray nuclei.[27] Postmortem studies have found noninflammatory diffuse brain edema as a result of hepatic encephalopathy.[27]

Despite numerous pathologic changes with chronic alcohol use, there is the additionally possibility of acute ethanol poisoning. Acute intoxication in severe cases can result in hemorrhage, specifically within the diencephalon and mesencephalon, and within the hemispheres, pons, and medulla.[27] Without hemorrhage, chronic alcohol use can result in a vasculopathy with apparent ischemic lesions.[27]

In addition, as result of ethanol-induced cerebellar damage, the incoordination between visual and motor systems may be the cause of the prominence of cerebellar signs, particularly ataxia and falls.[29]

Diagnosis

Imaging with computed tomography and MRI has shown morphologic changes of the brain associated with long-term ethanol use, including dilatation of ventricles with associated cerebral and cerebellar atrophy.[26]

Acute effects of ethanol toxicity on electroencephalograms (EEGs) are variable. With low doses of ethanol, a slow alpha rhythm or decrease of the alpha peak frequency has been observed.[30] However, with increasing doses of ethanol, slow alpha and theta are observed.[30] With chronic alcohol intake, there is increased resting theta activity, with less prevalent and lower alpha frequencies with low-voltage recordings commonly found.[30,31] Although there is some evidence to support changes in EEG patterns with both acute and chronic alcohol use, to date there are no specific changes that are known to be exclusively related to ethanol use. In states of alcohol withdrawal, the EEG changes can vary from normal to mild or diffuse slowing, outside of the periods of generalized seizures.[31]

Treatment

In terms of alcohol abuse, the treatment is focused on cessation; however, in the acute setting, management is initially mainly systemic support with a focus on airway, breathing, and circulation. In ethanol intoxication, in particular, there may be an associated malnutrition state. Intravenous thiamine supplementation is important because chronic ethanol use in association with thiamine deficiency can present with dementia-type symptoms, and therefore supplementation is important.[32] Subsequent focus on addiction treatment and ongoing counseling is important to reducing future exposure and reducing risk of irreversible neurologic changes.

SUMMARY

There are numerous environmental and industrial agents and medications, as well as ethanol, that, through either accidental or intentional use, can result in neurotoxicity (**Table 1**). The variability in presentation is important to recognize so that early cessation in exposure, use, or abuse can be initiated to reduce the severity of symptoms. Although numerous agents seem to have neurotoxic effects, the cerebellum seems to be particularly sensitive to injury.

DISCLOSURE

The authors have no commercial or financial conflicts of interest to disclose.

REFERENCES

1. Harris JB, Blain PG. Neurotoxicology: what the neurologist needs to know. J Neurol Neurosurg Psychiatry 2004;75(suppl 3):iii29–34.
2. Manto M. Chapter 12 - Toxic agents causing cerebellar ataxias. In: Subramony SH, Dürr A, editors. Handbook of clinical Neurology, vol. 103. Elsevier; 2012. p. 201–13.
3. Kano M, Watanabe M. Chapter 5 - Cerebellar Circuits. In: Rubenstein JLR, Rakic P, editors. Neural circuit development and function in the brain. Oxford: Academic Press; 2013. p. 75–93.

4. Camara-Lemarroy CR, Rodriguez-Gutierrez R, Monreal-Robles R, et al. Acute toluene intoxication–clinical presentation, management and prognosis: a prospective observational study. BMC Emerg Med 2015;15:19.

5. Clough SR. Toluene. In: Wexler P, editor. Encyclopedia of toxicology. 3rd edition. Oxford: Academic Press; 2014. p. 595–8.

6. Filley CM, Halliday W, Kleinschmidt-Demasters BK. The effects of toluene on the central nervous system. J Neuropathol Exp Neurol 2004;63(1):1–12.

7. Jain R, Verma A. Laboratory approach for diagnosis of toluene-based inhalant abuse in a clinical setting. J Pharm Bioallied Sci 2016;8(1):18–22.

8. Anderson CE, Loomis GA. Recognition and prevention of inhalant abuse. Am Fam Physician 2003;68(5):869–74.

9. Clarkson TW, Magos L, Myers GJ. The toxicology of mercury — current exposures and clinical manifestations. N Engl J Med 2003;349(18):1731–7.

10. Posin SL, Sharma S. Mercury Toxicity. In: StatPearls [Internet]. Treasure Island (FL): StatPearls Publishing; 2020. Available at: https://www.ncbi.nlm.nih.gov/books/NBK499935/.

11. Ekino S, Susa M, Ninomiya T, et al. Minamata disease revisited: An update on the acute and chronic manifestations of methyl mercury poisoning. J Neurol Sci 2007; 262(1):131–44.

12. Itoh K, Korogi Y, Tomiguchi S, et al. Cerebellar blood flow in methylmercury poisoning (Minamata disease). Neuroradiology 2001;43(4):279–84.

13. Suddock JT, Cain MD. Barbiturate Toxicity. In: StatPearls [Internet]. Treasure Island (FL): StatPearls Publishing; 2020. Available at: https://www.ncbi.nlm.nih.gov/books/NBK499875/.

14. Lewis CB, Adams N. Phenobarbital. In: StatPearls [Internet]. Treasure Island (FL): StatPearls Publishing; 2020 Jan-. Available at: https://www.ncbi.nlm.nih.gov/books/NBK532277/.

15. Kwan P, Brodie MJ. Phenobarbital for the treatment of epilepsy in the 21st century: a critical review. Epilepsia 2004;45(9):1141–9.

16. Iivanainen M, Savolainen H. Side effects of phenobarbital and phenytoin during long-term treatment of epilepsy. Acta Neurol Scand Suppl 1983;97:49–67.

17. Alekseeva N, McGee J, Kelley RE, et al. Toxic-metabolic, nutritional, and medicinal-induced disorders of cerebellum. Neurol Clin 2014;32(4):901–11.

18. Iorga A, Horowitz BZ. Phenytoin Toxicity. In: StatPearls [Internet]. Treasure Island (FL): StatPearls Publishing; 2020 Jan-. Available at: https://www.ncbi.nlm.nih.gov/books/NBK482444/.

19. Shanmugarajah PD, Hoggard N, Aeschlimann DP, et al. Phenytoin-related ataxia in patients with epilepsy: clinical and radiological characteristics. Seizure 2018; 56:26–30.

20. Ney GC, Lantos G, Barr WB, et al. Cerebellar atrophy in patients with long-term phenytoin exposure and epilepsy. Arch Neurol 1994;51(8):767–71.

21. De Marcos FA, Ghizoni E, Kobayashi E, et al. Cerebellar volume and long-term use of phenytoin. Seizure 2003;12(5):312–5.

22. Craig S. Phenytoin poisoning. Neurocrit Care 2005;3(2):161–70.

23. Al Khalili Y, Sekhon S, Jain S. Carbamazepine Toxicity. In: StatPearls [Internet]. Treasure Island (FL): StatPearls Publishing; 2020. Available at: https://www.ncbi.nlm.nih.gov/books/NBK507852/.

24. Xu W, Chen YL, Zhao Y, et al. A clinical study of toxication caused by carbamazepine abuse in adolescents. Biomed Res Int 2018;2018:3201203.

25. Specht U, May TW, Rohde M, et al. Cerebellar atrophy decreases the threshold of carbamazepine toxicity in patients with chronic focal epilepsy. Arch Neurol 1997; 54(4):427–31.
26. United States National Institute on Alcohol Abuse and Alcoholism (U.S.). 10th special report to the U.S. Congress on alcohol and health: highlights from current research from the Secretary of Health and Human Services. Rockville (MD): U.S. Dept. of Health and Human Services, Public Health Service, National Institutes of Health, National Institute on Alcohol Abuse and Alcoholism; 2000.
27. de la Monte SM, Kril JJ. Human alcohol-related neuropathology. Acta Neuropathol 2014;127(1):71–90.
28. Luo J. Effects of ethanol on the cerebellum: advances and prospects. Cerebellum 2015;14(4):383–5.
29. Sullivan EV, Rosenbloom MJ, Deshmukh A, et al. Alcohol and the cerebellum: effects on balance, motor coordination, and cognition. Alcohol Health Res World 1995;19(2):138–41.
30. Rangaswamy M, Porjesz B. Understanding alcohol use disorders with neuroelectrophysiology. Handb Clin Neurol 2014;125:383–414.
31. Krauss GL, Fisher RS. Alcohol and the EEG. Am J EEG Technol 1992;32(2):118–26.
32. Vonghia L, Leggio L, Ferrulli A, et al. Acute alcohol intoxication. Eur J Intern Med 2008;19(8):561–7.

Toxin-Induced Parkinsonism

Steven McKnight, MD[a,b], Nawaz Hack, MD[a,b,c],*

KEYWORDS

- Parkinsonism • MPTP • Mercury • Rotenone • Paraquat • Manganese
- Agent orange

KEY POINTS

- Toxin-induced parkinsonism is a clinical syndrome of resting tremors, bradykinesia, and rigidity with postural instability resembling Parkinson disease but caused by toxins or drugs.
- Mercury has been implicated as having an association with Parkinson disease risk.
- The effects of Agent Orange on the development of parkinsonism are still being investigated, although more evidence seems to show a possible connection between the two.

There are several toxins that have been identified as causing parkinsonism and being related to overall idiopathic Parkinson disease (PD) risk. These compounds range from heavy metals to pesticides to contaminants in synthetic heroin. Several of the compounds and metals described in this article exhibit significant oxidative stress on the neurons of the central nervous system (CNS) and have a particular predilection toward damage of dopaminergic neurons.[1] Although many of these toxins have well-established connections with PD risk, a few continue to be studied with data still being produced (eg, Agent Orange). The parkinsonisms caused by these agents have variable responses to dopaminergic therapies. The toxins discussed in detail here include manganese, mercury, 1-methyl-4-phneyl-1,2,5,6-tetrahydropyridine (MPTP), organochlorines, organophosphates, paraquat, rotenone, and Agent Orange.

MANGANESE

Manganese exposure may occur in certain occupations, including miners, welders, steel work, battery manufacturing, intravenous (IV) drug use, long-term parenteral

ª Neurology Department, Walter Reed National Military Medical Center, America Building #19, 6th Floor, Room 6146, 4954 North Palmer Road, Bethesda, MD 20889-5630, USA; ᵇ Department of Defense, Walter Reed National Military Medical Center, America Building #19, 6th Floor, Room 6146, 4954 North Palmer Road, Bethesda, MD 20889-5630, USA; ᶜ Department of Neurology, Armed Forces University of the Health Sciences
* Corresponding author. Neurology Department, Walter Reed National Military Medical Center (WRNMMC), America Building #19, 6th Floor, Room 6146, 4954 North Palmer Road, Bethesda, MD 20889-5630.
E-mail address: Nawaz.k.hack.mil@mail.mil

Neurol Clin 38 (2020) 853–865
https://doi.org/10.1016/j.ncl.2020.08.003
0733-8619/20/© 2020 Elsevier Inc. All rights reserved.

nutrition (IV sources of manganese are almost entirely retained),[2,3] and the manufacture/use of Maneb (fungicide and polymeric complex that includes manganese).[4,5] Ingestion of foods with manganese is the primary nonoccupational exposure source. These food sources include grains, dried fruit, vegetables, nuts, and tea.[6–8] Ingestion of foods with manganese generally does not cause symptoms, although in patients with liver failure, there may be decreased excretion. Dietary intake of high levels of manganese and iron may play a role in PD risk. A small percentage of patients with occupational exposure to manganese for more than 20 years have been shown in at least one study to have a higher risk of idiopathic PD.[9] There is some conflicting evidence regarding occupational welding exposure and idiopathic PD risk, although overall evidence largely suggests no clear association between the two.[10–12] Many of the studies did not differentiate well between manganese-induced parkinsonism and idiopathic PD.

Pathophysiology

There are two reactive forms of manganese that each have a different effect on the CNS. Divalent manganese tends to act as an antioxidant. Trivalent manganese can have a significant damaging effect by generating toxic free radicals. Divalent manganese is quickly oxidized into trivalent manganese in areas of the brain that have higher neuromelanin content (subtantia nigra and basal ganglia).[1,13] Neuromelanin has a high affinity for manganese, iron, and lipids. Neurotoxicity occurs when manganese is taken up by mitochondria, at which point it drives calcium accumulation and decreases oxidative phosphorylation. Manganese further inhibits glutamate transport, thus causing elevated glutamate levels within the cell. This cascade of events ultimately leads to initiation of apoptosis and cell death. Manganese tends to cause cell loss particularly in the pars reticulata of the substantia nigra. This cell loss tends to be less than that of idiopathic PD. Loss of autoreceptor-mediated control of the dopamine release tends to be the initial driver behind the symptoms of manganese toxicity. This is then followed subacutely by depletion in brain dopamine and increased dopamine synthesis and release. The more chronic symptoms of manganese toxicity are driven by neuron loss in the globus pallidus.[1,13]

Clinical Symptoms

There are a few features to manganese toxicity that differentiate it from idiopathic PD. The patient's symptoms generally include acute psychosis (which may be the only symptom initially).[1] Acutely, patients may also exhibit headache, vomiting, and hepatic dysfunction. The patient's acute psychosis eventually begins to subside while several extrapyramidal symptoms emerge. These symptoms include loss of balance, dyscoordination, dystonia, kinetic tremor, and a high-stepping dystonic gait (as opposed to the classic shuffling gait appreciated with PD).[2,14] Patients with manganese toxicity may not have a robust response to dopaminergic therapy, whereas there is generally a strong response in patients with idiopathic PD.[5,15] Symptoms of manganese toxicity may be progressive after the source of exposure is removed, although the rate of progression tends to be slower than that of idiopathic PD.

Diagnosis

Diagnosis of manganese toxicity is primarily based off of clinical and historical features. A strong history is important in these cases because manganese exposure may be easily missed unless the appropriate questions are asked, such as occupational history. MRI and serum manganese levels may lend supporting data, although these are not specific.[16]

Diagnostic Testing

Although diagnosis is primarily clinical, there are some supporting features that may be helpful to objectively distinguish manganese neurotoxicity. T1 MRI features include hyperintensity in the striatum and globus pallidus. Dopamine transporter scan is generally normal.[13] There are no established biomarkers for manganese toxicity. Although serum and whole-blood manganese levels may be measured and elevated levels may be associated with T1 signal changes on MRI, there is no clear clinical correlation.[16]

MERCURY

Per a 2013 report, there were 1300 mercury exposures in the United States during that year with only 24 being classified as having moderate to major effects.[17] Internationally, these rates are higher. There have been two large-scale exposures over the course of the last century, including incidents in Minamata Bay, Japan (1956) and in Iraq (1971).[18] During the incident in Minamata Bay, mercury was dumped into the water and any ingested fish during that time contained methylmercury. In total, there were 2252 symptomatic patients and 1043 deaths during the event. Patients exhibited what was deemed Minamata disease, which was a combination of sensory disturbances, ataxia, dysarthria, constriction of visual field, auditory disturbances, and tremor. The second exposure event occurred in Iraq in 1971 in which grain that had been treated with a methylmercury-based fungicide was used to make bread. In total, there were 6148 symptomatic patients and 452 deaths during the event. These patients exhibited symptoms of paresthesia, ataxia, dysarthria, and visual disturbances.

Mercury has been implicated as having an association with PD risk. A study from 1990 to 2008 showed an association between airborne mercury exposure and PD risk, particularly in female nurses (hazard ratio, 1.33; confidence interval, 0.99–1.79; P value = .10).[19] Within this study, the PD risk was higher among the nonsmoking group (hazard ratio, 1.68; confidence interval, 1.11–1.25; P value = .04).

There are several sources of possible mercury exposure. These sources include mercury mining in China, gold mining, and mercury-contaminated food sources. The primary source of mercury exposure is the ingestion of mercury-contaminated fish. Fish with a high mercury content include shark, tilefish, tuna, swordfish, king mackerel, pike, walleye, muskellunge, and bass. Sources for inorganic elemental mercury include devices that contain mercury, such as thermometers. Inorganic mercury salts may be encountered with disc battery ingestion or certain laxatives. Organic mercury may be encountered in contaminated seafood, paints with mercury, or ingestion and injections of thimerasol.[20] The route of exposure tends to be either ingestion (inorganic mercury salts) or inhalation (elemental mercury).

Clinical Signs and Symptoms

Systemic signs of mercury toxicity may vary depending on the type of mercury and the route of exposure. Patients with inhalation of elemental mercury generally show symptoms of shortness of breath, cough, fever, nausea, vomiting, diarrhea, headache, metallic taste, salivation, and visual disturbance.[21,22] If the inhalation of elemental mercury is severe, the patient may have respiratory distress/failure. Ingestion of elemental mercury tends to show similar symptoms as inhaled elemental mercury, although with a few added symptoms. These additional symptoms include decreased peripheral nerve conduction velocity, short-term memory issues, decreased color vision, difficulty with visual acuity, ataxia, tremor, difficulties with facial expression, emotional lability, polyarthritis, dermatitis, and a syndrome mimicking pheochromocytoma.[23] Ingestion of organic mercury salts acutely causes a metallic taste, graying of the oral mucosa, abdominal pain, hemorrhagic gastroenteritis, acute tubular necrosis, and shock. Subacute symptoms include gastrointestinal (GI) issues, neurologic issues, and renal symptoms to include loose teeth, salivation, burning sensations in the mouth, tremors, erethism, nephrotic syndrome, proteinuria, and acrodynia (paresthesia/burning in hands/feet with associated pink discoloration).[20] Toxic symptoms may also occur weeks to months after exposure and include orofacial paresthesia, headaches, tremors, and fatigue. Severe cases may have ataxia, blindness, movement disorders, and dementia. If a patient survives the initial exposure, they may have acute renal failure.

Neurologic Complications

There are multiple neurologic complications associated with mercury exposure. Some data suggest that there may be a correlation of mercury exposure with development of Alzheimer disease, particularly in in vitro and in vivo studies, although not all data seem to agree. Multiple processes may be involved in the development of PD. These processes include loss of dopamine receptors, glutathione depletion in the substantia nigra, increases in glutamate, and mitochondrial dysfunction. Mutated forms of the PARK7 gene that encode for the DJ-1 protein tend to show a loss of ability to properly bind metal ions and therefore may lead to an increased toxicity presentation in this group. Erethism, which has been described as the mad hatter disease or mad hatter syndrome, includes symptoms of behavioral changes (irritability, low self-confidence, depression, apathy, shyness, and timidity), possible delirium, generalized weakness, headaches, pain, and tremors.[24] Several animal studies implicate mercury exposure as a possible contributor to the development of amyotrophic lateral sclerosis. Development of the inflammatory processes of multiple sclerosis has also been associated with mercury exposure.[18]

Mercury confers neurotoxicity through multiple processes. The N-methyl-D-aspartate (NMDA) receptors become activated by exposure, possibly through direct interaction with the sulfhydryl group on NMDA receptors. Rat models show that overactivation at the post-synaptic NMDA receptors leads to increase in intracellular $Ca2+$ levels, altered membrane excitability, and altered cytoskeletal protein disassembly. Methylmercury also induces oxidative stress and free radical accumulation, decreases glutathione concentration, causes mitochondrial damage, and inhibits the nuclear factor-κB pathway.

Diagnostic Tests

Laboratory studies in patients with suspected mercury exposure include several different sources. Blood mercury levels may be obtained and are often detectable six times more frequently in patient with PD than in healthy control subjects.[18] Blood and urine levels correlate well to each other, although do not correlate well to total body burden. Mercury may be tested in blood, hair, and urine and can reflect recent exposure, although not total burden. Provocation with a chelator has been proposed as a mechanism to estimate total body burden. A chelator, such as 2,3 dimercapto-1-propanesulfonate, may be administered and then urine output collected to estimate total body mercury burden.[23]

The diagnosis of mercury exposure is primarily clinical, although laboratory studies may be helpful to confirm. There is no clear consensus criteria on diagnosis at this time. Testing and diagnosis are generally considered positive for mercury toxicity if the provoked metal output is more than two standard deviations higher than the National Health and Nutrition Examination Survey reference range.

Treatment

Treatment of mercury toxicity includes chelation with an agent, such as 2,3 dimercapto-1-propanesulfonate. Chelation therapy often leads to improvement in symptoms of hypomimia, coordination, tremor, fine motor movements, memory, insomnia, metallic taste, fatigue, anxiety, and paresthesias. EDTA may also be used as a chelation agent, which has a high affinity for removing lead, cadmium, nickel, and several other toxic metals. If chelation therapy is achieved early in the course of acute toxicity, there are improved outcomes.[25] Often there is only limited improvement with chronic mercury exposures. Chelating agents do not redistribute mercury that has already deposited in the brain, although they may be able to decrease risk of renal injury.

1-METHYL-4-PHNEYL-1,2,5,6-TETRAHYDROPYRIDINE
History and Exposure

MPTP is the chemical that has been the most researched in regard to parkinsonism.[1] The first reported exposures leading to parkinsonism were described in users of "synthetic heroin," specifically 1-methyl-4-phenyl-4-propionoxypiperidine (MPPP).[13] MPTP was found to be a by-product of the synthesis of MPPP and some of the MPPP in use at the time was contaminated with it. Historically, study of MPTP suggested for the first time that environmental factors may play a role in the development of idiopathic PD. This was the first recognized chemical that led to an animal model of parkinsonism. Aside from synthetic heroin, there are few sources for exposure to MPTP.

Pathophysiology

MPTP exhibits neurotoxicity on the cells of the substantia nigra pars compacta. Monoamine oxidase B plays a role in creating 1-methyl-4-phenyl pyridine, which results in free radicals and oxidative stress. 1-Methyl-4-phenyl pyridine is transported intracellularly through the dopamine transporter into dopaminergic neurons where it collects inside the mitochondria and inhibits Complex I of the mitochondrial electron transport chain, alters calcium homeostasis, and causes endoplasmic reticulum stress.[1,13] Although MPTP tends to affect the substantia nigra pars compacta, it largely spares other areas, unlike idiopathic PD.

Clinical Symptoms

Symptoms were first described in young IV drug users in Northern California. These drug users developed rapid onset, severe parkinsonism. These patients exhibited the classic features of parkinsonism, to include bradykinesia, rigidity, and resting tremor.

Diagnosis

Diagnosis of MPTP-induced parkinsonism is largely based on clinical and historical features. The rapidity of onset sets MPTP toxicity apart from idiopathic PD. Historical features of IV drug use may also be somewhat helpful in these cases. Because MPTP exposure is so rare and only seen in niche situations, there are no clear established biomarkers for exposure.

Treatment

If exposure to MPTP is detected early enough within the course of the exposure, treatment may be pursued to help mitigate some of the damage. Nonselective monoamine oxidase inhibitors may be used to help prevent neurotoxicity in patients with MPTP exposure.[1] Symptomatically, these patients tend to respond well to dopaminergic treatment.

ORGANOCHLORINES AND ORGANOPHOSPHATES
History and Exposure

Organochlorines and organophosphates make up a significant portion of historical and current pesticides. Organochlorides were used regularly from the 1940s to the 1970s, although most of these have since been banned in the United States secondary to their neurotoxic effects. There are a few of these compounds still registered for use in the United States. One of the most well-known organochlorines is dichlorodiphenyl-trichloroethane (DDT), which has not been consistently linked with PD risk. Of the organochlorides, there are two compounds that have been particularly associated with PD risk, dieldrin and β-hexachlorocyclohexane.[13] Exposure to organochlorines is generally via inhalation or ingestion of contaminated fish, dairy products, or certain fatty foods. There are multiple organophosphates that have been associated with an increased risk of PD. These compounds also have known acute neurotoxic effects. There are 36 currently registered organophosphate pesticides in use in the United States, although several have been discontinued. These compounds are highly regulated and controlled, although occasional exposures continue to occur, particularly in occupational settings. Exposures tend to occur in agricultural settings, homes, gardens, and veterinary medicine. The route of organophosphate exposure tends to be inhalation or ingestion, although certain compounds also have variable dermal penetration and absorption.[26]

Pathophysiology

Organochlorine compounds are thought to cause neurotoxicity by impairment of mitochondrial function and production of reactive oxygen species leading to oxidative stress. These compounds may also disrupt calcium homeostasis, particularly of dopaminergic cells. The substantia nigra is particularly susceptible to these effects. Certain genetic polymorphisms that cause a decreased ability to clear toxins in the CNS, in combination with organochlorine exposure, may confer a significant increase in PD risk. Some postmortem analyses of PD striatum have shown higher than normal organochlorine levels compared with non-PD controls. Organochlorine also acts as a γ-aminobutyric acid antagonist. Organophosphate compounds have been shown to cause dopaminergic cell loss and microglial activation. Several organophosphate compounds are converted into a toxic form called oxon in the bloodstream. Many of these oxon compounds are filtered through the liver, although those that are not filtered may be hydrolyzed in circulation by serum paraoxonase (PON1) before they have an opportunity to cross the blood-brain barrier. Some patients have a genetic variability in PON1 activity, making them more vulnerable to neurotoxicity with organophosphate exposure. The hypercholinergic effects of organophosphates are caused by phosphorylation and inactivation of acetylcholinesterase (AChE) at nerve endings.[13]

Clinical Symptoms

Patients with acute organochlorine toxicity may exhibit seizures, headache, vertigo, nausea, vomiting, tremor, confusion, weakness, slurred speech, and hypersecretion. Chronic exposure may lead to hepatotoxicity, renal damage, CNS involvement, thyroid toxicity, and bladder damage. Acute organophosphate toxicity may result in multiple hypercholinergic symptoms, including headache, hypersecretion, fascicula-tions, nausea, diarrhea, vomiting, miosis, respiratory depression, seizures, tachy-cardia/bradycardia, anxiety, confusion, and restlessness. Choreiform movements have been described in some cases. Seizures tend to be more common in childhood exposure than in adult exposure. Symptoms of toxicity tend to be faster in onset after inhalation exposures. If death occurs in the acute period, it tends to be secondary to acute respiratory failure.[26]

Diagnosis

Diagnosis of organochlorine and organophosphate toxicity is based on history and ex-amination features. History of work in pesticides may be helpful in these cases. If the patient is exhibiting significant hypercholinergic symptoms, organophosphate toxicity should be considered, although organochlorine toxicity symptoms are similar in na-ture. Organochlorine levels may be tested easily in serum and urine samples, although may also be found in fat, semen, and breast milk.[27] The levels seen in these samples do not correlate with the extent of exposure or help prognosticate outcomes. Organ-ophosphate levels may be tested by measuring plasma butyrylcholinesterase and red blood cell AChE levels. Patients with organophosphate toxicity generally have lower levels of plasma butyrylcholinesterase and RBC AChE.[28] These changes tend to occur at doses much lower than that needed to cause symptoms. Organophosphates are metabolized into alkyl phosphates and phenols, which may be detected in urine during an acute toxicity and up to 48 hours after. Urine detection is more sensitive than the plasma/RBC studies and may help to narrow the specific agent that the patient was exposed to.

Treatment

Treatment of organochlorine toxicity tends to be primarily supportive because there are no antidotes available. Airway protection should be one of the first elements of treatment of patients with organochlorine toxicity. Multiple dose activated charcoal may help with fecal elimination and cholestyramine may be helpful to find some of the compound. Acute treatment of organophosphate toxicity includes securing the patient's airway and administration of atropine sulfate, which is an anticholinergic agent. Atropine treatment has a primary end point of clear breath sounds and absent pulmonary secretions. Glycopyrrolate use may also be considered in some cases.[26]

PARAQUAT
History and Exposure

Paraquat is a bipyridyl herbicide that has been associated with idiopathic PD through several case-control studies.[13,29] The chemical structure of paraquat is quite similar to MPTP. The chemical is widely used primarily for weed and grass control. The Environ-mental Protection Agency classifies this chemical as "restricted use," making it only available to those that are licensed. In the United States, there are several safeguards in place with this chemical, including a blue dye, an added intense odor, and an added vomiting agent, although this is not the case for all sources of paraquat throughout the world. It is still commonly used worldwide as an herbicide. Exposure typically occurs through ingestion, although may also occur via prolonged skin exposure or inhalation. Historically, paraquat has been found in some marijuana in the United States, leading to occasional inhalation exposure. Those that are commercially licensed to apply paraquat are at highest risk of exposure.[30] The incidence of PD disease and extent of paraquat exposure has been found in several studies to correlate well, although there have been a minority of studies that have not shown this correlation.

Pathophysiology

Paraquat has multiple mechanisms that contribute to its overall neurotoxicity effect. Paraquat goes through multiple conversions and ultimately alters cell membrane permeability to disrupt cellular function. Paraquat is metabolized by NADPH-dependent reduction, resulting in a free radical that reacts with molecular oxygen and forms a superoxide free radical.[1] This superoxide anion reacts with superoxide dismutase to result in hydrogen peroxide. The resulting hydrogen peroxide and the original superoxide anion react with lipids in the cell membrane to cause lipid peroxidation. Paraquat has also been shown to stimulate glutamate efflux, leading to excitatory cytotoxicity. Animal studies have shown that paraquat may also cause α-synuclein upregulation, aggregate formation, and microglial activation.[13] These effects tend to have a predisposition toward the dopaminergic neuronal cells in the basal ganglia.

Clinical Symptoms

Symptoms of paraquat ingestion acutely tend to affect the GI system. Initially, patients tend to have erythema of the mouth and throat, followed by further GI symptoms, including nausea, vomiting, abdominal pain, and/or diarrhea. Downstream effects include dehydration, hyponatremia, hypokalemia, and hypotension. Within hours to days of a large ingestion, patients may exhibit confusion, coma, acute kidney failure, tachycardia, myopathy, liver failure, lung scarring, weakness, pulmonary edema, respiratory failure, and/or seizures. If the amount ingested is smaller, effects may not be appreciated until days to weeks later, at which point patients may exhibit heart failure, kidney failure, liver failure, and/or lung scarring.[30]

Diagnosis

Paraquat exposure and toxicity is diagnosed primarily based on history of exposure and clinical examination findings that are consistent with the diagnosis. Often oropharyngeal burns in patients with ingestion are quite prominent.[30] Late findings may include liver failure, kidney failure, heart failure, and lung scarring. Some diagnostic testing also may be supportive of the diagnosis. Paraquat may be measured in the urine and in the serum. Urine paraquat levels are primarily used to confirm or exclude exposure status.[31,32] Qualitative urine testing is performed when a solution of dithionite is added to urine, resulting in a blue color change.[33] A green color change suggests diquat is present instead of paraquat. It is possible to perform a semiquantitative test in this way because the darker blue is on testing, the higher the concentration of paraquat. Serum paraquat levels may be measured and compared with time since exposure to help with prognosis. Quantitative testing may be challenging because several laboratories do not perform it. Alternatively, qualitative testing may be pursued using the same technique as urine testing with dithionite looking for a blue color change.[34]

Treatment

Initial treatment after a known ingestion should include activated charcoal or Fuller earth, removal of any contaminated articles of clothing, and washing exposed skin/eyes. If the ingestion occurred within an hour, nasogastric suction may be helpful to remove some of the chemical from the GI tract.[30] Most other acute measures are supportive, including IV fluids, vasopressors, ventilation, and dialysis if needed. Excess oxygen administration is best avoided in the acute period because it may overall worsen the paraquat toxicity.

ROTENONE
History and Exposure

Rotenone is a naturally occurring pesticide that is regularly used as an insecticide and as an agent to kill fish.[13] The compound is found is several plant species, including barbasco, cub, haiari, nekoe, and timbo.[35] This compound was the first used as an insecticide in the 1840s.[36] Rat models have shown that rotenone may cause elements of PD, including bradykinesia, postural instability, and rigidity. The effect is reproducible to the extent that rotenone-exposed animals have become the standard animal model for PD. Epidemiologic studies have shown higher rates of PD in patients that have worked with rotenone than in those that have not.[37] This effect was seen whether those being studied had used protective gloves or not.[29] Exposure may be via inhalation, ingestion, or via dermal penetration/absorption.

Pathophysiology

The primary mechanism of the neurotoxicity exhibited by rotenone is inhibition of Complex I of the electron transport chain in the mitochondria, causing mitochondrial toxicity. Both dopaminergic and nondopaminergic neurons are affected by the resulting oxidative damage. Aggregates of α-synuclein and polyubiquitin have been found in dopamine neurons in the substantia nigra and enteric nervous systems of rat models that have been exposed to rotenone.[13] Some animal studies have shown that motor decline related to rotenone exposure is not always associated with dopaminergic cell loss, making other central, nondopaminergic effects on motor function likely.

Clinical Symptoms

Patients with acute rotenone toxicity exhibit local reactions that include conjunctivitis, dermatitis, sore throat, and congestion. Ingestion may lead to GI irritation and vomiting. Inhalation may lead to tachypnea, then depressed respiratory function and convulsions.[35] More chronic features are parkinsonian in nature and include bradykinesia, rigidity, and postural instability.

Diagnosis

Acute toxicity with rotenone is based on clinical history and examination. A strong history should be obtained to include any history of occupational exposures.

Treatment

Parkinsonism secondary to rotenone has been shown to be responsive to dopaminergic agents. Rotenone-based rat models have been used to pursue further options regarding treatment. Dietary phytocannabinoid has been shown in rat models to decrease oxidative damage, glial activation, and dopaminergic cell loss when given before rotenone exposure.[38] An adenosine receptor antagonist increased midbrain dopamine concentrations in rat models and decreased motor slowing.[39]

AGENT ORANGE
History and Exposure

The effects of Agent Orange on the development of parkinsonism are still being investigated, although more evidence seems to show a possible connection between the two. Agent Orange was an herbicide and defoliant chemical that was most notably used by the US military as an herbicidal warfare tactic in the Vietnam War. Agent Orange was a mixture of two compounds, 2,4-D and 2,4,5-T. These compounds are both chlorinated phenoxy acids. The potentially dangerous compound in Agent Orange is actually an impurity that is present in 2,4,5-T called 2,3,7,8-tetrachlorodibenzo-p-dioxin.[40] This compound is colloquially known as dioxin or TCDD. There are multiple different dioxins (polychlorinated biphenyls), although TCDD is the most toxic of these compounds.[41] The US Environmental Protection Agency classifies TCDD as a carcinogen. Exposure to TCDD can occur via ingestion, inhalation, or skin contact. Several studies have suggested that the oxidative stress caused by polychlorinated biphenyls, such as TCDD, may increase risk of neurodegenerative disease, such as PD. One retrospective mortality study of 17,321 polychlorinated biphenyl–exposed workers showed a subgroup analysis of highly exposed women that had increased rates of PD and dementia.[42] Although there are some studies showing a correlation between polychlorinated biphenyls and PD risk, there are several others that do not agree with these findings. One nested case-control study performed in Finland in 2012 did not show any significant correlation between exposure and increased PD risk and in fact trended toward a decreased PD risk in these patients without reaching statistical significance.[43] Further research is necessary in these patients to draw a more definitive conclusion.

Pathophysiology

The mechanism of dioxin toxicity is mediated by the aryl-hydrocarbon receptor (AhR), which is a transcriptional regulator of cell growth, differentiation, and migration. Dioxin binds to AhR in the cytoplasm, after which AhR then translocates to the nucleus where it undergoes dimerization with the Ah receptor nuclear translocator (Arnt). This interaction results in a heterodimeric transcription factor that plays a role in increased expression of numerous genes within the cell that contribute to the effects of dioxin toxicity. There is some further evidence that TCDD also may play a role in the modification of epigenetic factors.[44] Animal models show decreased dopamine levels in patients exposed to TCDD.[2]

Clinical Symptoms

TCDD has a well-documented carcinogenic effect including increased risk of prostate cancer, soft tissue sarcomas, and non-Hodgkin lymphoma.[45] It has further been associated with numerous other health issues, including reproductive issues, miscarriage, childhood developmental issues, liver damage, damage to the immune system, and interference with the endocrine system.[41]

Diagnostic Tests

Dioxin is no longer in use, although it was used in the United States in the 1960s and 1970s. These compounds are highly persistent in the environment. Polychlorinated biphenyls may be detectable in the blood of approximately 80% of Americans older than the age of 50.[42] This has been used to perform epidemiologic studies of long-term effects of polychlorinated biphenyl exposure.

CLINICS CARE POINTS

1. Acute-onset tremors, bradykinesia (slowing of movements), and rigidity should always be investigated as a toxin exposure.
2. Isolate and stop the offending toxin.
3. Hospitalize until a cause is known or the person is medically stable.

4. Parkinsonism secondary to toxin exposure does not usually progress once the agent is stopped.
5. Parkinsonism may not improve after stopping the agent; however, 10% to 20% may have improvement.

DISCLOSURE

The views expressed in this article are those of the author and do not reflect the official policy of the Department of Army/Navy/Air Force, Department of Defense, or US Government.

REFERENCES

1. Ratner MH, Feldman RG. Environmental toxins and Parkinson's disease. In: Ebadi MS, Pfeiffer RF, editors. Parkinson's disease. Boca Raton (FL): CRC Press; 2005. p. 51–62.
2. Masumoto K, Suita S, Taguchi T, et al. Manganese intoxication during intermittent parenteral nutrition: report of two cases. JPEN J Parenter Enteral Nutr 2001; 25(2):95–9.
3. Aschner JL, Aschner M. Nutritional aspects of manganese homeostasis. Mol Aspects Med 2005;26(4–5):353–62.
4. University of Hertfordshire. Maneb. PPDB: pesticide properties DataBase 2018. Available at: http://sitem.herts.ac.uk/aeru/ppdb/en/Reports/426.htm. Accessed January 10, 2020.
5. Feldman RG. Occupational and environmental neurotoxicology. Philadelphia: Lippincott-Raven; 1999.
6. Food and Nutrition Board of the Institute of Medicine. Dietary reference intakes for vitamin A, vitamin K, arsenic, boron, chromium, copper, iodine, iron, manganese, molybdenum, nickel, silicon, vanadium, and zinc. Washington, DC: National Academies Press; 2000. Available at: https://www.nap.edu/catalog/10026/dietary-reference-intakes-for-vitamin-a-vitamin-k-arsenic-boron-chromium-copper-iodine-iron-manganese-molybdenum-nickel-silicon-vanadium-and-zinc. Accessed January 10, 2020.
7. Egan SK, Tao SS, Pennington JA, et al. US Food and Drug Administration's Total Diet Study: intake of nutritional and toxic elements, 1991-96. Food Addit Contam 2002;19(2):103–25.
8. Powell JJ, Burden TJ, Thompson RP. In vitro mineral availability from digested tea: a rich dietary source of managanese. Analyst 1998;123(8):1721–4.
9. Gorell JM, Johnson CC, Rybicki BA, et al. Occupational exposures to metals as risk factors for Parkinson's disease. Neurology 1997;48(3):650–8.
10. Mortimer JA, Borenstein AR, Nelson LM. Associations of welding and manganese exposure with Parkinson disease: review and meta-analysis. Neurology 2012; 79(11):1174–80.
11. Racette BA, Searles Nielsen S, Criswell SR, et al. Dose-dependent progression of parkinsonism in manganese-exposed welders. Neurology 2017;88(4):344–51.
12. Park J, Yoo CI, Sim CS, et al. Occupations and Parkinson's disease: a case-control study in South Korea. Ind Health 2004;42(3):352–8.
13. Nandipati S, Litvan I. Environmental exposures and Parkinson's disease. Int J Environ Res Public Health 2016;13(9):881.
14. Chandra SV. Neurological consequences of manganese imbalance. In: Dreosti IE, Smith RM, editors. Neurobiology of the Trace elements, Vol. 2:

Neurotoxicology and Neuropharmacology. Clifton (NJ): Humana Press; 1983. p. 167–96.

15. Lu CS, Huang CC, Chu NS, et al. Levodopa failure in chronic manganism. Neurology 1994;44(9):1600–2.

16. Dickerson RN. Manganese intoxication and parenteral nutrition. Nutrition 2001; 17(7–8):689–93.

17. Posin SL, Sharma S. Mercury toxicity. In: StatPearls. Treasure Island (FL): Stat-Pearls Publishing; 2020. Available at: https://www.ncbi.nlm.nih.gov/books/NBK499935/.

18. Cariccio VL, Samà A, Bramanti P, et al. Mercury involvement in neuronal damage and in neurodegenerative diseases. Biol Trace Elem Res 2019;187(2):341–56.

19. Palacios N, Fitzgerald K, Roberts AL, et al. A prospective analysis of airborne metal exposures and risk of Parkinson disease in the nurses' health study cohort. Environ Health Perspect 2014;122(9):933–8.

20. Mercury Factsheet. Centers for Disease Control and Prevention. 2017. Available at: https://www.cdc.gov/biomonitoring/Mercury_FactSheet.html. Accessed January 5, 2020.

21. Kanluen S, Gottlieb CA. A clinical pathologic study of four adult cases of acute mercury inhalation toxicity. Arch Pathol Lab Med 1991;115(1):56–60.

22. Asano S, Eto K, Kurisaki E, et al. Review article: acute inorganic mercury vapor inhalation poisoning. Pathol Int 2000;50(3):169–74.

23. Bernhoft RA. Mercury toxicity and treatment: a review of the literature. J Environ Public Health 2012;2012:460508.

24. Bluhm RE, Bobbitt RG, Welch LW, et al. Elemental mercury vapour toxicity, treatment, and prognosis after acute, intensive exposure in chloralkali plant workers. Part I: history, neuropsychological findings and chelator effects. Hum Exp Toxicol 1992;11(3):201–10.

25. Kosnett MJ. The role of chelation in the treatment of arsenic and mercury poisoning. J Med Toxicol 2013;9(4):347–54.

26. Reigart JR, Roberts JR, editors. Recognition and management of pesticide poisonings. 6th edition. Washington, DC: Environmental Protection Agency; 2013.

27. Organochlorine pesticides. Delaware health and social services. Available at: https://www.dhss.delaware.gov/dph/files/organochlorpestfaq.pdf. Accessed January 20, 2020.

28. Kim JH, Stevens RC, MacCoss MJ, et al. Identification and characterization of biomarkers of organophosphorus exposures in humans. Adv Exp Med Biol 2010;660:61–71.

29. Tanner CM, Kamel F, Ross GW, et al. Rotenone, paraquat, and Parkinson's disease. Environ Health Perspect 2011;119(6):866–72.

30. Facts about Paraquat. Centers for Disease Control and Prevention. 2018. Available at: https://emergency.cdc.gov/agent/paraquat/basics/facts.asp. Accessed January 20, 2020.

31. Scherrmann JM, Houze P, Bismuth C, et al. Prognostic value of plasma and urine paraquat concentration. Hum Toxicol 1987;6(1):91–3.

32. Berry DJ, Grove J. The determination of paraquat (I,I'-dimethyl-4,4'-bipyridylium cation) in urine. Clin Chim Acta 1971;34(1):5–11.

33. Koo JR, Yoon JW, Han SJ, et al. Rapid analysis of plasma paraquat using sodium dithionite as a predictor of outcome in acute paraquat poisoning. Am J Med Sci 2009;338(5):373–7.

34. Kuan CM, Lin ST, Yen TH, et al. Paper-based diagnostic devices for clinical paraquat poisoning diagnosis. Biomicrofluidics 2016;10(3):034118.

35. Rotenone. Extoxnet. 1993. Available at: http://pmep.cce.cornell.edu/profiles/extoxnet/pyrethrins-ziram/rotenone-ext.html. Accessed January 25, 2020.

36. Metcalf RL. The mode of action of organic insecticides. Washington, DC: National Research Council; 1948.

37. Dhillon AS, Tarbutton GL, Levin JL, et al. Pesticide/environmental exposures and Parkinson's disease in East Texas. J Agromedicine 2008;13(1):37–48.

38. Ojha S, Javed H, Azimullah S, et al. β-Caryophyllene, a phytocannabinoid attenuates oxidative stress, neuroinflammation, glial activation, and salvages dopaminergic neurons in a rat model of Parkinson disease. Mol Cell Biochem 2016;418(1–2):59–70.

39. Fathalla AM, Soliman AM, Ali MH, et al. Adenosine A2A receptor blockade prevents rotenone-induced motor impairment in a rat model of parkinsonism. Front Behav Neurosci 2016;10:35.

40. Buckingham WA. The Air Force and herbicides in Southeast Asia 1961-1971. Office of Air Force history. Washington, DC: United States Air Force; 1982.

41. Dioxins: Your Environment, Your Health | National Library of Medicine." U.S. National Library of Medicine, National Institutes of Health. 2017. Available at: Toxtown.nlm.nih.gov/chemicals-and-contaminants/dioxins. Accessed October 17, 2019.

42. Steenland K, Hein MJ, Cassinelli RT 2nd, et al. Polychlorinated biphenyls and neurodegenerative disease mortality in an occupational cohort. Epidemiology 2006;17(1):8–13.

43. Weisskopf MG, Knekt P, O'Reilly EJ, et al. Polychlorinated biphenyls in prospectively collected serum and Parkinson's disease risk. Mov Disord 2012;27(13):1659–65.

44. Patrizi B, Siciliani de Cumis M. TCDD toxicity mediated by epigenetic mechanisms. Int J Mol Sci 2018;19(12):4101.

45. Kogevinas M, Becher H, Benn T, et al. Cancer mortality in workers exposed to phenoxy herbicides, chlorophenols, and dioxins. An expanded and updated international cohort study. Am J Epidemiol 1997;145(12):1061–75.

Toxin-Induced Seizures

Haley N. Phillips, MD[a],*, Laura Tormoehlen, MD[a,b]

KEYWORDS

• Toxin • Seizure • Mechanism • Clinical management

KEY POINTS

• Many toxins can cause seizure in overdose and are changing over time, with new toxins always emerging; the authors outline common toxins resulting in seizure.

• Mechanisms for toxins are outlined to assist in identification of future toxins with similar mechanisms of action that may result in seizure.

• Toxidromes of selected toxins are outlined, along with treatment approaches unique to each toxin.

INTRODUCTION

An important distinction in seizure management is the identification of a provoked versus an unprovoked seizure. This distinction allows for proper treatment of seizures and avoidance of unnecessary side effects of treatments that would not reduce risk of seizure recurrence. Toxicity and withdrawal of medications, chemicals, and environmental toxins can result in seizure with some substances' effects more widely known than others.[1,2] The national incidence of toxin-induced seizures is unclear, but select population studies indicate the most common toxins that result in seizure have evolved over time as prescribing practices evolve and new illicit substances become more widely available (**Fig. 1**).[3–5] The basic mechanism of seizure activity resulting from chemicals, medications, or toxins (referred to as toxins throughout this paper) involves stimulation of central nervous system (CNS) excitatory pathways, or inhibition of inhibitory pathways within the CNS, or withdrawal of long-term CNS depressants. It is important to distinguish and identify toxin-induced seizure from epilepsy as the long- and short-term treatments differ.[4,6,7] The authors have identified and outline the mechanisms and specific examples of toxins that result in seizure in 6 main categories. These categories include stimulants, cholinergics, gamma-aminobutyric acid (GABA) antagonists including GABA agonist withdrawal, glutamate agonists,

[a] Department of Neurology, Indiana University, Indiana University Neuroscience Center, 355 West 16th Street, Suite 4700, Indianapolis, IN 46202, USA; [b] Department of Emergency Medicine-Toxicology, Indiana University, Indiana University Neuroscience Center, 355 West 16th Street, Suite 4700, Indianapolis, IN 46202, USA
* Corresponding author.
E-mail address: haleykathol@gmail.com

Neurol Clin 38 (2020) 867–879
https://doi.org/10.1016/j.ncl.2020.07.004
0733-8619/20/© 2020 Elsevier Inc. All rights reserved.

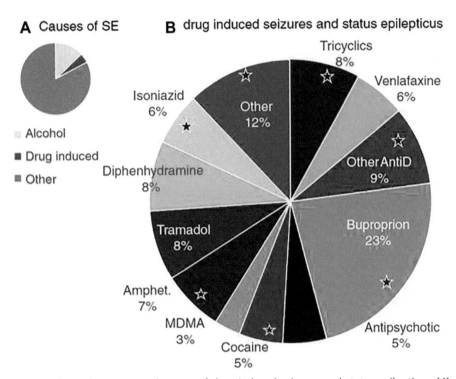

A Causes of SE

Alcohol

Drug induced

Other

B drug induced seizures and status epilepticus

Tricyclics 8%
Venlafaxine 6%
Isoniazid 6%
Other 12%
Other AntiD 9%
Diphenhydramine 8%
Buproprion 23%
Tramadol 8%
Amphet. 7%
Antipsychotic 5%
MDMA 3%
Cocaine 5%

Fig. 1. Relative frequency and causes of drug-induced seizures and status epilepticus. (*A*) Data from a prospective population-based study of status epilepticus (SE) (n = 204 cases). (*B*) Data from a retrospective review of cases (n = 386) where seizures were reported as an outcome reported to the California State Poisons Registry in 2003; proportion (%) by drug/drug class. 3.6% of cases overall had status epilepticus (indicated by a star) and 27.7% had 2 or more seizures. amphet, amphetamine; AntiD, antidepressants; MDMA, 3,4-methylenedioxy-methamphetamine. (*From* Cock, HR. Drug-induced status epilepticus. *Epilepsy & Behavior*. 2015; 49. 76-2; with permission.)

histamine antagonists, and adenosine antagonists. There are many other drugs and toxins that cause seizures that are outside the scope of this paper (**Table 1**) (PLASTICs Mnemonic).[8] Also outside the scope of this paper are drug-induced metabolic derangements that cause seizures (eg, insulin and hypoglycemia or carbon monoxide and hypoxia).

The basic mechanism by which toxins cause seizure activity involve (1) increased excitation, (2) decreased inhibition, or (3) withdrawal of depressants. Excitatory neuronal activity can be caused by glutamate agonists, stimulants/sympathomimetics, and cholinergic agonists.[9] Excitation is the result of increased cellular sodium influx and decreases in chloride influx and potassium efflux. CNS depression results from GABA, adenosine, and histamine action; antagonizing the activity of these neurotransmitters results in decreased CNS inhibitory activity, thus shifting the balance toward CNS activation with seizure as a potential result.[10,11]

STIMULANTS

Stimulants are substances that shift the excitation-inhibition balance in the brain toward excitation, resulting in an agitated delirium. Many stimulants are

Table 1 PLASTIC mnemonic	
PLASTIC Mnemonic[a] for Partial Listing of Drugs and Chemicals that May Cause Acute Seizures	
P	Phencyclidine, pesticides, phenol, propoxyphene
L	Lead, lithium, lindane, local anesthetics
A	Antidepressants, antipsychotics, anticonvulsants, antihistamines, abstinence syndromes
S	Salicylate, sympathomimetics, strychnine, solvents, shellfish (domoic acid)
T	Theophylline, tricyclic antidepressants, thallium, tobacco (nicotine)
I	Isoniazid, insulin (and other causes of hypoglycemia), insecticides
C	Camphor, cocaine, cyanide, carbon monoxide, chloroquine, cyclonite (C4 plastic explosive), cicutoxin

[a] The authors would like to acknowledge Dr James R. Roberts for being the first to develop and teach this mnemonic at The Poison Control Center, Phila.

From Osterhoudt KC, Henretiq FM. A 16-Year-Old With Recalcitrant Seizures. Pediatric Emergency Care 2012;28(3):304-306; with permission.

sympathomimetic substances that increase the release of dopamine (DA), serotonin (5-HT), norepinephrine (NE), and epinephrine while also blocking their reuptake from the synaptic space, resulting in increased extracellular concentrations of these neurotransmitters. Sympathomimetic syndrome is characterized by anxiety, delusions, diaphoresis, hypertension, tachycardia, hyperreflexia, mydriasis, paranoia, piloerection, and seizures. Complications of severe poisoning include status epilepticus and uncoupling of oxidative phosphorylation.

Cocaine is a sympathomimetic that blocks the DA transporter, thereby increasing synaptic levels of biogenic amines (DA, 5-HT, and NE), and is also a sodium channel blocker. The result is a toxidrome that includes hypertension but can also result in hypotension, QRS prolongation, and malignant cardiac dysrhythmia from sodium channel blockade.[12] Acute cocaine intoxication can be complicated by seizure, acidosis, hyperthermia, and uncoupling. Cocaine-induced hypertension generally should not be treated with beta blockers, which could result in unopposed alpha-adrenergic action. The benzodiazepines used for the agitated delirium and seizures will be useful in lowering heart rate and blood pressure.

Amphetamines and phenethylamines are sympathomimetics that diffuse into presynaptic vesicles, causing monoamine release. In addition, they block monoamine oxidase (MAO) and the dopamine reuptake transporter, which results in DA excess. At higher doses, receptors and synaptic clefts are flooded after increased vesicle release and blockade of 5-HT reuptake. Amphetamine and methamphetamine block metabolism by inhibiting MAO and increasing the concentration of monoamines in the presynaptic nerve terminal, thereby promoting their release and directly activating postsynaptic receptors. Psychotic symptoms occur in overdose from excess 5-HT and DA activity; designer phenethylamines have variable psychoactive properties including hallucinations from 5-HT receptor agonism.[13] Serotonin syndrome is also possible, and clinical features are hyperthermia, mydriasis, clonus, rigidity, and agitated delirium.

Synthetic cathinones or "bath salts" are a newer drug of abuse that can result in seizure, with notable prevalence in both pediatric and adult populations.[14,15] Seizure likely results from sympathomimetic toxicity with increased NE, 5-HT, and DA activity. Hyperthermia and seizure activity have been found to be associated in some studies.[14,15] Hyponatremia can also result, and the mechanism is unclear but may be similar to that of 3,4-methylenedioxy-methamphetamine (MDMA), resulting from syndrome of inappropriate antidiuretic hormone (SIADH), outlined in the following section.[16]

Other psychostimulant designer drugs that are reported to result in seizure include benzylpiperazine (BZP), trifluoromethylphenylpiperazine (TFMPP), and MDMA. BZP and TFMPP enhance release of DA, NE, and 5-HT at the nerve terminals. BZP primarily increases DA and NE, whereas TFMPP has more 5-HT agonist activities that increase activity at postsynaptic cell receptors.[17] MDMA acts to increase 5-HT activity by promoting its release into the synaptic cleft, inhibiting reuptake, which promotes prolonged 5-HT concentration in the synaptic cleft, resulting in increased binding to postsynaptic 5-HT2a receptors. MDMA also has been shown to reduce glutamic acid decarboxylase in the hippocampus, resulting in the increase of extracellular glutamate within the hippocampus that can lead to seizure, as well as resulting in GABAergic neuronal cell death.[18] The toxidrome for MDMA includes hypertension, hyperthermia, tachycardia, and hepatotoxicity. The serotonergic toxicity can cause serotonin syndrome. SIADH may also be seen, with serum sodium monitoring warranted in addition to seizure treatment with benzodiazepines and correction of hyponatremia if present.

Atypical antidepressants bupropion and venlafaxine are responsible for toxin-related seizures in 23% and 6% of a toxin-induced seizure cohort, respectively.[3] Bupropion, a monocyclic antidepressant, inhibits presynaptic DA and NE reuptake transporters as well as increases DA, NE, and 5-HT vesicular transport into presynaptic vesicles and promotes their release to the synaptic space.[19–21] This results in a toxidrome including tremors, agitation, or tachycardia, but seizure can occur without other signs of CNS toxicity and may be delayed up to 24 hours. QRS prolongation caused by bupropion is due to blockade of cardiac gap junctions.[22] QTc interval prolongation may also result from potassium channel blockade, especially if taken with other agents that can prolong QT intervals, and this should be monitored, as Torsade de Pointes can occur. Venlafaxine inhibits 5-HT and NE reuptake. It is also associated with QRS prolongation from sodium channel blockade, and seizure occurs at a higher rate than in selective serotonin reuptake inhibitors (SSRIs) or tricyclic antidepressant (TCA) overdose.[23]

Synthetic cannabinoids (SCs) (eg, "K2" and "Spice") cause psychoactive effect by complete cannabinoid receptor-1 (CB_1R) agonism in the CNS. Although not directly sympathomimetic, these drugs do produce a stimulant syndrome. A higher binding affinity for CBRs has been noted in most SCs compared with Δ9-tetrahydrobannabinol (Δ9-THC); it is also known that SCs have full agonist activity compared with the partial agonist activity of Δ9-THC.[24] The toxidrome other than seizures for SCs include anxiety, psychosis, agitation, and tachycardia and are felt to be secondary to the high affinity of SC metabolites for CB_1R and CB_2R, increased direct activity on the receptors, as well as possible upregulation of 5HT-2 receptors from CB_2R activation.[24,25] A potentially additive mechanism for seizure is prolonged or exaggerated effect, as the metabolites of SC parent compounds bind with much higher affinity to CBRs than Δ9-THC does.[26]

Phencyclidine (PCP) is an N-methyl-D-aspartate (NMDA) receptor antagonist with high affinity for receptors in the limbic system, as well as a DA, NE, and 5-HT reuptake inhibitor. It has a stimulant toxidrome that is often marked by significant agitation, seizure, psychosis, and alteration in awareness.[27] Overall, the primary clinical treatment of stimulant toxicity is benzodiazepines. The mechanism of this is increased GABA activity to combat sympathomimetic toxidromes and for seizure treatment. Frequent monitoring of serum electrolytes (particularly sodium, potassium, and glucose) and cardiac monitoring for QRS and QTc prolongation, arrhythmias, and cardiac ischemia are important in the supportive care for patients with stimulant/sympathomimetic toxidromes. Primary treatment of cardiac dysrhythmias is sodium bicarbonate for QRS prolongation and potassium repletion (to keep >4.0 mEq/L) and magnesium supplementation for QTc prolongation. Avoidance of beta-blockers in some settings may be warranted depending on the toxins involved. In general, no methods of enhanced elimination or antidotes are indicated, although cyproheptadine may be considered as a second-line treatment of serotonin syndrome.[1,16]

CHOLINERGIC AGENTS

Acetylcholine (Ach) agonists stimulate directly by binding nicotinic or muscarinic receptors to promote their activity. Alternatively, some agents inhibit acetylcholinesterase, resulting in an increased amount of acetylcholine at the nerve terminal by preventing its intrasynaptic breakdown. The increased acetylcholine binds to nicotinic and muscarinic receptors. Different studies have shown muscarinic or nicotinic receptors may both be responsible for seizures depending on the region of the brain (basal forebrain by nicotinic receptors or zona incerta by muscarinic).[28,29]

Pilocarpine, (RS)-propan-2yl methylphosphonofluoridate (Sarin), and O-ethyl S-[2-(diisopropylamino)ethyl]methylphosphonothioate (VX) have been observed in vivo to result in seizures and status epilepticus by increasing muscarinic receptor action in the entorhinal cortex-hippocampus complex.[30] In nerve agent poisoning, animal models have also shown an initial response to atropine, an antimuscarinic agent, stopping seizures in the acute setting, but prolonged seizure activity results in neuropathology that causes recurrent seizure activity. This seems to be due to prolonged cholinergic action resulting in NMDA receptor stimulation and glutamatergic excitation and resultant cellular damage.[6,31] VX and Sarin bind to serine residues at the active site of the acetylcholinesterase enzyme, resulting in seizure from excessive ACh activity in the CNS.[32] Associated symptoms from neuromuscular junction nicotinic ACh activity include weakness, fasciculations, and respiratory depression. The muscarinic symptoms of cholinergic toxicity can be represented by the mnemonic DUMBBELS: defecation, urination, miosis, bradycardia, bronchospasm, emesis, lacrimation, and salivation. Treatment with pralidoxime may be warranted to treat and/or prevent nicotinic symptoms, specifically weakness. Atropine is the treatment of muscarinic symptoms and is typically dosed to resolution of broncorrhea.[33] Seizures should be treated with benzodiazepines.

Organophosphate pesticides have the same basic mechanism as nerve gases and can result in convulsions as well, with early seizure resulting from nicotinic ACh receptor hyperstimulation, followed by a mixed cholinergic and noncholinergic phase, then finally into a noncholinergic phase with associated glutamatergic excitotoxicity resulting in permanent damage to neurons.[33] They have a DUMBBELS toxidrome from hyperstimulation of muscarinic Ach receptors.[34] Benzodiazepines have primarily been used to treat seizure in these cases. It has been proposed that cholinergic stimulation may cause increased central glutamatergic activity, and thus treatment with glutamate receptor antagonists, adenosine receptor agonists, or antimuscarinics with antiglutamatergic action could hypothetically play a role in future treatment.[34,35] Otherwise, treatment recommendations mirror those for the nerve gases.

Nicotine acts on the central and peripheral nervous systems to result in gastrointestinal, respiratory, cardiovascular, and neurologic effects. One proposed mnemonic is the days-of-the-week "MTWTFSS," for Mydriasis, Tachycardia, Weakness, Tremors, Fasciculations, Seizures, and Somnolence, to recall the nicotinic toxidrome.[36] Seizure is hypothesized to result from nicotine by activation of central nicotinic acetylcholine receptor. Several hypotheses of the mechanism include excitatory amino acid transporter 3 activity reduction by nicotine, resulting in glutamate accumulation. Other hypotheses include enhancing NO production through glutamate release and NMDA receptor activation, reducing GABAergic signal to the hippocampus, oxidative stress from nicotine causing glutathione depletion, and oxidative stress causing increased reactive oxygen and nitrogen species leading to epileptogenesis.[37]

Treatment of seizures resulting from excess cholinergic activity rely on benzodiazepines and support for additional associated symptoms with antimuscarinics and/or oximes as described. There are no indicated methods of enhanced elimination other than activated charcoal in pesticide ingestion.

GAMMA-AMINOBUTYRIC ACID ANTAGONISTS

The GABA-A receptor is a chloride ion (Cl-) channel. GABA-ergic neurons have postsynaptic GABA-A receptors and presynaptic GABA-B receptors. When bound to the GABA-A receptor, GABA results in chloride ion influx into the cell resulting in hyperpolarization and thus inhibits action potentials. GABA-A agonists (ie, benzodiazepines and barbiturates) reduce cerebral activity, and toxicity from these drugs results in coma. Withdrawal states can precipitate seizures as well as status epilepticus.[4] GABA-B receptors are metabotropic and have second messenger systems; binding of presynaptic GABA-B results in prevention of release of GABA. Postsynaptic GABA-B receptor activation induces a slower and longer inhibition than GABA-A.[38] GABA-B activity results in muscle relaxation, decreased cognitive function, pain relief, bronchiolar relaxation, nausea, reduced intestinal peristalsis, and dizziness.[39]

A commonly used analgesic that is known to cause seizure is the partial *mu*-opioid agonist tramadol.[3] It is notable that therapeutic levels of tramadol have been known to result in seizure, with single exposure overdose ingestion in up to 52.5% of patients in one population. Another state reported 13.7% of toxin-induced seizures were from tramadol over 2.5 years.[40,41] The exact mechanism for seizure is unknown but likely results from decreased GABA-A antagonism, 5-HT inhibition, and NE reuptake.[42–44]

Baclofen is a known GABA-B receptor agonist that results in seizure from abrupt withdrawal as well as intoxication.[3] Baclofen binds to the GABA-B receptor and promotes presynaptic GABA release by potassium efflux as well as decreased calcium conductance. This hyperpolarizes neurons, resulting in diminished release of neurotransmitters but can result in a paradoxic seizure in high doses.[45] It is thought that baclofen in toxic doses becomes a GABA-A and -B receptor agonist in the brain and spinal cord and via unknown mechanisms causes seizure.[46] Abrupt withdrawal of the GABA-B agonist can also precipitate seizure, see section on withdrawal.[47]

Antimicrobials

A key mechanism in toxin-induced seizures is that GABA synthesis requires glutamate to be converted to GABA via glutamic acid decarboxylase, a reaction that requires pyridoxine as a coenzyme. Depletion of pyridoxine (vitamin B6) can result in excess glutamate activity and GABA depletion. The resulting GABA deficiency will prevent the GABA-A channel from opening, that is GABA itself is required for receptor function. Thus, benzodiazepines alone will not be successful in treating seizure in the setting of pyridoxine deficiency, the deficiency must be treated.

Isoniazid (INH) is an inhibitor of pyridoxine phosphokinase by hydratization of pyridoxal-5-phosphate, which results in depletion of active B6, so GABA synthesis from glutamate is unable to proceed. This results in excessive glutamatergic action and absence of GABA tone; pyridoxine and benzodiazepines are both needed to treat seizures resulting from INH.[38,48]

Penicillin, cephalosporins (particularly cefepime), carbapenems, and fluoroquinolones all bind to and inhibit the GABA-A receptor, which results in a reduction of Cl- influx, allowing for convulsive activity to be promoted and not inhibited. Penicillin and aztreonam can also bind the channel to block influx of chloride resulting in decreased GABA tone. Penicillin has also been postulated to directly bind to the benzodiazepine site on the GABA-A receptor to produce convulsions.[21,49]

Withdrawal of Gamma-Aminobutyric Acid Agonists

Acute or abrupt withdrawal from various sedatives can precipitate in seizures via mechanisms of the GABA pathways, which were outlined earlier. Acute withdrawal from GABA agonists has been shown to result in seizure in the literature and sedative withdrawal has increased as a cause for toxin-induced seizure.[3] Chronic use of GABA agonists such as benzodiazepines, ethanol, gamma-hydroxybutyrate, barbiturates, and baclofen result in decreased GABA receptor density in the brain. Then, the abrupt discontinuation of the medication results in seizure from relative unopposed excitatory action with less GABA tone to promote inhibitory action. The medication flumazenil is a partial agonist at the GABA receptor. It is a medication sometimes used as a reversal agent in overdose but is known to precipitate an acute GABA withdrawal by competitively binding to the receptors, decreasing overall GABA tone, and thus resulting in seizure.[3,50]

Baclofen is a GABA-B receptor agonist that in withdrawal can precipitate seizures and status epilepticus. Seizure has been documented to occur with baclofen toxicity, outlined previously, and withdrawal precipitates seizure from lack of GABA tone that was previously maintained with chronic baclofen administration.[51,52]

Antidepressants and Antipsychotics

TCAs are medications often prescribed and have been noted in one study to represent nearly 8% of drug-induced seizures, which is less than previously reported, but still the third leading cause of seizure reported to a poison control center.[3] The primary mechanism of inducing seizure is from GABA-A antagonism. TCAs possess antimuscarinic and antihistaminergic properties, as well as cause sodium channel blockade. Hyperthermia, flushing, mydriasis, ileus, and urinary retention occur as a result of antimuscarinic toxicity, QRS prolongation from sodium channel blockade, as well as QTc prolongation from potassium efflux blockade. Physostigmine is contraindicated in TCA toxicity, as it has been associated with cardiac arrest in TCA overdose, regardless of the prominent anticholinergic toxidrome.[53]

Other antidepressants including SSRIs and selective serotonin and norepinephrine reuptake inhibitors have been shown to result in seizure.

Venlafaxine increases 5-HT and NE to result in seizure activity alone or with combination of other serotonergic agents. Citalopram has been cited to more likely cause seizure than escitalopram given its racemic mixture of R- and S-enantiomers. SSRIs in overdose can lead to serotonin syndrome as well as hyponatremia, with paroxetine use at therapeutic doses also leading to seizure from hyponatremia.[54–56] Glutamate release increase, α-amino-3-hydroxy-5-methyl-4-isoxazolepropionic acid (AMPA) receptor expression increase, and NMDA receptor interaction postsynaptically may also play a role in antidepressant overdose, resulting in seizure.[54,57,58]

Antipsychotics in particular have been reported to have a 2-fold increase in seizure when used in combination with other antipsychotic drugs, tricyclic antidepressants, or lithium in an inpatient psychiatric population.[3,57] Phenothiazine antipsychotics are also known to result in seizure in toxicity or overdose—common examples include chlorpromazine, prochlorperazine, thioridazine, and perphenazine, although true incidence of these rates are unclear. Clozapine particularly has been reported to cause seizures, often in concomitant use with other antidepressants or antipsychotics as well as in high therapeutic doses. Potassium and sodium channel blockade can result in cardiac dysrhythmia, DA and muscarinic receptor imbalance can result in dystonic reactions, and antidopaminergic effect can result in neuroleptic malignant syndrome.[20,54,58]

Treatment of GABA agonist withdrawal or GABA antagonists involve maintaining or improving GABA tone with benzodiazepines. Pyridoxine should be given in cases of pyridoxine deficiency, as benzodiazepines will not be effective without the presence of GABA. Barbiturates may be required for treatment as well if the benzodiazepine site is blocked by an antagonist or as adjunctive therapy in severe cases.[6]

GLUTAMATE AGONIST

Glutamate agonists bind 3 subgroups of receptors to induce seizure activity: (1) NMDA, (2) AMPA, and (3) kainite. They promote Na + influx and K+ efflux from neurons to further perpetuate action potentials and promote hyperactivity. Glutamate transporter inhibition also results in excess glutamate in the synaptic cleft and promotes neruoexcitability, resulting in seizure.[2,9,11] Domoic acid is produced by algae consumed by shellfish, bioaccumulated in the shellfish, and is ingested by humans who consume the shellfish. Seizures result from glutaminergic AMPA receptor activation. This can result in mesial temporal sclerosis; thus patients may develop recurrent complex partial seizures even after acute toxicity has resolved.[59] Amanita muscaria mushrooms, with large red caps and white spots, are ingested for hallucinogenic effects or by accidental ingestion. Ibotenic acid and muscimol are the toxins concentrated in the caps of the mushroom. Ibotenic acid results in CNS excitation, whereas muscimol promotes CNS depression. Ibotenic acid results in excitatory effects at glutamic acid receptors in the CNS, which is responsible for causing seizure. Toxidrome of ingestion of A. muscaria include somnolence or coma (from action of muscimol to promote GABA action), hallucinations, seizure, nausea and vomiting, diarrhea, and salivation. Treatment of delirium, agitation, or seizures is primarily with benzodiazepines, and toxicity generally resolves after 24 hours.[60,61] Treatment of glutamate agonist toxicity include counteraction with benzodiazepines to promote GABA activity.

HISTAMINE ANTAGONISTS

Histamine can inhibit seizure by binding to its G protein–coupled receptors to promote several intracellular pathways that play a role in GABA, glutamate, DA, 5-HT, and ACh pathways. Seizures result from excitotoxicity from antagonism at histamine receptor 1. Dysregulation of the sodium/hydrogen pump has been shown to be caused by HRs. How the loss of HR function lowers seizure threshold is not fully understood. One theory is the sodium/hydrogen pump loss of function causes neuronal cells to have an inability to regulate pH changes and reduce the threshold for cellular signaling, resulting in propagation of epileptic discharges.[62,63]

Diphenhydramine is perhaps the most common antihistamine to result in seizure, the causative agent in 8% of a cohort study population of drug-induced seizures.[3,64] Other examples of antihistamines than can cause seizures include doxylamine, hydroxyzine, and chlorpheniramine. Sodium channel blockade also contributes to the toxidrome, leading to QRS prolongation and wide complex tachycardia. Status epilepticus is less common.[4,65] Anticholinergic syndrome is characterized by confusion, ataxia, disorientation, hallucinations, agitated delirium, psychosis, dry mucous membranes, and mydriasis. Treatment of seizures include benzodiazepines, but overall, seizures are usually self-limited and avoidance of further antihistamines is encouraged.[4]

ADENOSINE ANTAGONISTS

Intracellular adenosine is used in the adenosine-diphosphate (ADP) conversion to adenosine-triphosphate for cellular energy, the base compound being mediated by adenosine kinase to help formulate adenosine monophosphate from adenosine. It is helpful to understand this as it outlines the relationship of adenosine to seizure activity from a cellular level. The uptake of adenosine by overactivity of adenosine kinase leads to low synaptic adenosine levels, which results in increased risk of seizure activity. The high likelihood of recurrent seizures or status epilepticus is likely due to adenosine's role in endogenous antiseizure effects.[3,66,67] Historically, theophylline is a common example of adenosine antagonism resulting in seizure, although its prevalence may be decreasing.[3] It is adenosine receptor antagonism that causes relative increases in cGMP while preventing cAMP increases. Seizure activity results from theophylline's action to block the brain's natural anticonvulsant adenosine; theophylline toxicity typically presents as focal and generalized seizures clinically, which do not respond to anticonvulsant drugs. Often, patients with theophylline-induced seizure have elevated serum levels of theophylline, but a therapeutic dose may also result in seizure. The physiology of chronic obstructive pulmonary disease (COPD) results in increased sympathetic response. This, combined with the adenosine antagonism of theophylline, puts patients with COPD taking this medication at a higher risk for seizure and toxicity, as there is a dual mechanism for CNS excitation.[66] Bronchodilation from phosphodiesterase antagonism is also seen with theophylline toxicity but seizure may be the only presenting symptom. Mortality from theophylline toxicity is as high as 10%, especially if seizures or cardiac dysrhythmia occur.[68]

Other methylxanthines, including caffeine, act via adenosine pathways to result in seizure in toxicity in a similar mechanism. Compared with other stimulants or theophylline, caffeine-induced seizure is less commonly cited in the literature among human studies but has been described in animal models.[69–71] It should be noted though, that some report a lowered seizure threshold in patients with underlying epilepsy during caffeine use.[72] Treatment of adenosine antagonist–mediated seizures in toxicity primarily involves discontinuing the offending agent and supportive treatment with benzodiazepines for seizure cessation. Barbiturates or propofol after initiation of mechanical ventilation may be required for prolonged seizures or status epilepticus.[68] Hemodialysis may be indicated for enhanced elimination.[73]

SUMMARY

Many toxins cause seizure in therapeutic use or overdose, as well as in withdrawal states, although the most common culprits change over time.[3] Although not a complete and exhaustive list, the reviews discussed earlier commonly reported toxins and mechanisms of seizure. Understanding the mechanism, characteristic toxidromes, and treatments of commonly reported toxins is essential to correctly identify and appropriately treat patients who present after a toxin induced seizure. Physician familiarity with the commonly known toxins that result in seizure is pivotal in comprehensive evaluation of seizure (see **Fig. 1**).[8] Physician awareness also helps in the ongoing reporting efforts to identify the evolution of toxin trends, as new toxins are continually emerging. The mechanisms understood to cause seizure in existing toxins can be helpful in predicting if new toxins will likely result in seizure in the setting of overdose, abuse, or poisoning, as well as therapeutic use.

CLINICS CARE POINTS

- Benzodiazepines are first-line therapy in the acute treatment of toxin-induced seizure. This is, in part, because they can treat other acute symptoms of some toxidromes (e.g. agitation, tachycardia).
- Electrocardiogram, along with electrolyte, renal, and hepatic function laboratories, are warranted to identify and treat resultant systemic effects of toxins. Acetaminophen and salicylate drug concentrations are important in any suspected ingestion due to the common co-ingestion of prescription and over-the-counter medications.
- Early identification of toxins is imperative and involves a detailed history, neurologic exam, and careful attention to clinical toxidromes to allow for proper care and treatment of the patient. This, in addition to the above ancillary studies, directs when antidotal therapy and enhanced elimination may be indicated. It also allows for monitoring for delayed complications and avoidance of drug interactions (i.e. avoiding beta-blockade in cocaine overdose).
- The American Association of Poison Control Centers (1-800-222-1222) is a valuable resource for clinicians who need guidance in the care of a potentially poisoned patient.

DISCLOSURE

The authors have nothing to disclose.

REFERENCES

1. Barry JD, Wills BK. Neurotoxic Emergencies. Neurol Clin 2011;29(3):539–63.
2. Alldredge BK, Lowenstein DH, Simon RP. Seizures associated with recreational drug abuse. Neurology 1989;39(8):1037–9.
3. Thundiyil JG, Kearney TE, Olson KR. Evolving epidemiology of drug-induced seizures reported to a Poison Control Center System. J Med Toxicol 2007;3(1):15–9.
4. Cock HR. Drug-induced status epilepticus. Epilepsy Behav 2015;49:76–82.
5. DeLorenzo RJ, Hauser WA, Towne AR, et al. A prospective, population-based epidemiologic study of status epilepticus in Richmond, Virginia. Neurology 1996;46(4):1029.
6. Chen H-Y, Albertson TE, Olson KR. Treatment of drug-induced seizures. Br J Clin Pharmacol 2016;81(3):412–9.
7. Lee T, Warrick BJ, Sarangarm P, et al. Levetiracetam in toxic seizures. Clin Toxicol (Phila) 2018;56(3):175–81.
8. Osterhoudt KC, Henretig FM. A 16-Year-Old With Recalcitrant Seizures. Pediatr Emerg Care 2012;28(3):304–6.
9. Chapman AG. Glutamate receptors in epilepsy. Prog Brain Res 1998;116:371–83.

10. Schlicker E, Kathmann M. Role of the Histamine H3 Receptor in the Central Nervous System. Handb Exp Pharmacol 2017;241:277–99.
11. Barker-Haliski M, White HS. Glutamatergic mechanisms in seizures and epilepsy. Cold Spring Harb Perspect Med 2015;5. a022863.
12. Sanchez-Ramos J. Neurologic Complications of Psychomotor Stimulant Abuse. Int Rev Neurobiol 2015;120:131–60.
13. Dean BV, Stellpflug SJ, Burnett AM, et al. 2C or not 2C: phenethylamine designer drug review. J Med Toxicol 2013;9(2):172–8.
14. Riley AL, Nelson KH, To P, et al. Abuse potential and toxicity of the synthetic cathinones (i.e., "Bath salts"). Neurosci Biobehav Rev 2019;110:150–73.
15. Tekulve K, Alexander A, Tormoehlen L. Seizures Associated With Synthetic Cathinone Exposures in the Pediatric Population. Pediatr Neurol 2014;51(1):67–70.
16. Prosser JM, Nelson LS. The toxicology of bath salts: a review of synthetic cathinones. J Med Toxicol 2012;8(1):33–42.
17. Schep LJ, Slaughter RJ, Vale JA, et al. The clinical toxicology of the designer "party pills" benzylpiperazine and trifluoromethylphenylpiperazine. Clin Toxicol (Phila) 2011;49(3):131–41.
18. Huff CL, Morano RL, Herman JP, et al. MDMA decreases glutamic acid decarboxylase (GAD) 67-immunoreactive neurons in the hippocampus and increases seizure susceptibility: Role for glutamate. Neurotoxicology 2016;57:282–90.
19. Foley KF, DeSanty KP, Kast RE. Bupropion: pharmacology and therapeutic applications. Expert Rev Neurother 2006;6(9):1249–65.
20. Grosset KA, Grosset DG. Prescribed drugs and neurological complications. J Neurol Neurosurg Psychiatry 2004;75(Suppl 3):iii2–8.
21. Wallace KL. Antibiotic-induced convulsions. Crit Care Clin 1997;13(4):741–62.
22. Caillier B, Pilote S, Castonguay A, et al. QRS widening and QT prolongation under bupropion: a unique cardiac electrophysiological profile. Fundam Clin Pharmacol 2012;26(5):599–608.
23. Buckley NA, Faunce TA. 'Atypical' antidepressants in overdose: clinical considerations with respect to safety. Drug Saf 2003;26(8):539–51.
24. Malyshevskaya O, Aritake K, Kaushik MK, et al. Natural ((9)-THC) and synthetic (JWH-018) cannabinoids induce seizures by acting through the cannabinoid CB1 receptor. Sci Rep 2017;7(1):10516.
25. Adamowicz P, Gieroń J, Gil D, et al. The effects of synthetic cannabinoid UR-144 on the human body—A review of 39 cases. Forensic Sci Int 2017;273:e18–21.
26. Tai S, Fantegrossi WE. Pharmacological and Toxicological Effects of Synthetic Cannabinoids and Their Metabolites. Curr Top Behav Neurosci 2017;32:249–62.
27. Bailey DN. Phencyclidine Abuse: Clinical Findings and Concentrations in Biological Fluids after Nonfatal Intoxication. Am J Clin Pathol 1979;72(5):795–9.
28. Browning R, Maggio R, Sahibzada N, et al. Role of brainstem structures in seizures initiated from the deep prepiriform cortex of rats. Epilepsia 1993;34(3):393–407.
29. Brudzynski SM, Cruickshank JW, McLachlan RS. Cholinergic Mechanisms in Generalized Seizures: Importance of the Zona Incerta. Can J Neurol Sci 1995; 22:116–20.
30. Friedman A, Behrens CJ, Heinemann U. Cholinergic Dysfunction in Temporal Lobe Epilepsy. Epilepsia 2007;48(s5):126–30.
31. McDonough JH Jr, Shih TM. Neuropharmacological mechanisms of nerve agent-induced seizure and neuropathology. Neurosci Biobehav Rev 1997;21(5): 559–79.
32. Albaret C, Lacoutière S, Ashman WP, et al. Molecular mechanic study of nerve agent O-ethyl S-[2-(diisopropylamino)ethyl]methylphosphonothioate (VX) bound

to the active site of Torpedo californica acetylcholinesterase. Proteins 1997;28(4): 543–55.

33. King AM, Aaron CK. Organophosphate and Carbamate Poisoning. Emerg Med Clin North Am 2015;33(1):133–51.

34. Kozhemyakin M, Rajasekaran K, Kapur J. Central cholinesterase inhibition enhances glutamatergic synaptic transmission. J Neurophysiol 2010;103(4): 1748–57.

35. Tattersall J. Seizure activity post organophosphate exposure. Front Biosci (Landmark Ed) 2009;14:3688–711.

36. Meehan TJ. Rosen's Emergency Medicine: Concepts and Clinical Practice. 2018;e2:1813–22.

37. Yoon HJ, Lim YJ, Zuo Z, et al. Nicotine decreases the activity of glutamate transporter type 3. Toxicol Lett 2014;225(1):147–52.

38. DeLorey TM, Olsen RW. Gamma-aminobutyric acidA receptor structure and function. J Biol Chem 1992;267(24):16747–50.

39. Bowery NG. GABAB receptor: a site of therapeutic benefit. Curr Opin Pharmacol 2006;6(1):37–43.

40. Murray BP, Carpenter JE, Dunkley CA, et al. Seizures in tramadol overdoses reported in the ToxIC registry: predisposing factors and the role of naloxone. Clin Toxicol (Phila) 2019;57(8):692–6.

41. Marquardt KA, Alsop JA, Albertson TE. Tramadol exposures reported to statewide poison control system. Ann Pharmacother 2005;39(6):1039–44.

42. Samadi M, Shaki F, Bameri B, et al. Caffeine attenuates seizure and brain mitochondrial disruption induced by Tramadol: the role of adenosinergic pathway. Drug Chem Toxicol 2019;1–7. https://doi.org/10.1080/01480545.2019.1643874.

43. Shadnia S, Brent J, Mousavi-Fatemi K, et al. Recurrent seizures in tramadol intoxication: implications for therapy based on 100 patients. Basic Clin Pharmacol Toxicol 2012;111(2):133–6.

44. Rehni AK, Singh I, Kumar M. Tramadol-induced seizurogenic effect: a possible role of opioid-dependent γ-aminobutyric acid inhibitory pathway. Basic Clin Pharmacol Toxicol 2008;103(3):262–6.

45. Rush JM, Gibberd FB. Baclofen-induced epilepsy. J R Soc Med 1990;83(2): 115–6.

46. Fakhoury T, Abou-Khalil B, Blumenkopf B. EEG changes in intrathecal baclofen overdose: a case report and review of the literature. Electroencephalogr Clin Neurophysiol 1998;107(5):339–42.

47. Perry HE, Wright RO, Shannon MW, et al. Baclofen overdose: drug experimentation in a group of adolescents. Pediatrics 1998;101(6):1045–8.

48. Sutter R, Ruegg S, Tschudin-Sutter S. Seizures as adverse events of antibiotic drugs: A systematic review. Neurology 2015;85(15):1332–41.

49. Naeije G, Lorent S, Vincent JL, et al. Continuous epileptiform discharges in patients treated with cefepime or meropenem. Arch Neurol 2011;68(10):1303–7.

50. Borowski TB, Kirkby RD, Kokkinidis L. Amphetamine and antidepressant drug effects on GABA- and NMDA-related seizures. Brain Res Bull 1993;30(5–6): 607–10.

51. Hyser CL, Drake ME Jr. Status epilepticus after baclofen withdrawal. J Natl Med Assoc 1984;76(5):533–8.

52. Triplett JD, Lawn ND, Dunne JW. Baclofen Neurotoxicity: A Metabolic Encephalopathy Susceptible to Exacerbation by Benzodiazepine Therapy. J Clin Neurophysiol 2019;36(3):209–12.

53. Kerr GW, McGuffie AC, Wilkie S. Tricyclic antidepressant overdose: a review. Emerg Med J 2001;18(4):236–41.
54. Judge BS, Rentmeester LL. Antidepressant Overdose–induced Seizures. Psychiatr Clin North Am 2011;36(2):245–60.
55. Corrington KA, Gatlin CC, Fields KB. A case of SSRI-induced hyponatremia. J Am Board Fam Pract 2002;15(1):63–5.
56. Kirchner V, Silver LE, Kelly CA. Selective serotonin reuptake inhibitors and hyponatraemia: review and proposed mechanisms in the elderly. J Psychopharmacol 1998;12(4):396–400.
57. Druschky K, Bleich S, Grohmann R, et al. Seizure rates under treatment with antipsychotic drugs: Data from the AMSP project. World J Biol Psychiatry 2019;20(9):732–41.
58. Jobe PC, Browning RA. The serotonergic and noradrenergic effects of antidepressant drugs are anticonvulsant, not proconvulsant. Epilepsy Behav 2005;7(4):602–19.
59. Ramsdell JS, Gulland FM. Domoic acid epileptic disease. Mar Drugs 2014;12(3):1185–207.
60. Benjamin DR. Muschroom poisoning in infants and children: the Amanita pantherina/muscaria group. J Toxicol Clin Toxicol (Phila) 1992;30(1):13–22.
61. Kondeva-Burdina M, Voynova M, Shkondrov A, et al. Effects of Amanita muscaria extract on different in vitro neurotoxicity models at sub-cellular and cellular levels. Food Chem Toxicol 2019;132:110687.
62. Cox GA, Lutz CM, Yang C-L, et al. Sodium/Hydrogen Exchanger Gene Defect in Slow-Wave Epilepsy Mutant Mice. Cell 1997;91(1):139–48.
63. Bhowmik M, Khanam R, Vohora D. Histamine H3 receptor antagonists in relation to epilepsy and neurodegeneration: a systemic consideration of recent progress and perspectives. Br J Pharmacol 2012;167(7):1398–414.
64. Yokoyama H, Onodera K, Iinuma K, et al. Proconvulsive effects of histamine H1-antagonists on electrically-induced seizure in developing mice. Psychopharmacology (Berl) 1993;112(2–3):199–203.
65. Jang DH, Manini AF, Trueger NS, et al. Status epilepticus and wide-complex tachycardia secondary to diphenhydramine overdose. Clin Toxicol (Phila) 2010;48(9):945–8.
66. Nakada T, Kwee IL, Lerner AM, et al. Theophylline-induced seizures: clinical and pathophysiologic aspects. West J Med 1983;138(3):371–4.
67. Weltha L, Reemmer J, Boison D. The role of adenosine in epilepsy. Brain Res Bull 2018;151:46–54.
68. Boison D. Methylxanthines, seizures, and excitotoxicity. Handb Exp Pharmacol 2011;200:251–66.
69. Morgan PF, Durcan MJ. Caffeine-induced seizures: Apparent proconvulsant action of n-ethyl carboxamidoadenosine (NECA). Life Sci 1990;47(1):1–8.
70. Chu N-S. Caffeine- and aminophylline-induced seizures. Epilepsia 1981;22(1):85–94.
71. Czuczwar SJ, Gasior M, Janusz W, et al. Influence of different methylxanthines on the anticonvulsant action of common antiepileptic drugs in mice. Epilepsia 1990;31(3):318–23.
72. Kaufman KR, Sachdeo RC. Caffeinated beverages and decreased seizure control. Seizure 2003;12(7):519–21.
73. Ghannoum M, Wiegand TJ, Liu KD, et al. Extracorporeal treatment for theophylline poisoning: systematic review and recommendations from the EXTRIP workgroup. Clin Toxicol (Phila) 2015;53(4):215–29.

Section III
Special Topics in Clinical Neurotoxicology

Neurochemical and Neurobiological Weapons

James J. Sejvar, MD

KEYWORDS

- Neurochemical • Neurobiological • Acetylcholinesterase inhibitor • Sarin • Anthrax
- Botulism

KEY POINTS

- Neurochemical and neurobiological weapons are among the most lethal of weapons. Although most countries have pledged not to develop them, rogue nations and terrorist groups may consider their use.
- Neurotoxic agents center around acetylcholinesterase (AChE) inhibitors. AChE inhibitors cause illness by preventing the breakdown of ACh in the neuromuscular junction, leading to flaccid weakness.
- Neurobiological weapons use organisms or toxins that can produce neurologic illness. Bacterial toxins include anthrax toxins and botulinum toxin; ricin is a plant-formed toxin.

INTRODUCTION

Since the unprecedented attacks on US civilians by weaponized anthrax in 2001, the landscape of the use of chemical and biological agents as weapons of mass destruction has taken on a renewed sense of urgency, concern, and strategy. Among the most lethal and debilitating agents that can be used as weapons, none are as poignant, frightening, and devastating as agents acting on the nervous system. The fact that the central and peripheral nervous systems are key to nearly every function of the body—intelligence, emotion, motor action, and higher thought—implies that anything that impairs on these functions is by nature devastating. And this is why, throughout history, nerve agents and neurobiological weapons have been the agents of choice for inflicting as much harm on fellow human beings as possible.

This article focuses on the nature, mechanism, and impact of various salient agents, both chemical and biological, that have been successfully weaponized in order to inflict as much harm as possible on populations, both military and civilian, in wartime or as terrorist actions. Although not a complete list, the most salient agents of use in the current age are reviewed.

Division of High-Consequence Pathogens and Pathology, National Center for Emerging and Zoonotic Infectious Diseases, Centers for Disease Control and Prevention, 1600 Clifton Road, Mailstop H24-12, Atlanta, GA 30033, USA
E-mail address: zea3@cdc.gov

Neurol Clin 38 (2020) 881–896
https://doi.org/10.1016/j.ncl.2020.07.007
0733-8619/20/Published by Elsevier Inc.

neurologic.theclinics.com

NEUROCHEMICAL WEAPONS

A discussion of nerve agents used as chemical weapons must begin with cholines-terase (ChE) inhibitors. Acetylcholine (ACh) is the key neurotransmitter involved with neuromuscular junction synaptic transmission that is responsible for relaying motor signals from motor neurons to effector muscles, as well as playing a key role in auto-nomic transmission. An interruption of ACh from nerve to muscle will result in essential paralysis of innervated muscle. Alternatively, an aberrant increase in the amount or the duration of presence of ACh can result in overstimulation of muscles, fasciculations, spasms, and, eventually, fatigue and flaccid paralysis due to muscle overstimulation. Thus, the discussion of nerve agents begins with acetylcholinesterase (AChE) inhibitors.

Acetylcholinesterase Inhibitors

As mentioned, ACh is the key neurotransmitter for postsynaptic neuromuscular trans-mission and the autonomic ganglia (nicotinic ACh) and the postganglionic parasympa-thetic fibers (innervating glands, respiratory and gastrointestinal systems, muscarinic ACh). Most cholinesterase-inhibiting compounds are either carbamates or organo-phosphorous compounds.[1–3] Among the carbamates, the most common are physo-stigmine and neostigmine (which was initially developed as a therapeutic for myasthenia gravis); pyridostigmine has also been used for years for the treatment of myasthenia gravis. Organophosphates include malathion, used as an insecticide. Or-ganophosphates used as weapons include tabun, sarin, soman, and VX.[1,4]

Sarin gas was famously used in 1995 on the Tokyo, Japan subway system in a bio-terrorism attack. During this episode, 13 persons died, more than 50 were injured, and more than 1000 persons were left with temporary visual problems. The domestic terrorist group Aum Shinrikyo had previously killed nearly 20 Aum dissidents and a po-litical foe with weaponized VX gas in 1994.

Pharmacology of Cholinesterase Inhibitors

Nerve agents exert their biological properties by inhibition of the enzyme AChEs. AChEs belong to a class of enzymes that catalyze the hydrolysis of esters.[5] The enzyme AChE is found at the receptor sites of tissues innervated by the cholinergic nervous system and hydrolyzes ACh rapidly.[6] Nerve agents act by inhibiting ChE, which then cannot hydrolyze ACh; the intoxicating effect of such nerve agents is directly related to the buildup of exogenous ACh within the synaptic junction. The 2 major efferents of the human nervous system include the adrenergic nervous system and the cholinergic nervous system.[5] The adrenergic system uses noradrenaline (norepinephrine) as the major neurotransmitter, whereas the cholinergic nervous system uses acetylcholine as the neurotransmitter. The cholinergic system can be further subdivided into the muscarinic and nicotinic systems. Muscarinic receptors are innervated by postgangli-onic parasympathetic fibers, innervate glands, pulmonary and gastrointestinal muscu-lature, and efferent organs of the cranial nerves. Nicotinic receptors are at the autonomic ganglia and skeletal muscle. In the cholinergic system, ChE hydrolyzes the neurotransmitter ACh to terminate its activity at the postsynaptic site.[7] Nerve agents inhibit AChE, which leads to a buildup of ACh and a resultant buildup of exog-enous ACh, leading to ongoing stimulation of the postsynaptic receptor.

There are in fact 2 forms of ChE in the blood: butyrocholinesterase (BuChE), which is found in plasma and serum, and erythrocyte, or red blood cell cholinesterase (RBC-ChE), which is found in or on erythrocytes. The enzyme BuChE is present in blood and in tissues; its physiologic role in humans is unclear.[8] RBC-ChE is synthesized with erythrocytes, and the activity of this enzyme is reduced in certain diseases and increased during periods of active reticulocytosis. Some ChE-inhibiting substances inhibit BuChE preferentially and some inhibit RBC-ChE preferentially; large doses of ChE inhibitors will completely inhibit both enzymes.[9,10] When ChE enzymes have been completely and irreversibly inhibited, recovery of ChE activity depends on production of new plasma enzymes or production of new erythrocytes. So, complete recovery BuChE activity will occur in about 50 days, and recovery of RBC-ChE will occur in about 120 days.[11]

Nerve Agents

Table 1 demonstrates the chemical, physical, environmental, and biological properties of the various nerve agents. Toxic nerve agents differ from more commonly used ChE inhibitors because they are more toxic (ie, a smaller dose will cause an effect on the organism). A biologically effective amount depends on the concentration (C) and the time (t) needed to cause death in 50% of the exposed population (lethal dose$_{50}$).[12] The lethal dose for anticholinergic nerve agents is referred to as the LCt$_{50}$. For a vapor or aerosol exposure the LCt$_{50}$ is as follows[1]:

Tabun vapor: 400mg-min/m^3
Sarin vapor: 100 mg-min/m^3
Soman vapor: 50 mg-min/m^3
VX vapor: 10mg-min/m^3

For percutaneous exposure (skin exposure to a liquid), the estimated LD$_{50}$ is as follows:

Tabun: 1000 mg
Sarin: 1700 mg
Soman: 350 mg
VX: 10 mg

Table 1
Chemical, physical, environmental, and biological properties of nerve agents

Properties	Tabun	Sarin	Soman	VX
Chemical/Physical				
Boiling point	230°C	158°C	198°C	298°C
Appearance	Colorless to brown liquid	Colorless liquid	Colorless liquid	Colorless to straw colored liquid
Odor	Fruity	No odor	Fruity	No odor
Persistency				
In soil	Half-life1 to 1.5 d	2–24 h	Persistent	2–6 d
On clothing	Unknown	Unknown	Unknown	Persistent
Biologically effective amount				
Vapor	LCt50 400 mg-min/m^3	LCt50 100 mg-min/mg^3	LCt50 50 mg-min/m^3	LCt50 10 mg-min/m^3
Liquid (on skin)	LD50 1.0 g	LD50 1.7 g	LD50 350 mg	LD50 10 mg

(*From* Sidell F, Takafuji ET, Franz DR, eds. Textbook of Military Medicine, Part I – warfare, weaponry, and the casualty; Medical Aspects of Chemical and Biological Warfare. Published by the Office of the Surgeon General, Department of the Army, United States of America; publication date 1997.)

Exposure Routes

The 4 nerve agents—tabun, sarin, soman, and VX—are liquids at moderate temperatures and in their pure state are clear, colorless, and generally tasteless.[6] At higher temperatures, they can become volatile and become vaporous. In an inhalational exposure to vapor, effects can begin seconds to minutes after exposure, depending on the concentration. The effects usually reach maximal severity within minutes if the individual is removed from exposure to the vapor, or if the exposure continues, the symptoms may continue to worsen. At low cycle threshold (Ct), the eyes, nose, and/or airway are first affected.[4] Because the eyes and nose are the most sensitive to vapor exposure, initial symptoms may include miosis, usually with painful conjunctival injection, and rhinorrhea. If exposure increases, a triad of eye, nose, and lung involvement will generally occur. Marked miosis, secretions of the nose and mouth, and ventilatory impairment are seen. In the case of a large exposure to nerve agent vapor, loss of consciousness, convulsions, generalized fasciculations, and flaccid paralysis may occur, as well as apnea.

In the case of dermal exposure to liquid nerve agent, the signs and symptoms will depend on several factors, including the amount of nerve agent, the site of the body exposed, temperature, and humidity.[13] For small exposures, localized sweating may occur at the site of the exposure; in addition, fasciculations of the muscle underlying the droplet may occur. Gastrointestinal symptoms, including nausea, vomiting, and diarrhea, are frequently the next noticed signs. For large cutaneous exposures, the time to onset of the effects is shorter and can include a combination of loss of consciousness, myoclonus, fasciculations, respiratory distress, and secretions.

Effects on the Nervous System

The nervous system effects of nerve agents can roughly be divided into those effects on the neuromuscular junction and on the central nervous system. Effects on other end organs are beyond the scope of this article but are summarized in **Table 2**. Regarding effects on the skeletal musculature, the effects are caused initially by stimulation of muscle fibers, then by stimulation of muscles and muscle groups, then eventually by fatigue and paralysis of muscle groups.[14] Fasciculations can be localized in the event of a small exposure or generalized in the scenario of a severe exposure. In the event of a severe exposure, hyperactivity is followed by severe muscle fatigue and flaccid paralysis.

Effects on the central nervous system are somewhat less delineated. Usually cognitive and behavioral changes will occur within a few hours and last from several days to several weeks.[3,15] Persons may complain of feelings of uneasiness and fatigue and may seem forgetful or slow to respond to simple questions or commands.[16] Exposure to sarin or tabun has been reported to produce symptoms such as difficulty with concentration, mental confusion, insomnia, and vivid/disturbing dreams.[17,18] Long-term effects on the human central nervous system have been reported but are even less clearly delineated. Reports of long-term effects have indicated that such changes can last weeks to several months.

Treatment of Nerve Agent Exposure

The general principles of treatment of nerve agent poisoning include termination of the exposure, maintenance of ventilation, administration of an antitoxin, and correction of cardiovascular problems.[11] Importantly, because a small amount of nerve agent can cause death within minutes, rapid decontamination is

Table 2 Effects of nerve agents in humans	
Organ/System	**Effect**
Eye	Miosis, conjunctival injection, pain in/around the eye, blurred vision, diplopia
Nose	Rhinorrhea
Mouth	Excessive salivation
Pulmonary tract	Bronchoconstriction and excessive secretions, cough, chest tightness, shortness of breath, wheezing, rhonchi
Gastrointestinal tract	Increase in secretions and gastrointestinal motility, nausea/vomiting, diarrhea, abdominal pain
Skin/sweat glands	Excessive sweating
Musculature	Fasciculations, flaccid paralysis, muscle "twitching", flaccid weakness
Cardiovascular	Labile heart rate, alternating tachy/bradycardia, hypertension
Central nervous system	Acute effects, severe exposure: loss of consciousness, seizures, depression of respiratory drive leading to apnea Acute effects, mild or moderate exposure: forgetfulness, irritability, decreased comprehension, feeling of uneasiness, depression, insomnia, frightening/vivid dreams

(*From* Sidell F, Takafuji ET, Franz DR, eds. Textbook of Military Medicine, Part I – warfare, weaponry, and the casualty; Medical Aspects of Chemical and Biological Warfare. Published by the Office of the Surgeon General, Department of the Army, United States of America; publication date 1997.)

tantamount. For vapor exposures, moving to an environment free of the toxic vapor and/or using a protective mask is necessary. For liquid agents on exposed skin or clothing, physical removal and chemical detoxification is necessary. Because nerve agents will penetrate clothing, simply removing clothing is inadequate, and the underlying skin should be decontaminated after clothing removal.

Atropine is the standard antidote to nerve agents. Atropine works by blocking the effects of excess acetylcholine at muscarinic receptors; thus, it does not block the direct effects of cholinesterase inhibition but rather binds to the ACh receptors and blocks the effects of the excess ACh.[19,20] A standard dose of 2 mg is used because it reverses the effects of nerve agents, and the associated side effects can be tolerated.[21] For an inhalational exposure to nerve agent vapor, signs and symptoms will come on quite rapidly, and aggressive atropine therapy is indicated. In military situations, service members at risk of exposure are issued so-called MARK I kits, which contain 2 autoinjectors—one containing 2 mg of atropine in 0.7 mL of diluent and one containing 600 mg of 2-pyridine-2-aldoxime methiodide (PAM) Cl in 2 mL of diluent.[22,23] In the setting of inhalational exposure, 2 MARK I kits are generally administered. For skin exposure, guidelines are somewhat less clear. Skin exposure has a less immediate onset, although the greater the amount of exposure, the sooner the onset of signs and symptoms. Asymptomatic persons should be medically monitored; persons developing signs/symptoms should be administered the contents of 1 or 2 MARK I kits.

BIOLOGICAL WARFARE AGENTS
Anthrax

Anthrax is a zoonotic disease caused by *Bacillus anthracis*, a large gram-positive spore-forming bacillus.[24,25] It occurs naturally in domesticated and wild animals. Humans become infected through contact with infected animals or contaminated animal products. Human infection is predominantly through the cutaneous route, but can also be transmitted through respiratory or gastrointestinal routes. Anthrax occurs worldwide and exists in the soil as spores.[26] Animals become infected when they ingest the spores while grazing on contaminated land or eating contaminated feed. Human anthrax infection is associated with agricultural or industrial exposure to infected animals/animal products, including handling of contaminated carcasses, hides, wool, and hair or ingesting contaminated meat. Contact with contaminated material results in cutaneous disease, whereas ingestion of infected meat leads to gastrointestinal anthrax. Inhalation of spores may lead to inhalational anthrax.[27–29]

B anthracis possesses 3 virulence factors, which include a capsule that prevents phagocytosis, and 2 exotoxins known as edema toxin and lethal toxin. The toxins share a protective, cell-binding domain; then each of the toxins are combined with a separate protein leading to the pathophysiologic effects of each of the toxins.[26,30,31] Human infection is caused by inoculation of spores through skin or mucosa. Spores are taken up by macrophages and then become vegetative bacilli producing the capsule and toxins. The bacteria proliferate at the inoculation site and produce edema and lethal toxins that interfere with host lymphocyte function and lead to edema, hemorrhage, and necrosis.

Most clinical anthrax illness is cutaneous in nature. After skin inoculation, there is an incubation period of 1 to 5 days. It first produces a papule that progresses over days to a vesicle containing serosanguinous fluid; this vesicle will then rupture, resulting in a necrotic ulcer.[25] Patients will also generally develop fever, headache, and malaise, as well as localized lymphadenitis. Ultimately a blackened eschar develops, which will then leave a scar. Overall, case fatality is low for cutaneous anthrax. Inhalational anthrax, however, is a much more severe infection. After an incubation period of 1 to 6 days, patients will develop fever, fatigue, and myalgias, as well as a nonproductive cough and chest discomfort.[28,32] This can then be followed by a rather rapid onset of respiratory distress, dyspnea, increased chest pain, and diaphoresis. Chest radiograph examination usually shows a characteristic widening of the mediastinum along with pleural effusions, which is nearly pathognomonic for inhalational anthrax.[33] A concomitant hemorrhagic meningitis can occur in up to 50% of cases (**Figs. 1** and **2**). Although rare, inhalational anthrax is severe, with case fatality approaching 100% despite treatment.

Gastrointestinal and oropharyngeal anthrax are due to ingestion of infected, undercooked meat. After an incubation period of 1 to 5 days, patients may present with severe sore throat, as well as local oral or tonsillar ulcers with fever and cervical/submandibular lymphadenopathy and edema. In gastrointestinal anthrax, patients will develop nausea, vomiting, and fever, as well as severe abdominal pain with hematemesis.[29,34] Mortality for both of these forms of anthrax can approach 50%.

Hemorrhagic meningitis can occur in the setting of bacteremia and can also be a complication of any of the other clinical presentations.[35,36] It is almost invariably fatal. In the anthrax attacks in the United States in 2001, the index case suffered from anthrax meningitis.[33]

The diagnosis of anthrax can be challenging, but cutaneous anthrax should be considered in the setting of development of a painless pruritic papule, vesicle, or ulcer

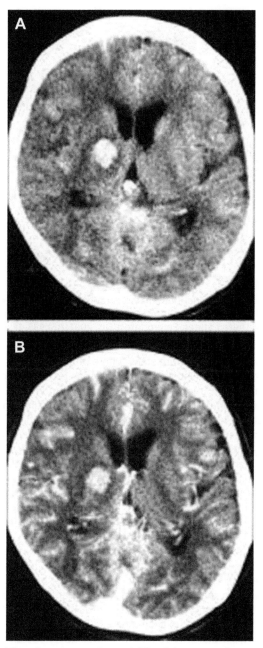

Fig. 1. Precontrast (*A*) and contrast-enhanced (*B*) axial computed tomography scans show diffuse subarachnoid hemorrhage and leptomeningeal enhancement. Mile ventriculomegaly is also seen. (*From* Kim HJ, Jun WB, Lee SH. CT and MR Findings of Anthrax Meningoencephalitis: Report of Two Cases and Review of the Literature. Am J Neuroradiol 2001:22;1303-1305; with permission.)

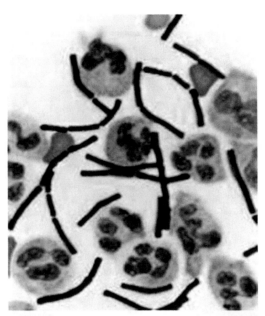

Fig. 2. Gram stain of cerebrospinal fluid, demonstrating *Bacillus anthracis*. (*From* Jernigan JA, Stephens DS, Ashford DA, et al. Bioterrorism-related inhalational anthrax: the first 10 cases reported in the United States. Emerg Infect Dis. 2001;7(6):933-44; with permission.)

with surrounding edema.[24,37,38] Gram stain/culture of the lesion will generally confirm the diagnosis. The diagnosis of inhalational anthrax can be quite hard to make, but the presence of a hemorrhagic mediastinitis along with hemorrhagic pleural effusions should lead to a suspicion of the diagnosis.[32,39] Gastrointestinal anthrax is rare, and the symptoms relatively nonspecific, but should be considered in the setting of consumption of undercooked meat along with severe acute abdomen. Anthrax meningitis is similar to other purulent meningitides but should be considered in the setting of gross hemorrhagic meningeal involvement. As far as treatment is concerned, penicillin is the drug of choice, although ciprofloxacin is increasingly used.[25] For cutaneous anthrax, oral doses will generally suffice, but for more severe manifestations, intravenous therapy with high doses is needed. Prophylaxis is offered by the anthrax vaccine, which is made from sterile filtrates of an attenuated, unencapsulated nonproteolytic strain of *B anthracis*.[40–42] The vaccine should be given to workers potentially exposed to contaminated animal products from countries where anthrax is endemic. It is also given to the military service members at risk of exposure to anthrax in the setting of a biological warfare setting.

The anthrax attacks in the United States in 2001 demonstrated the potential for anthrax to be weaponized and used as an agent of bioterrorism. Altogether, a total of 5 deaths and 17 others afflicted with anthrax occurred. The attacks involved anthrax spores in a white powder that was sent to most victims by postal service. Half of the cases were inhalational anthrax, and the index case suffered from anthrax meningitis.[33]

Variola Virus (Smallpox)

Variola virus, of the *Poxviridae* family, is a large, enveloped DNA virus. More specifically, it is an Orthopoxvirus, which has one of the largest genomes of any virus-causing illness in humans.[43,44] It is a very stable virus and can remain infective for long periods outside of the host, of which humans are the only known ones. It is spread through aerosolized droplets and requires close contact for person-to-person transmission.[45,46] After exposure, the virus travels from the upper or lower respiratory tract to local lymph nodes, replicates, and leads to viremia. Following an incubation period of about 12 days, a characteristic rash appears. Prodromal symptoms include fever, malaise, vomiting, and headache. The rash initially appears on the extremities, then spreads centrally to the trunk. The lesions progress from macules to papules to pustular vesicles; the lesions largely remain at the same stage on the body as they develop. Later in the course of infection, the pustules scab over; during this time variola virus can be isolated from the scabs.[47]

Two distinct types of smallpox have been recognized—variola major and variola minor. Variola major was the prevalent type of smallpox in Asia and parts of Africa. Variola minor, which was associated with milder illness and fewer pox lesions, was found in Africa, South America, and parts of Europe.[48,49] Although most cases of variola major were associated with typical lesions, variations in clinical syndromes, associated with higher case fatality rates and more severe illness, were recognized. Several other complications from variola infection, including arthritis, orchitis, bronchitis, and encephalitis, were rarely reported. Keratitis and corneal ulcers, however, were an important complication.[50]

The diagnosis of smallpox is complicated by the fact that it is not seen anymore and has clinical similarities to other viral exanthems including chickenpox (varicella) and allergic contact dermatitis.[51] The typical method of laboratory diagnosis is identification of characteristic virions on electron microscopy of vesicular scrapings.[43,52] Another characteristic feature observed under light microscopy, aggregations of variola virus particles called Guarnieri bodies, may be seen. Polymerase chain reaction (PCR) of skin lesions is very specific for various Orthopoxviruses; an immunoglobulin G (IgG) and IgM enzyme-linked immunosorbent assay (ELISA) exists but is for Orthopoxviruses in general.

As far as medical management is concerned, any confirmed case of smallpox should be considered a public health emergency. Strict quarantine measures with respiratory isolation for 17 days should be applied to anyone having direct contact with the case.[53] Immediate vaccination should also be applied for all persons potentially exposed to smallpox. The ultimate eradication of smallpox rested on aggressive case identification, as well as quarantine and immunization of contacts.[54] Vaccinia virus, which is a related Orthopoxvirus and is essentially nonpathogenic to humans, has been used for years as the vaccination against smallpox.[44] The vaccinia vaccine has been associated with some adverse events, including inadvertent inoculation to other skin and mucous membrane sites (known as autoinoculation) or infection of other persons (secondary inoculation). Other serious adverse events associated with vaccinia vaccination include eczema vaccinatum and *postvaccinal encephalitis*.[44,55–59] This latter complication, although rare, was associated with mortality and ongoing neurologic morbidity in up to 25% of persons. Thus, despite current eradication of smallpox, it continues to pose a military and bioterrorism threat.

The weaponization of smallpox is an old concept. Before and during World War II, the Japanese military investigated the use of smallpox as a biological weapon. There are currently 2 repositories of smallpox/variola virus—one at the US Centers for Disease Control and Prevention in Atlanta, Georgia, USA and the second one at the Vector Laboratories in Russia. There is an ongoing debate as to whether these remaining lots of smallpox should be destroyed. There are arguments for and against preserving these specimens.

Botulinum Toxins

Neurotoxins due to *Clostridium* species are among the most potent toxins known.[60] *Clostridium tetani* is the agent causing tetanus; although rare in the resource-rich world due to widespread vaccination, it remains a significant public health problem in many low- and middle-income countries. *Clostridium botulinum*, the agent of botulism, remains a substantial public health threat in much of the world. Because humans are not protected against botulinum toxins, and because of their relative ease of production, botulinum toxins remain likely biowarfare agents.[61] The extreme toxicity of botulinum toxin made it one of the first agents to be considered as a biological weapon. During World War II, both the United States and Germany attempted to develop botulinum toxin as a weapon of warfare and efforts were made to purify the toxin.

Both *C botulinum* and *C tetani* are anaerobic, spore-forming bacteria found worldwide in soil.[60] However, the mechanism of action of the toxins is quite different (**Table 3**). *C tetani* executes its clinical features by inhibition of GABAergic inhibitory interneurons to the anterior horn cell. Tetanus toxin is taken up into the presynaptic terminus of the neuromuscular junction, then undergoes retrograde transport to the neuron cell body. Once there, it crosses the synaptic terminus and is taken up by inhibitory interneurons, where it prevents the release of inhibitory GABA neurotransmitter.[62–64] This causes the anterior horn cell to become disinhibited, resulting in overactive excitatory activity at the neuromuscular junction. The resultant clinical syndrome is spasticity, hyperreflexia, and opisthotonus (severe spasms of axial muscles along the back and neck, resulting in an arching position)[60] (see an illustration of opisthotonus: https://museum.rcsed.ac.uk/the-collection/search-the-museum-collections-adlib). Botulism has a very different mechanism of action and causes a very different clinical scenario. Spores from *C botulinum* produce botulinum toxin; there are 7 recognized serotypes of botulinum toxin, with nomenclature A—G.[65] Human illness is most frequently due to serotypes A, B, E, and F. The toxin is taken up into the presynaptic terminal at the neuromuscular junction, where it interacts and inactivates, by an enzymatic reaction, several key proteins involved with permitting the fusion of the vesicles containing the neurotransmitter acetylcholine, including

Table 3
Clinical and pathophysiologic features of tetanus and botulism

	Tetanus	Botulism
Bacterial Agent	*Clostridium tetani*	*Clostridium botulinum*
Toxin	Tetanospasmin	Botulinum toxin (types A-G)
Location of toxin action	Inhibitory interneurons of spinal cord, brainstem	Presynaptic terminals of neuromuscular junction
Mode of acquisition	Wound; injection; unhygienic birth; abortion; unhygienic umbilical practices	Home-canned food; injection drug use; honey; iatrogenic
Major clinical features	Muscular rigidity; painful spasms; trismus; risus sardonicus; opisthotonus	Pentad of dry mouth; nausea/vomiting; dysphagia; diplopia; fixed dilated pupils, followed by cranial nerve and extremity weakness

synaptophysin, syntaxin, and SNAP-25.[66,67] Thus, the acetylcholine vesicles are unable to fuse with the presynaptic membrane, and as a result acetylcholine, the neurotransmitter responsible for activation of skeletal muscle and some autonomic innervation, is unable to be released. This leads to essential chemical denervation of muscle, producing flaccid, areflexic weakness. Botulinum toxins are essentially the most poisonous substances known, with a LD_{50} of 1 ng/kg.[63,68]

Clinical illness with botulinum toxin takes several forms. The most common form of clinical illness is infant botulism, in which the infant gut is colonized by *Clostridium* bacteria or bacterial spores, due to the immaturity of the infant gut flora.[69,70] A similar syndrome can rarely be seen in adults who have altered gastrointestinal flora due to medical procedures. Perhaps the most familiar form of botulism is foodborne botulism, in which food contaminated with bacteria or germinated spores is ingested.[71,72] Wound botulism occurs with the infection of skin wounds by bacteria and germination of spores; it can frequently be seen among intravenous heroin users.[73,74] Inhalational botulism is the most likely syndrome to be seen in warfare or bioterrorism but is very rare.[61] Regardless of route of exposure, clinical illness begins with cranial nerve findings including ptosis/ophthalmoplegia, dysarthria, dysphagia, and dilated pupils. If severe, weakness can go on to involve the respiratory musculature, resulting in respiratory insufficiency, as well as weakness in extremities in a descending fashion.[65,75] Diagnosis of botulism largely rests on the use of a mouse bioassay using serum or stool, although a PCR assay also exists. Testing of foods suspected of leading to the botulism exposure can also be tested. Treatment of botulism involves aggressive supportive care with airway protection and respiratory support, along with the use of botulinum antitoxin (BAT).[76–78] BAT must be given very early in the course of intoxication to be maximally effective, and as such, in cases of clinically suspected botulism, treatment should be rendered before confirmatory testing is completed, because the mouse bioassay can take several days.

Ricin

Ricin toxin is found in the bean of the castor plant *Ricinus communis* and is one of the most toxic of plant toxins.[79,80] Castor beans were used for producing an oil with lubricating properties during World War I and II for aircraft, and although this industrial purpose is no longer used, castor beans and castor oil are still produced throughout the world.[81] The toxin itself is within the castor pulp after the oil has been extracted and may be extracted through a salting-out procedure, a method for protein purification.[82] Its mechanism of action is to block protein synthesis by eukaryotic ribosomes; after being endocytosed into cells, it enzymatically cleaves the 28S ribosomal subunit, thereby blocking protein synthesis.[83,84]

Clinical signs and symptoms of ricin intoxication vary by the dose and route of exposure. Inhalation results in respiratory distress and airway lesions; ingestion leads to gastrointestinal signs and hemorrhage with liver and spleen necrosis[85]; and intramuscular intoxication produces localized signs, pain, and muscle and lymph node necrosis. Oral intoxication with ricin is less toxic than by other routes due to poor absorption and digestion of some of the protein.[86] Case fatality from oral ingestion is generally low, and symptoms include rapid onset of nausea/vomiting, abdominal pain, bloody diarrhea, and vascular compromise/shock. Oral ingestion results in ulcerations and hemorrhage of gastric mucosa and necrosis of mesenteric lymph nodes. Detailed human data on inhalational exposure is limited but has been recognized in workers exposed to castor bean dust in castor oil processing plants, where it produced an allergic respiratory syndrome. However, inhalation exposure in rats and rhesus monkeys is associated with a diffuse necrotizing pneumonia with interstitial and alveolar inflammation.[87] Cause of death in ricin intoxication is probably due to vascular leakage resulting in hypoalbuminemia and edema leading to hypoxemia. Ricin can cause either miosis or mydriasis and has been associated with central nervous system signs and symptoms including lethargy and confusion, disorientation, and somnolence.

Diagnosis of ricin inhalation intoxication can be established by ELISA of a nasal swab or by serologic assay for circulating antibody.[84,88] Medical management of a ricin exposure is complicated because it is rapidly and irreversibly distributed to lung parenchyma or vital organs. Therefore, immunization or preexposure prophylaxis is the most effective medical countermeasure. There are currently no Food and Drug Administration–approved prophylactic or postexposure therapies for ricin toxin exposure. A vaccine candidate using an inactivated segment of the A-chain of the ricin molecule is currently being developed.[89–91]

SUMMARY

Neurochemical and neurobiological agents are the most dangerous weapons used for mass destruction or tools of terrorism. Most countries have ceased investigating and/or manufacturing these weapons under the Biological Weapons Ban, which prohibits member states from producing, manufacturing, and stockpiling biological and chemical weapons. However, rogue nation-states and terrorist groups continue to try to develop these weapons to exert their aims. Neurotoxins and neurobiological weapons are among the most deadly of these agents, due to their adverse effects on the central and peripheral nervous system. In the future, progresses in genetic engineering and molecular biology will raise the specter of more lethal biological and chemical weapons. Enhanced pathogenicity through genetic splicing, bioengineered toxin production, and "genetic weapons" are all real possibilities. This will necessitate ongoing assessment of states and organizations that intend to develop these weapons and require ongoing development of countermeasures.

CLINICS CARE POINTS

- Nerve agents work by blocking Acetylcholinesterase, which leads to overstimulation of muscles, and resultant flaccid paralysis.
- Nerve agents can affect multiple organ systems, including the central nervous system.
- Atropine is the standard antidote to nerve agents, and acts by blocking excess acetylcholine at muscarinic receptors.
- For treatment of anthrax, penicillin is the drug of choice, though ciprofloxacin is being increasingly used.
- Smallpox is transmitted through respiratory droplets; the lesions in smallpox begin in the extremities and spread centrally to the trunk.
- The lesions in smallpox progress from macules to papules to pustular vesicles; later in the course the vesicles scab over, and variola virus can be isolated from scab material.
- Treatment of botulism involves careful medical management, and administration of botulism antitoxin (BAT). BAT prevents progression of disease, and must be given early in the course of illness.
- The mechanism of ricin toxicity is to block protein synthesis by eukaryotic ribosomes.
- Ricin can be inhaled, ingested orally, or can be administered intramuscularly; inhalation ricin exposure is the most deadly form.

DISCLOSURE

The author has nothing to disclose.

REFERENCES

1. Greathouse B, Zahra F, Brady MF. Acetylcholinesterase inhibitors (Sarin, Soman, VX) toxicity. In: StatPearls. Treasure Island (FL): StatPearls Publishing LLC; 2019.
2. Holstege CP, Kirk M, Sidell FR. Chemical warfare. Nerve agent poisoning. Crit Care Clin 1997;13(4):923–42.
3. Grob D. Manifestations and treatment of nerve gas poisoning in man. U S Armed Forces Med J 1956;7(6):781–9.
4. Koelle GB. Organophosphate poisoning–an overview. Fundam Appl Toxicol 1981;1(2):129–34.
5. Koelle GB. Acetylcholine–current status in physiology, pharmacology and medicine. N Engl J Med 1972;286(20):1086–90.
6. Koelle GB, Gilman A. Anticholinesterase drugs. J Pharmacol Exp Ther 1949;95 Pt. 2(4):166–216.
7. Pohanka M. Inhibitors of Cholinesterases in Pharmacology: The Current Trends. Mini Rev Med Chem 2020;20(15):1532–42.
8. Koelle GB, Koelle WA, Smyrl EG. Effects of inactivation of butyrylcholinesterase on steady state and regenerating levels of ganglionic acetylcholinesterase. J Neurochem 1977;28(2):313–9.
9. Williams A, Zhou S, Zhan CG. Discovery of potent and selective butyrylcholinesterase inhibitors through the use of pharmacophore-based screening. Bioorg Med Chem Lett 2019;29(24):126754.
10. Mukhametgalieva AR, Aglyamova AR, Lushchekina SV, et al. Time-course of human cholinesterases-catalyzed competing substrate kinetics. Chem Biol Interact 2019;310:108702.
11. Grob D, Harvey AM. The effects and treatment of nerve gas poisoning. Am J Med 1953;14(1):52–63.
12. Koelle GB, Volle RL, Holmstedt B, et al. Anticholinesterase Agents. Science 1963; 141(3575):63–5.
13. Grob D. The manifestations and treatment of poisoning due to nerve gas and other organic phosphate anticholinesterase compounds. AMA Arch Intern Med 1956;98(2):221–39.
14. Rickett DL, Glenn JF, Beers ET. Central respiratory effects versus neuromuscular actions of nerve agents. Neurotoxicology 1986;7(1):225–36.
15. Bowers MB Jr, Goodman E, Sim VM. Some behavioral changes in man following anticholinesterase administration. J Nervous Ment Dis 1964;138:383–9.
16. Levin HS, Rodnitzky RL. Behavioral effects of organophosphate in man. Clin Toxicol 1976;9(3):391–403.
17. Levin HS, Rodnitzky RL, Mick DL. Anxiety associated with exposure to organophosphate compounds. Arch Gen Psychiatry 1976;33(2):225–8.
18. Rodnitzky RL. Occupational exposure to organophosphate pesticides: a neurobehavioral study. Arch Environ Health 1975;30(2):98–103.
19. Ketchum JS, Sidell FR, Crowell EB Jr, et al. Atropine, scopolamine, and ditran: comparative pharmacology and antagonists in man. Psychopharmacologia 1973;28(2):121–45.
20. Weissman BA, Raveh L. Therapy against organophosphate poisoning: the importance of anticholinergic drugs with antiglutamatergic properties. Toxicol Appl Pharmacol 2008;232(2):351–8.

21. Sidell FR. Chemical agent terrorism. Ann Emerg Med 1996;28(2):223–4.
22. Clair P, Wiberg K, Granelli I, et al. Stability study of a new antidote drug combination (Atropine-HI-6-Prodiazepam) for treatment of organophosphate poisoning. Eur J Pharm Sci 2000;9(3):259–63.
23. Friedl KE, Hannan CJ Jr, Schadler PW, et al. Atropine absorption after intramuscular administration with 2-pralidoxime chloride by two automatic injector devices. J Pharm Sci 1989;78(9):728–31.
24. Brachman PS. Anthrax. Ann N Y Acad Sci 1970;174(2):577–82.
25. Kanj SS, Kanafani ZA, Ghossain A. Anthrax: a review. Lebanese Med J 2003; 51(1):29–37.
26. Moayeri M, Leppla SH, Vrentas C, et al. Anthrax Pathogenesis. Annu Rev Microbiol 2015;69:185–208.
27. Abramova FA, Grinberg LM, Yampolskaya OV, et al. Pathology of inhalational anthrax in 42 cases from the Sverdlovsk outbreak of 1979. Proc Natl Acad Sci U S A 1993;90(6):2291–4.
28. Brachman PS. Inhalation anthrax. Ann N Y Acad Sci 1980;353:83–93.
29. Beatty ME, Ashford DA, Griffin PM, et al. Gastrointestinal anthrax: review of the literature. Arch Intern Med 2003;163(20):2527–31.
30. Brossier F, Weber-Levy M, Mock M, et al. Role of toxin functional domains in anthrax pathogenesis. Infect Immun 2000;68(4):1781–6.
31. Sirard JC, Mock M, Fouet A. The three Bacillus anthracis toxin genes are coordinately regulated by bicarbonate and temperature. J Bacteriol 1994;176(16): 5188–92.
32. Kuehnert MJ, Doyle TJ, Hill HA, et al. Clinical features that discriminate inhalational anthrax from other acute respiratory illnesses. Clin Infect Dis 2003;36(3): 328–36.
33. Jernigan JA, Stephens DS, Ashford DA, et al. Bioterrorism-related inhalational anthrax: the first 10 cases reported in the United States. Emerg Infect Dis 2001;7(6):933–44.
34. Ozer V, Gunaydin M, Pasli S, et al. Gastrointestinal and cutaneous anthrax: Case series. Turkish J Emerg Med 2019;19(2):76–8.
35. Parlak E, Parlak M, Atli SB. Unusual cause of fatal anthrax meningitis. Cutan Ocul Toxicol 2015;34(1):77–9.
36. Sejvar JJ, Tenover FC, Stephens DS. Management of anthrax meningitis. Lancet Infect Dis 2005;5(5):287–95.
37. Brachman PS. Bioterrorism: an update with a focus on anthrax. Am J Epidemiol 2002;155(11):981–7.
38. Doganay M, Demiraslan H. Human anthrax as a re-emerging disease. Recent Pat Antiinfect Drug Discov 2015;10(1):10–29.
39. Grinberg LM, Abramova FA, Yampolskaya OV, et al. Quantitative pathology of inhalational anthrax I: quantitative microscopic findings. Mod Pathol 2001;14(5): 482–95.
40. Ivins BE, Welkos SL. Recent advances in the development of an improved, human anthrax vaccine. Eur J Epidemiol 1988;4(1):12–9.
41. Iacono-Connors LC, Welkos SL, Ivins BE, et al. Protection against anthrax with recombinant virus-expressed protective antigen in experimental animals. Infect Immun 1991;59(6):1961–5.
42. Head BM, Rubinstein E, Meyers AF. Alternative pre-approved and novel therapies for the treatment of anthrax. BMC Infect Dis 2016;16(1):621.
43. Moore ZS, Seward JF, Lane JM. Smallpox. Lancet 2006;367(9508):425–35.

44. Booss J, Davis LE. Smallpox and smallpox vaccination: neurological implications. Neurology 2003;60(8):1241–5.
45. Fleischauer AT, Kile JC, Davidson M, et al. Evaluation of human-to-human transmission of monkeypox from infected patients to health care workers. Clin Infect Dis 2005;40(5):689–94.
46. Dales S, Pogo BG. Biology of poxviruses. Virol Monogr 1981;18:1–109.
47. Mitra AC, Sarkar JK, Mukherjee MK. Virus content of smallpox scabs. Bull World Health Organ 1974;51(1):106–7.
48. Sarkar JK, Mitra AC. Virulence of variola virus isolated from smallpox cases of varying severity. Indian J Med Res 1967;55(1):13–20.
49. Marsden JP. Variola minor. Mon Bull Minist Health Public Health Lab Serv 1952; 11:74–7.
50. Sarkar JK. Smallpox–mild and severe. Bull Calcutta Sch Trop Med 1966; 14(2):57–8.
51. Sarkar JK, Mitra AC, Mukherjee MK, et al. Concurrent smallpox and chickenpox. Bull World Health Organ 1976;54(1):119–20.
52. Sarkar JK, Mitra AC, Mukherjee MK. The minimum protective level of antibodies in smallpox. Bull World Health Organ 1975;52(3):307–11.
53. Noble J Jr, Rich JA. Trsmission of smallpox by contact and by aerosol routes in Macaca irus. Bull World Health Organ 1969;40(2):279–86.
54. Breman JG, Arita I. The confirmation and maintenance of smallpox eradication. N Engl J Med 1980;303(22):1263–73.
55. Feery BJ. Adverse reactions after smallpox vaccination. Med J Aust 1977;2(6): 180–3.
56. Gurvich EB, Vilesova IS. Vaccinia virus in postvaccinal encephalitis. Acta Virol 1983;27(2):154–9.
57. Melekhin VV, Karem KL, Damon IK, et al. Encephalitis after secondary smallpox vaccination. Clin Infect Dis 2009;48(1):e1–2.
58. Miravalle A, Roos KL. Encephalitis complicating smallpox vaccination. Arch Neurol 2003;60(7):925–8.
59. Rockoff A, Spigland I, Lorenstein B, et al. Postvaccinal encephalomyelitis without cutaneous vaccination reaction. Ann Neurol 1979;5(1):99–101.
60. Berkowitz AL. Tetanus, botulism, and diphtheria. Continuum (Minneapolis, Minn) 2018;24(5, Neuroinfectious Disease):1459–88.
61. Cenciarelli O, Riley PW, Baka A. Biosecurity threat posed by botulinum toxin. Toxins 2019;11(12):681.
62. Link E, Blasi J, Chapman ER, et al. Tetanus and botulinal neurotoxins. Tools to understand exocytosis in neurons. Adv Second Messenger Phosphoprotein Res 1994;29:47–58.
63. Habermann E, Dreyer F. Clostridial neurotoxins: handling and action at the cellular and molecular level. Curr Top Microbiol Immunol 1986;129:93–179.
64. Dong M, Masuyer G, Stenmark P. Botulinum and Tetanus Neurotoxins. Annu Rev Biochem 2019;88:811–37.
65. Carrillo-Marquez MA. Botulism. Pediatr Rev 2016;37(5):183–92.
66. Rummel A. The long journey of botulinum neurotoxins into the synapse. Toxicon 2015;107(Pt A):9–24.
67. Blasi J, Chapman ER, Link E, et al. Botulinum neurotoxin A selectively cleaves the synaptic protein SNAP-25. Nature 1993;365(6442):160–3.
68. Rossetto O, Montecucco C. Tables of Toxicity of Botulinum and Tetanus Neurotoxins. Toxins (Basel) 2019;11(12):686.

69. Lyons-Warren AM, Risen SR, Clark G. Infant Botulism With Asymmetric Cranial Nerve Palsies. Pediatr Neurol 2019;92:71–2.

70. Van Horn NL, Street M. Infantile botulism. In: StatPearls. Treasure Island (FL): StatPearls Publishing LLC; 2019.

71. Palma NZ, da Cruz M, Fagundes V, et al. Foodborne botulism: neglected diagnosis. Eur J Case Rep Intern Med 2019;6(5):001122.

72. Scalfaro C, Auricchio B, De Medici D, et al. Foodborne botulism: an evolving public health challenge. Infect Dis 2019;51(2):97–101.

73. Kuehn B. Wound botulism outbreak. JAMA 2019;321(6):538.

74. Martin SJ, Penrice G, Amar C, et al. Wound botulism, its neurological manifestations, treatment and outcomes: A case series from the Glasgow outbreak, 2015. Scott Med J 2017;62(4):136–41.

75. Jeffery IA, Karim S. Botulism. In: StatPearls. Treasure Island (FL): StatPearls Publishing LLC; 2019.

76. Ni SA, Brady MF. Botulism Antitoxin. In: StatPearls. Treasure Island (FL): StatPearls Publishing LLC; 2019.

77. Chalk CH, Benstead TJ, Pound JD, et al. Medical treatment for botulism. Cochrane Database Syst Rev 2019;(4):CD008123.

78. Long SS. BabyBIG has BIG advantages for treatment of infant botulism. J Pediatr 2018;193:1.

79. Balint GA. Ricin: the toxic protein of castor oil seeds. Toxicology 1974;2(1):77–102.

80. Rauber A, Heard J. Castor bean toxicity re-examined: a new perspective. Vet Hum Toxicol 1985;27(6):498–502.

81. Schep LJ, Temple WA, Butt GA, et al. Ricin as a weapon of mass terror–separating fact from fiction. Environ Int 2009;35(8):1267–71.

82. Lord JM, Roberts LM, Robertus JD. Ricin: structure, mode of action, and some current applications. FASEB J 1994;8(2):201–8.

83. Lord JM, Gould J, Griffiths D, et al. Ricin: cytotoxicity, biosynthesis and use in immunoconjugates. Prog Med Chem 1987;24:1–28.

84. Spivak L, Hendrickson RG. Ricin Crit Care Clin 2005;21(4):815–24, viii.

85. Balint GA, Halasz N. Ricin-induced injury of the liver ultrastructure. Acta Physiol 1972;42(2):169–75.

86. Lopez Nunez OF, Pizon AF, Tamama K. Ricin Poisoning after Oral Ingestion of Castor Beans: A Case Report and Review of the Literature and Laboratory Testing. J Emerg Med 2017;53(5):e67–71.

87. Wilhelmsen CL, Pitt ML. Lesions of acute inhaled lethal ricin intoxication in rhesus monkeys. Vet Pathol 1996;33(3):296–302.

88. Poli MA, Rivera VR, Hewetson JF, et al. Detection of ricin by colorimetric and chemiluminescence ELISA. Toxicon 1994;32(11):1371–7.

89. Pittman PR, Reisler RB, Lindsey CY, et al. Safety and immunogenicity of ricin vaccine, RVEc, in a Phase 1 clinical trial. Vaccine 2015;33(51):7299–306.

90. Poli MA, Rivera VR, Pitt ML, et al. Aerosolized specific antibody protects mice from lung injury associated with aerosolized ricin exposure. Toxicon 1996;34(9):1037–44.

91. Roy CJ, Brey RN, Mantis NJ, et al. Thermostable ricin vaccine protects rhesus macaques against aerosolized ricin: Epitope-specific neutralizing antibodies correlate with protection. Proc Natl Acad Sci U S A 2015;112(12):3782–7.

Women's and Fetal Issues in Neurotoxicology

Amy Hessler, DO

KEYWORDS

- Pregnancy • Lactation • Medication in pregnancy • Multiple sclerosis • Epilepsy
- Headache

KEY POINTS

- The FDAs Pregnancy and Lactation Labeling Rule replaced the pregnancy category system. The intent was for practitioners to not rely on the letter system but to weigh the potential risks.
- Multiple sclerosis often stabilizes during pregnancy but can relapse postpartum. It is recommended that disease-modifying therapies be discontinued before conception.
- Preconception seizure freedom before pregnancy is probably associated with a high likelihood of remaining seizure-free during pregnancy. The North American AED Pregnancy Registry continues to prospectively follow women with epilepsy on AEDs to determine the risk of major congenital malformations.
- Primary headache disorders often improve during pregnancy. Symptomatic versus prophylactic medications are important to consider with the least potential toxic risk to the infant during pregnancy and postpartum.

INTRODUCTION

Management of the pregnant patient with neurologic disease is challenging. Ideally, preconception planning can optimize the women's neurologic condition before pregnancy. More than half of pregnancies are unplanned which makes careful consideration of medications vitally important.

This article focuses on the potential toxic risk to the fetus of medications deemed necessary to manage several common maternal neurologic issues: multiple sclerosis (MS), epilepsy, and headache during pregnancy and postpartum. Because the Food and Drug Administration (FDA) has recently changed the pregnancy category system, it is important for the practitioner to have an understanding beyond the category system to understand the potential toxic risks to the fetus.

For a full monograph of diagnosis, evaluation, and management of neurologic issues during pregnancy, see the issue *of Neurologic Clinics of North America* devoted to neurology of pregnancy (February 2019, volume 37).

Neurology, University of Kentucky, 740 South Limestone, Lexington, KY 40536, USA
E-mail address: Amy.Hessler@uky.edu

Neurol Clin 38 (2020) 897–912
https://doi.org/10.1016/j.ncl.2020.08.004
0733-8619/20/© 2020 Elsevier Inc. All rights reserved.

neurologic.theclinics.com

MEDICATION CLASSIFICATION IN PREGNANCY

The FDA labeling of medications in pregnancy is important to briefly discuss because the pregnancy designations have changed. The Pregnancy Category System adopted in 1979, *Labeling for Prescriptions Used in Man*, gave guidance of potential risk during pregnancy (A, B, C, D, and X) (**Table 1**). Historically, it was assumed that pregnant women did not need medication with the main goal "to inform counseling between a physician and a patient planning pregnancy – to provide evidence-based, risk/benefit guidance prospectively, before an embryo fetal exposure occurred."[1] Twenty five years later in 2004, a study found that 64% of women were on at least one medication during pregnancy.[2]

The Content and Format of Labeling for Human Prescription Drug and Biological Products: Requirements for Pregnancy and Lactation Labeling or simply, "Pregnancy and Lactation Labeling Rule" (PLLR) was published in December 2014.[3] The new "Final Rule" was adopted June 30, 2015 with plans for a 3 to 5 year phase-in for older medications. The FDA Deputy Director of the Office of New drugs, Dr Sandra Kweder stated, "Prescribing decisions during pregnancy and lactation are individualized and involve complex maternal, fetal and infant risk-benefit considerations. The letter category system was overly simplistic and was misinterpreted as a grading system, which gave an oversimplified view of product risk."[4]

The FDA developed the PLLR after input from public hearings, focus groups, and advisory committees. Overall, the groups reported that letter categories did not provide clinical information about drug exposure during pregnancy and lactation nor the potential maternal or fetal concerns of stopping medications during pregnancy. Interestingly, 60% of medications were classified as category C. Within a Category C designation were medications with data supporting adverse effects in animals as well as medication with no data from animal studies. Therefore, it was not the severity or incidence of risk but the amount and quality of available data. In 2009, the FDA did a mental-model research study to understand how health care professionals prescribed

Table 1
1979 pregnancy category system

Drug Category	Associated Risk
A	Adequate and well-controlled studies have failed to demonstrate a risk to the fetus in the first trimester of pregnancy (and there is no evidence of risk in later trimesters).
B	Animal reproduction studies have failed to demonstrate a risk to the fetus and there are no adequate and well-controlled studies in pregnant women.
C	Animal reproduction studies have shown an adverse effect on the fetus and there are no adequate and well-controlled studies in humans, but potential benefits may warrant use of the drug in pregnant women despite potential risks.
D	There is positive evidence of human fetal risk based on adverse reaction data from investigational or marketing experience or studies in humans, but potential benefits may warrant use of the drug in pregnant women despite potential risks.
X	Studies in animals or humans have demonstrated fetal abnormalities and/or there is positive evidence of human fetal risk based on adverse reaction data from investigational or marketing experience, and the risks involved in use of the drug in pregnant women clearly outweigh potential benefits.

Adapted from https://chemm.nlm.nih.gov/pregnancycategories.htm.

medications to pregnant and lactating women. A total of 54 providers were queried by telephone and the study found that they relied heavily on the letter category system rather than additional information on the product labeling.[5]

The PLLR changes (**Fig. 1**) include combining 8.1 Pregnancy and 8.2 Labor and Delivery into one section 8.1 Pregnancy with subsections of: "Pregnancy Exposure Registry," "Risk Summary," "Clinical Considerations," and "Data." "Pregnancy Exposure Registry" is to be included only if a registry exists and includes information of how to enroll in the registry. The "Risk Summary" subsection is a narrative and includes any human or animal risk data. It also includes the risk of major birth defects and miscarriages in the United States. "Clinical Considerations" details disease associated maternal/fetal risk, necessary dose adjustments, maternal/fetal adverse reactions, and labor and delivery considerations. Section 8.3 "Nursing Mothers" has become 8.2 "Lactation" with subsections of "Risk Summary," "Clinical Considerations," and "Data." The "Risk Summary" indicates the presence of the drug in the breast milk, and the effect on milk production and breastfed infant and risk/benefit of use. "Clinical Considerations" includes data on minimizing exposure and monitoring for adverse reactions. Lastly, there is a new section 8.3 "Females and Males of Reproductive Potential." This includes recommendations on pregnancy testing and/or contraception before, during, or post drug therapy and any animal or human data on effecting fertility.[6] The PLLR also requires that medication labeling must be updated when new animal or human data become available.

A small randomized trial assessing the effect of removal of pregnancy category on prescribing was presented as a platform presentation at the 2018 American College of Obstetrics and Gynecology annual meeting. During a 1-year period (October 2015–October 2016) a convenience sample of providers were recruited into a survey-based study. They were all given four clinical vignettes, one for each drug letter category (A, B, C, and D). Each vignette described a pregnant patient and indication for a drug and provided detailed drug information. There were two forms of the vignettes distributed: the vignettes were identical but one included the drug letter category and the detailed drug information, and the other included only the detailed drug information. A total of 162 respondents were asked to complete a five-point Likert scale of the likelihood to prescribe the medication based on the information provided. The study found that providers were less likely to prescribe category B or C medications if the drug letter category was not provided. Analysis of the data showed that being provided with the

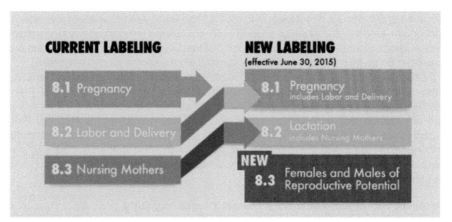

Fig. 1. Prescription drug labeling sections 8.1-8.3 Use in Specific Populations. (*From* https://www.fda.gov/drugs/labeling-information-drug-products/pregnancy-and-lactation-labeling-drugs-final-rule.)

drug letter category affected the providers' decision to prescribe category B ($P<.001$) and category C medications ($P<.008$). After controlling for covariates (ie, age, gender, specialization) the significance persisted ($P <.001$). The authors concluded that without the drug letter category, providers were less likely to prescribe category B and C medications. The concern was raised that without the drug letter category that pregnant women would be restricted from medication.[7]

NEUROTOXICOLOGY AND MULTIPLE SCLEROSIS
Natural History of Multiple Sclerosis in Pregnancy

Multiple Sclerosis (MS) affects 2.5 million people worldwide. This disease has a female predominance with 70% to 75% having clinical symptoms during childbearing years, most commonly in the mid-20s. Up until the late twentieth century, many neurologists feared that pregnancy would worsen the MS disease course and counseled patient to avoid pregnancy completely.[8]

The landscape changed with the publication of the landmark Pregnancy in Multiple Sclerosis (PRIMS) study in the New England Journal of Medicine, 1998 by Confavreux and colleagues.[9] This was the first large, prospective study of the natural history of MS in pregnancy. A total of 254 women were followed with 269 pregnancies (12 European countries) and they were followed for 2 years postpartum. There was approximately 70% decrease in the relapse rate in the third trimester (0.2 ± 1.0) compared with the year before pregnancy (0.7 ± 0.9). However, there was a significant increase in relapse in 3 months postdelivery (1.2 ± 2.0).[9] Following the PRIMS study, it was noted that 72% did not have 3-month postpartum relapses. It was determined the three predictors of relapse of the 25% that did relapse included: (1) increase in relapse the year before pregnancy, (2) increase in relapse during pregnancy, and (3) higher expanded disability status score at pregnancy onset.[10] Overall, the 21-month annualized relapse rate did not differ from the prepregnancy relapse rate. Additionally, breastfeeding was not predictive of relapse or worsening disability.[10] These findings have been replicated in numerous studies.

Treatment of Relapses in Pregnancy

As clarified by the PRIMS study, MS relapses more often do not occur during pregnancy. However, if they occur it tends to occur during the first and second trimester. These relapses do need proper evaluation and management.[9] MRI in pregnancy is likely safe; however, no FDA guidelines exist. FDA guidance has been to use MRI if clinically indicated and there is a direct benefit to mother and fetus. Animal studies have shown gadolinium entering the fetal circulation with associated miscarriage and developmental anomalies, therefore it is not recommended in pregnancy.[11] New lesions are visualized on an MRI without gadolinium particularly if baseline study is available.

If a clinical relapse is severe enough to warrant treatment, methylprednisolone is the steroid of choice because of being metabolized before crossing the placenta. There has been long-standing concern about the risk of steroid use during the first trimester and association with oral clefts. Fortunately, two recent studies, the National Birth Defect Prevention Study[12] and a large Danish study,[13] showed no increased oral clefts or congenital malformations in children of greater than 1000 women exposed to steroids during the first trimester. Additionally, intravenous immunoglobulin is thought to be safe during pregnancy.[14]

Treatment with Disease-Modifying Therapy During Pregnancy

The position statement of the FDA and the MS Society (https://www. nationalmssociety.org/Living-Well-With-MS/Diet-Exercise-Healthy-Behaviors/

Womens-Health/Pregnancy) is that none of the disease-modifying therapies are FDA approved during pregnancy. It is generally recommended that these medications be discontinued before conception. However, the timing of discontinuation needs to be an individualized decision between the patient and the neurologist. Based on medication half-lives, it is recommended to complete a washout before attempting to conceive. Longer washout periods are required for the oral disease-modifying therapies and the infusions, and a specific protocol is suggested for teriflunomide with rapid elimination.[15]

In keeping with the PLLR, it is important for the practitioner to counsel their patients on potential risks of medication. The US general population estimated background risk of major congenital malformations (MCMs) is 2% to 4% and miscarriage is 15% to 20%.[16] The pregnancy data in **Table 2** have been collected on patients exposed to medications during early pregnancy. Because of the safety profiles of certain

Table 2
Disease-modifying therapies and recommendations postpartum

Drug/Route	Pregnancy Category	Last Dose Before Conception	Data in Human Exposures	Breastfeeding
Interferons (SQ/IM)	C	2 mo	No miscarriages or malformations[15]	Likely safe
Glatiramer acetate (SQ)	B	1–2 mo	No miscarriages or malformations[15]	Likely safe
Natalizumab (IV)	C	2 mo	No miscarriages or malformations Mild to moderate hematologic abnormalities[17]	Not Recommended Excreted into milk
Fingolimod (PO)	C	2 mo	Birth defects reported, no pattern[18]	Contraindicated Excreted into milk
Teriflunomide (PO)	X	Elimination protocol with cholestyramine for early pregnancy or d/c plasma concentration <0.02 mg/L	Teratogenic in animals No spontaneous abortions or birth defects reported Drug detected in male semen[16]	Contraindicated Excreted into milk
Dimethyl fumerate (PO)	C	Few days or weeks prior	No miscarriages or malformations[19]	No data Avoid breastfeeding
Alemtuzamab (IV)	C	4 mo	No miscarriages or malformations Maternal thyroid monitoring[20]	Avoid breastfeeding within 4 mo
Ocrelizumab (IV)	C	6 mo	Limited data Potential hematologic concerns (rituximab data)[21]	No data Avoid breastfeeding
Cladribine (PO)		6 mo	Teratogenic in animals Limited human data[22]	Contraindicated No human data

Abbreviations: IM, intramuscularly; IV, intravenous; PO, by mouth; SQ, subcutaneously.

medications, particularly glatiramer and possibly interferons, some practitioners may elect to treat women with fragile disease throughout the pregnancy with medication.[15]

NEUROTOXICOLOGY AND EPILEPSY
Seizures During Pregnancy

Epilepsy is common in the United States including 1.5 million women of childbearing age and each year 24,000 give birth.[23] A recent observational cohort study, Women with Epilepsy Outcomes and Delivery (WEPOD), studied the fertility of 89 women with epilepsy (WWE) to 108 age-matched control subjects and was comparable.[24]

WWE and practitioners are concerned about the risk of maternal seizure recurrence during pregnancy. Unlike MS, there is not a natural history of epilepsy. The 2009 American Academy of Neurology/American Epilepsy Society Practice Parameter reviewed all available studies and concluded that seizure freedom for 9 months to 1 year before pregnancy is probably associated with a high likelihood (84%–92%) of remaining seizure-free during pregnancy (level B evidence).[25] The International Registry of Antiepileptic Drugs and Pregnancy (European Union Registry of Antiepileptic and Pharmaceuticals [EURAP]) data showed that of all cases, 66.6% were seizure-free throughout pregnancy (3806 pregnancies in 3451 women). Notable was that 15.2% of pregnancies were complicated by generalized tonic-clonic seizures. Women with idiopathic generalized epilepsies were more likely to remain seizure-free (73.6%) throughout the duration of their pregnancies when compared with women with an underlying focal epilepsy (59.5%). Seizure worsening occurred from first to second trimester or third trimester in 15.8% of pregnancies.[26]

The reason for breakthrough seizures during pregnancy is most often multifactorial. There is often a misconception that the antiepileptic drugs (AEDs) will be toxic to the fetus and on becoming pregnant, the WWE abruptly stops her AEDs. Hormone fluctuations especially in Weeks 8 to 16 of pregnancy, sleep deprivation, and psychosocial factors all contribute. The most common reason for breakthrough seizures, however, is reduced plasma concentrations of AEDs because of changes in metabolism.[27] Two commonly used AEDs in pregnancy because of their safety profiles include lamotrigine and levetiracetam. However, the serum clearance of these two medications is as high as 200% higher than nonpregnant baseline; therefore, establishing a prepregnancy baseline and monthly monitoring of AED levels is recommended.[28,29]

There are several large pregnancy registries including the North American AED Pregnancy Registry (NAAPR) and the EURAP (45 countries in Europe, Oceania, Asia, Latin America, and Africa). These pregnancy registries prospectively collect date of WWE or women on AEDs for other medical conditions and compare this with healthy, age-matched control subjects.

Treatment with Antiepileptic Drugs and Major Congenital Malformations During Pregnancy

The NAAPR has reported out data on MCMs in 2012, 2016, The most recent data is shown in (Fig. 2). MCMs are defined as structural abnormalities of surgical, functional, or cosmetic significance. This was in comparison with a reference population with the risk of malformations (approximately 1 per 1000). The 2016 data was collected between February 1997 and December 2015 in which 9294 women taking AEDs (for any reason) were enrolled and 5962 were taking AEDs as monotherapy in the first trimester. MCMs were highest for valproate (8.9%), phenobarbital (5.9%), topiramate (4.4%), carbamazepine (3.0%), phenytoin (2.8%), lamotrigine (2.1%), and levetiracetam (2.0%). The EURAP reported out prospective data on 7555 pregnancies reporting

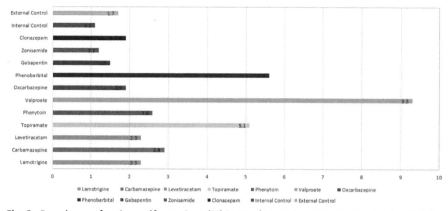

Fig. 2. Prevalence of major malformations (%) in North American pregnancy registry: October 2019. (*Data from* the North American Antiepileptic Drug Pregnancy Registry http://www. aedpregnancyregistry.org/for-health-care-providers-introduction/; with permission.)

similar findings of MCMs in valproate of 10.3% with the lowest being 2.8% for levetiracetam. Lower total daily dosages were seen to have lower MCMs.[30]

It has been well established since 1984 that valproate has the highest teratogenic potential of neural tube defects. The risk of MCMs is 8.9% and has been associated with dosage. The risk of greater than 1500 mg/day is associated with a 24% risk of MCM versus 700 mg/day with a 5% to 6% risk.[31] These malformations include spina bifida, brain malformations, and hypospadias and limb defects. There is an association with autism and autism spectrum disorder with valproate use even without maternal epilepsy.[32] The Neurodevelopmental Effects of Antiepileptic Drugs (NEAD) study found that fetal valproate exposure was associated with a lower IQ at 3 and 6 years of age compared with the other three AEDs studied (carbamazepine, lamotrigine, and phenytoin). However, the use of folic acid 0.4 mg per day as well as breastfeeding was associated with an improved cognitive outcome.[33] Other teratogenic effects are listed in **Table 3**. Risk of MCMs with lamotrigine have consistently been low in numerous studies compared with older AEDs and the risk does not seem to change with escalation in dosages of lamotrigine. The risk associated with oxcarbazepine, gabapentin, and zonisamide was unknown because of small sample sizes, therefore conclusions could not be drawn.[34]

Table 3 lists commonly used antiepileptic medications and toxic risk during pregnancy clarified with associated risk based on NAAPR data.[34] Specific MCM (>0.2%) are included recalling that the reference population risk (~1 per 1000 = 0.1%) are reported. Because of small numbers and wide confidence intervals, risks of MCMs for oxcarbazepine, gabapentin, and zonisamide could not be made. NAAPR data also demonstrated low birth weight for those infants exposed to topiramate and zonisamide in utero compared with lamotrigine.[35,36]

Treatment with Antiepileptic Drugs and Lactation

In general breastfeeding is considered safe and recommended in WWE. Infants are exposed to AEDs through breast milk. Mothers are counseled to monitor the infant for excessive sleepiness, irritability, and weight loss. The relative infant dose is calculated by dividing the infant's dose through breast milk by the maternal dose in mg/kg/d. This determines the amount the infant is ingesting. A relative infant dose less than 10% of maternal dose is thought to pose a low risk to the infant. Of the commonly used

Table 3
AEDs and MCMs

Antiepileptic	Pregnancy Category	MCMs Overall MCMs from 10/2019, Specific % from 2012 Data
Gabapentin	C	MCM = 1.5%/n = 207
Zonisamide	C	MCM = 1.2%/n = 166
Oxcarbazepine	C	MCM = 1.9%/n = 265
Levetiracetam	C	MCM = 2.3%/n = 1029 Neural tube defects (0.22%), cardiac (0.22%) Reflux (>2 g/d), inguinal hernia (>4 g/d) EURAP data
Lamotrigine	C	MCM = 2.3%/n = 2179 Oral cleft (0.45%)
Clonazepam	D	MCM = 1.9%/n = 104
Phenytoin	D	MCM = 2.6%/n = 431 Oral clefts (0.46%) and cardiac (0.96%)
Carbamazepine	D	MCM = 2.9%/n = 2179 Neural tube defects (0.29%), cardiac (0.29%), oral clefts (0.48%)
Topiramate	D	MCM = 5.1%/n = 489 Cardiac (0.28%), oral clefts (1.4%), hypospadias (1.1%)
Phenobarbital	D	MCM = 5.6%/n = 195 Oral clefts (2.0%), cardiac (2.5%), and hypospadias (0.97%)
Valproic acid	D	MCM = 9.3%/n = 335 Neural tube defects (1.2%), hypospadias (3.1%), oral clefts (1.2%), cardiac (2.5%), limb defects, neurodevelopmental

AEDs, phenobarbital, topiramate, and ethosuximide have a potentially high relative infant dose. Additionally, lamotrigine is 9.2% to 18.3%, making this moderately safe.[30] Practitioners can reference LactMed, http://www.mothertobaby.org/, and Hal's Medications and Mothers' Milk for more information.

The Maternal Outcomes and Neurodevelopmental Effects of Antiepileptic Drug (MONEAD) prospective cohort study followed 351 women with 345 infants, throughout their pregnancies and 9 months postpartum. Of the 345 infants, 222 (64.3%) were breastfed. Blood levels of AEDs were collected from mother and infants, 5 to 20 weeks after birth. The study found the AED blood levels in breastfed infants was substantially lower than maternal blood concentrations.[36]

NEUROTOXICOLOGY AND HEADACHE
Natural History of Headaches in Pregnancy

The International Classification of Headache Disorders-3 (https://www.ichd-3.org/)[37] defines a primary headache disorder as the headache is the disorder itself and caused by independent pathology and not by other disorders. Examples of primary headache disorders include tension, migraine, and trigeminal autonomic cephalgias. A secondary headache disorder results as a cause of a symptom from another disorder. Examples of secondary headache include meningitis, medication overuse, or trauma.[37]

The most important initial question that a practitioner needs to ask is if a pregnant women has a primary headache or a secondary headache during pregnancy and during the postpartum period. A retrospective study done by Robbins and colleagues[38] considered headaches in pregnant women. Of the 140 women studied, 65% were primary headaches and 35% were secondary headaches. Most importantly was analyzing the "red flags" for headaches in this pregnant population. This small study found that elevated blood pressure (55%), lack of a headache history (36%), seizures (12%), fever (8%), and abnormal neurologic examination (35%) were the most important factors in considering a secondary headache diagnosis. In contrast to most women having primary headache disorders during pregnancy, in the postpartum period, there is a high likelihood of a secondary headache. Vgontzas and Robbins[39] found that in 63 women presenting with acute postpartum headache, defined as 6 weeks postdelivery, 27% were primary headaches and 76.5% were secondary headaches. The secondary headaches included postdural puncture (45.7%), postpartum preeclampsia (26.1%), and cerebrovascular disorders (26.1%). An easy way to remember the incidence is that the percentages flip in the postpartum period. Most headaches during pregnancy were primary, whereas most headaches postpartum were secondary. A detailed discussion of secondary headaches is beyond the scope of this article and is well covered elsewhere.[40,41]

In counseling a patient before pregnancy, it is important to discuss the natural history of primary headache disorders. Tension-type headaches often improve during pregnancy. Migraines without aura and menstrual migraines often improve. Migraines with aura are variable in their course during pregnancy. Unfortunately, migraines often persist if there has been no improvement by the end of the first trimester of pregnancy.[41] Many of the primary headache disorders improve throughout the course of pregnancy; often only limited symptomatic treatment is needed because the headache improves.

In considering primary headache disorders, a large prospective study, the Norwegian Mother and Child Cohort, followed 60,435 women to determine the prevalence of headache in pregnancy. In the 6099 mothers with migraine in the 6 months before pregnancy, 2999 (49%) had migraines during pregnancy, whereas 3100 (51%) had resolution of their migraines during pregnancy. In the original group, 54,336 had no migraines before pregnancy and only 481 (0.8%) had new onset of migraines during pregnancy.[42]

Treatment of Migraines During Pregnancy and Postpartum

Preconception counseling needs to include nonpharmacologic approaches before pharmaceutical interventions. These should include sleep hygiene and duration, cessation of nicotine, aerobic exercise, stretching, intraoral appliances, and massage. Additionally, biofeedback demonstrated a 78% reduction in headaches in pregnant women compared with 29% with attention control. Biofeedback continued to have a sustained benefit of 68% decrease in postpartum headaches.[43]

The medication management of migraine, the most common primary headache disorder, is shown in **Tables 4** and **5** including drug, former pregnancy category system, and potential toxic exposure risk to the fetus during pregnancy. It is important to be aware that treatment can vary by trimester because of the potential risks to the fetus.

Table 4
Acute treatment of migraine during pregnancy

Drug	Pregnancy Category	Data in Exposed Humans
Acetaminophen	B	ADHD in children exposed antepartum, case reports of PDA closure with 3rd trimester use, childhood asthma with frequent use.
Metoclopramide	B	Likely safe. Potential maternal cardiac conduction changes and extrapyramidal symptoms.
Ondansetron	B	No MCMs. Conflicting studies on possible congenital cardiac malformations, cleft palate.
Aspirin	C	1st and 2nd trimester but avoided in 3rd trimester risk of prolonged labor, hemorrhage and neonatal bleeding, perinatal mortality by IUGR. Possible closure of PDA in 3rd trimester.
Butalbital	C	Traditionally second-line treatment. Mixed data: 1 large study showed possible increase in fetal heart defects when used preconception. Another large study showed no increased risk. Can have withdrawal seizures with barbiturate withdrawal. Infant withdrawal if used in 3rd trimester.
NSAIDS (Diclofenac, Ibuprofen, Ketoprofen, Naproxen and Indomethacin)	B (1st/2nd) D (3rd)	Ibuprofen is the NSAID of choice during 2nd trimester ONLY. First trimester many increase risk of miscarriages. 3rd trimester but CONTRAINDICATED after 30 wk d/t PDA closure and oligohydramnios.[35]
Codeine	C	Cardiac, respiratory, cleft defects.
Narcotics (Morphine, Tramadol and Meperidine)	C	Safe in 1st/2nd trimester. Use with caution in 3rd trimester. Could aggravate nausea and reduce gastric motility. Chronic use associated with neonatal withdrawal and neonatal abstinence if used in late pregnancy.
Prochlorperazine Promethazine	C	Other antiemetics preferred. Platelet aggregation inhibition, irritability, extrapyramidal symptoms, and infant withdrawal if used 3rd trimester.
Triptans	C	No increased risk of MCMs. Ongoing pregnancy registries. Best evidence for sumatriptan, naratriptan, rizatriptan.
Ergots	X	Uterine hypertonicity and vascular disruption increase risk of miscarriage.

Abbreviations: ADHD, attention-deficit/hyperactivity disorder; IUGR, intrauterine growth restriction; NSAID, nonsteroidal anti-inflammatory drug; PDA, Patent Ductus Arteriosus.

Data from MacGregor AE. Migraine in pregnancy and lactation. Neurol Science. 2014. 35, Suppl 1. S61-64.

Treatment with triptans during pregnancy remains unresolved. However a recent meta-analysis looked at six studies and more than 4208 exposed infants and found no increase risks for MCM, prematurity, or spontaneous abortions compared with

Table 5
Prophylactic treatment of migraine during pregnancy

Drug	Pregnancy Category	Data in Exposed Humans
Propranolol/metoprolol Pindolol	C B (Pindolol)	Drug of choice 3rd trimester stop 2–3 d before delivery to reduce fetal bradycardia. Watch for hypotension and hypoglycemia. Small increase in risk of IUGR, small placenta, and congenital abnormalities.
TCA (amitriptyline/nortriptyline) More data for amitriptyline than nortriptyline	C	Second-line choice Low-dose amitriptyline 10–25 mg/day. High dose has been associated with limb deformities. Taper 3–4 wk before delivery to avoid adverse effects in infant. Monitor for infant irritability, urinary retention, or constipation with late-term exposure.
CCB (Verapamil)	C	Tocolytic effect on the uterus so avoid late pregnancy. No congenital anomalies; may cause fetal bradycardia, hypotension, heart block; case report of congenital cardiomyopathy after IV x 2.
SSRI/SNRI	C	Conflicting data of congenital malformations. BMJ 2015 birth defects 2–3.5 times higher with paroxetine and fluoxetine in late use in pregnancy can result in neonatal withdraw period.
Gabapentin	C	Limited data; no increase in fetal congenital malformations; possible increased risk of preterm birth, can cross placenta.
Pregabalin	C	Limited data; possible increase in major congenital malformations.
Memantine	B	Animal studies showed no teratogenic effects.
Cyclobenzaprine	B	Animal studies showed no teratogenic effects.
Lidocaine SQ (ONB)	B	Limited data; existing studies show no increased risk of major congenital malformations; animal studies showed no teratogenic effects.
Magnesium	A D (IV >5 d)	Prolonged IV magnesium sulfate caused skeletal deformities. PO forms (oxide and citrate) not associated with MCMs, skeletal not assessed.[35]

(continued on next page)

Table 5
(continued)

Drug	Pregnancy Category	Data in Exposed Humans
ARB (Candesartan)	D	Avoid use Case reports of malformations and fetal death with 2nd/3rd trimester use. May cause oligohydramnios, renal failure lung hypoplasia, skull ossification defects; may cause hypotension, oliguria, hyperkalemia in exposed infants.
ACE-I (Lisinopril)	D	Avoid use Same risks as ARB.
Topiramate	D	Avoid use FDA changed designation in 2014 d/t North American AED pregnancy registry reporting higher incidence of cleft lip or palate, small for gestational age; concern for metabolic acidosis. Hypospadias, low birth weight.
Valproic acid	X	Contraindicated Increased risk of neural tube defects, craniofacial defects, cardiovascular malformations, autism, decreased IQ, and other teratogenic effects.
Botox	C	Studies at cosmetic doses, which are lower than PREEMPT, 20.9% fetal loss and 2.7% MCMs.[44,45] Do not attempt conception for 12 wk after use.
CGRP	N/A	No data in humans. Ongoing registries.
Co-Q-10	N/A	Limited data. A single randomized controlled trial of 200 mg/d in second half of pregnancy did NOT show increased risk of adverse fetal outcomes.
Vitamin B$_2$	N/A	Safe at physiologic doses, no evidence for use at supraphysiologic doses.
Feverfew	N/A	Contraindicated May cause uterine contraction and spontaneous abortions.

Abbreviations: ACE-I, angiotensin-converting enzyme inhibitor; ARB, angiotensin receptor blocker; CCB, calcium channel blocker; CGRP, calcitonin gene related peptide; IV, intravenous; N/A, non-applicable; ONB, occipital nerve block; PO, by mouth; SNRI, serotonin and norepinephrine reuptake inhibitor; SSRI, selective serotonin reuptake inhibitor; TCA, tricyclic antidepressant.

Data from MacGregor AE. Migraine in pregnancy and lactation. Neurol Science. 2014. 35, Suppl 1. S61-64.

migraineurs without use of triptans.[46] An American Headache Society guideline found level A evidence for use of triptans in pregnancy compared with level C evidence for butalbital combinations; these have traditionally been thought as second-line treatment of migraines during pregnancy.[47,48]

Table 6
Acute medication for migraine during breastfeeding

Drug	Data in Exposed Humans
NSAIDs	Drugs of choice
Triptans	Choose short-acting triptan Eletriptan has lowest concentration in milk Avoid long-acting triptans (naratriptan or frovatriptan)
Metoclopramide	Safe Actually can increase milk production
Diphenhydramine	Safe Actually can decrease milk production

Data from Burch, Rebecca. Headache in Pregnancy and Puerperium. Neurol Clinics; 2018; 31-51.

Rescue medications of the pregnant patient with status migrainosus often includes intravenous fluids and antiemetics; either intravenous or rectal suppositories are used. If steroids are required, prednisone is often preferred to dexamethasone because the former is less likely to cross the placenta.

Migraines often return in the postpartum period; therefore, consideration of medications during that period is needed (**Tables 6** and **7**). Breastfeeding mothers have a lower migraine recurrence than nonbreastfeeding mothers. However, one-half of breastfeeding mothers experience migraine recurrence within 1 month.[10] Several drug references are useful during lactation; these include LactMed (https://toxnet. nlm.nih.gov/newtoxnet/lactmed.htm) and Hale's Medication and Mothers' Milk.

Table 7
Preventative medications during breastfeeding

Drug	Data in Exposed Humans
Propranolol/metoprolol	Drug of choice Watch for sedation in infant
CCB (Verapamil)	Excreted into milk
ACE-I (Lisinopril)	Insufficient data
ARB (Candesartan)	Insufficient data
TCA	Low levels in milk Watch for sedation in infant
SSRI/SNRI	Variable (fluoxetine high)
Gabapentin	Low levels, monitor
Topiramate	Low levels, monitor
Valproic acid	Low levels, watch for jaundice
Low-dose aspirin	Low risk
Botox	Insufficient data

Abbreviations: ACE-I, angiotensin-converting enzyme inhibitor; ARB, angiotensin receptor blocker; CCB, calcium channel blocker; SNRI, serotonin and norepinephrine reuptake inhibitor; SSRI, selective serotonin reuptake inhibitor; TCA, tricyclic antidepressant.
Data from MacGregor AE. Migraine in pregnancy and lactation. Neurol Science. 2014. 35, Suppl 1. S61-64.

SUMMARY

The management of the pregnant and postpartum woman is challenging. With the recent FDA change to the PLLR classification, it is important for the practitioner to not rely solely on the letter category system but to weigh the available evidence to make the best management decision for the pregnant and postpartum woman with neurologic disease.

This review article presents the currently available evidence concerning the natural history and pharmacologic management of MS, epilepsy, and headache during pregnancy and postpartum. The ultimate goal is to optimally manage the maternal neurologic disease while minimizing the potential toxic risk to the fetus.

REFERENCES

1. Feibus KB. FDA's proposed rule for pregnancy and lactation labeling: improving maternal child health through well-informed medicine use. J Med Toxicol 2008; 4(4):284–8.
2. Andrade SE, Gurwitz JH, Davis RL, et al. Prescription drug use in pregnancy. Am J Obstet Gynecol 2004;191(2):398–407.
3. Food and Drug Administration. Content and format of labeling for human prescription drug and biological products: requirements for pregnancy and lactation labeling. Fed Regist 2014;79(233):72064–103. Available at: www.gpo.gov/fdsys/pkg/FR-2014-12- 04/pdf/2014-28241.pdf.
4. Food and Drug Administration. FDA issues final rule on changes to pregnancy and lactation labeling information for prescription drug and biological products. 2014. Available at: http://www.fda.gov/NewsEvents/Newsroom/PressAnnouncements/%20ucm425317.htm. Accessed January 22, 2020.
5. Decision Partners, LLC. Evaluation of how best to communicate to healthcare providers about the risks and benefits of prescription drug use for pregnant and nursing women: a mental models research report. 2009. Available at: http://www.fda.gov/AboutFDA/ReportsManualsForms/Reports/EconomicAnalyses/%20default.htm. Accessed January 22, 2020.
6. Pernia S, DeMaagd G. The new pregnancy and lactation labeling rule. P T 2016; 41(11):713–5.
7. Robinson A, Atallah F. Effect of removal of pregnancy category on prescribing in pregnancy: a randomized trial [abstract]. In: American College of Obstetrics and Gynecology meeting. Austin, TX, April 27–29, 2018. [5OP].
8. Coyle PK. Pregnancy and multiple sclerosis. Neurol Clin 2012;30(3):877–88.
9. Confavreux C, Hutchinson M, Hours MM, et al. Rate of pregnancy-related relapse in multiple sclerosis. N Engl J Med 1998;339(5):285–91.
10. Vukusic S, Hutchinson M, Hours M, et al. Pregnancy and multiple sclerosis (the PRIMS study): clinical predictors of post partum relapse. Brain 2004;127: 1353–60.
11. Stenick L, Hsu Liangge. Imaging considerations in pregnancy. Neurol Clin 2019; 37:1–16.
12. Skuladottir H, Wilcox AJ, Ma C, et al. Corticosteroid use and risk of orofacial clefts. Birth Defects Res A Clin Mol Teratol 2014;100(6):499–506.
13. Bay Bjorn AM, Ehrenstein V, Hundborg HH, et al. Use of corticosteroids in early pregnancy is not associated with risk of oral clefts and other congenital malformations in offspring. Am J Ther 2014;21(2):73–80.
14. Kaplan T. Management of demyelinating disorders in pregnancy. Neurol Clin 2019;37:17–30.

15. Lu E, Wang BW, Guimond C, et al. Disease-modifying drugs for multiple sclerosis in pregnancy: a systematic review. Neurology 2012;79(11):1130–5.

16. Haghikia A, Langer-Gould A, Rellensmann G, et al. Natalizumab use during third trimester of pregnancy. JAMA Neurol 2014;71(7):891–5.

17. Karlsson G, Francis G, Koren G, et al. Pregnancy outcomes in the clinical development program of fingolimod in multiple sclerosis. Neurology 2014;82(8):674–80.

18. AUBAGIO (teriflunomide). Full Prescribing Information. 2019. Available at: http://products.sanofi.us/aubagio/aubagio.html. Accessed January 22, 2020.

19. TECFIDERA (dimethyl fumerate) Full Prescribing Information. 2019. Available at: https://www.tecfidera.com/content/dam/commercial/tecfidera/pat/en_us/pdf/full-prescribing-info.pdf. Accessed January 22, 2020.

20. Oh J, Achiron A, Chambers C, et al. Pregnancy outcome in patients with RRMS who received alemtuzumab in clinical development program. (S24.008). Neurology 2016;86(16 Supplement):S24.

21. OCREVUS (ocrelizumab). Full Prescribing Information. 2019. Available at: https://www.ocrevus.com/hcp/dosing.html. Accessed January 22, 2020.

22. MAVENCLAD (cladribine. Full Prescribing Information. 2019. Available at: https://www.mavenclad.com. Accessed January 22, 2020.

23. Ngugi AK, Bottomley C, Kleinschmidt I, et al. Estimation of the burden of active and life-time epilepsy: a meta –analytic approach. Epilepsia 2010;51(5):883–90.

24. Pennell PB, French JA, Harden CL, et al. Fertility and birth outcomes in women with epilepsy seeking pregnancy. JAMA Neurol 2018;75(8):962–9.

25. Harden CL, Hopp J, Ting TY, et al. Practice parameter update: management issues for women with epilepsy–focus on pregnancy (an evidence-based review): obstetrical complications and change in seizure frequency: report of the Quality Standards Subcommittee and Therapeutics and Technology Assessment Subcommittee of the American Academy of Neurology and American Epilepsy Society. Neurology 2009;73(2):126–32.

26. Battino D, Tomson T, Bonizzoni E, et al, EURAP Study Group. Seizure control and treatment changes in pregnancy: observations from the EURAP epilepsy pregnancy registry. Epilepsia 2013;54(9):1621–7.

27. Sazgar M. Treatment of women with epilepsy. Continuum (Minneap Minn) 2019; 25(2):408–30.

28. Patel SI, Pennell PB. Management of epilepsy during pregnancy: an update. Ther Adv Neurol Disord 2016;9(2):118–29.

29. Harden CL, Hopp J, Ting TY, et al. Practice parameter update: management issues for women with epilepsy–focus on pregnancy (an evidence-based review): vitamin K, folic acid, blood levels and breast feeding: report of the Quality Standards Subcommittee and Therapeutics and Technology Assessment Subcommittee of the American Academy of Neurology and American Epilepsy Society. Neurology 2009;73(2):142–9.

30. Holmes LB, Hernandez-Diaz S, Quinn M, et al. Update on monotherapy findings: comparative safety of 11 antiepileptic drugs used during pregnancy. The North American Pregnancy Registry Newsletter 2016. Available at: www.aedpregnancyregistry.org/wp-content/uploads/2016-newsletter-Winter-2016.pdf.

31. Tomson T, Battino D, Bonizzon E, et al. Dose-dependent teratogenicity of valproate in mono- and polytherapy: an observational study. Neurology 2015;85:866–72.

32. Christensen J, Groborg TK, Sorensen MJ, et al. Prenatal valproate exposure and risk of autism spectrum disorder and childhood autism. JAMA 2013;309: 1696–703.

33. Meador KJ, Baker GA, Browning N, et al, NEAD Study Group. Fetal antiepileptic drug exposure and cognitive outcomes at age 6 years (NEAD study): a prospective observational study. Lancet Neurol 2013;12(3):244–52.

34. Hernandez-Diaz S, Smith CR, Shen A, et al. Comparative safety of antiepileptic drugs during pregnancy. Neurology 2012;78:1692–9.

35. Hernandez-Diaz S, Mittendorf R, Smith CR, et al. Association between topiramate and zonisamide use during pregnancy and low birth weight. Obstet Gynecol 2014;123:21–8.

36. Birbaum AK, Meador KJ, Karanam A, et al. Antiepileptic drug exposure in infants of breastfeeding mothers with epilepsy. JAMA Neurol 2019. https://doi.org/10. 1001/jamaneurol.2019.4443.

37. International Classification of Headache Disorders version 3. Available at: https:// www.ichd-3.org. Accessed January 22, 2020.

38. Robbins MS, Farmakidis C, Dayal AK, et al. Acute headache diagnosis in pregnant women: a hospital based study. Neurology 2015;85:1024–30.

39. Vgontzas A, Robbins M. A hospital based retrospective study of acute postpartum headache. Headache 2018;58:845–51.

40. Burch R. Headache in pregnancy and puerperium. Neurol Clin 2019;37:31–51.

41. Robbins M. Headache in pregnancy. Continuum 2018;28(4):1092–107.

42. Nezalova-Herriksen K, Spigset O, Nordeng H, et al. Maternal characteristics and migraine pharmacotherapy during pregnancy: cross-sectional analysis of data from large cohort study. Cephalagia 2009;29:1276.

43. Scharff L, Marcus DA, Turk DC. Maintenance of effects in nonmedical treatment of headaches during pregnancy. Headache 1996;36:285–90.

44. Brin MF, Kirby RS, Slavotinek A, et al. Pregnancy outcomes following exposure to onabotulinum toxin A. Pharmacoepidemiol Drug Saf 2016;25(2):179–87.

45. Hoshiyama E, Tatsumoto M, Iwanami H. Postpartum migraines: a long term prospective study. Intern Med 2012;51(22):3119–23.

46. MacGregor AE. Migraine in pregnancy and lactation. Neurol Science 2014; 35(Suppl 1):S61–4.

47. Marchenko A, Etwel F, Olutunfese O, et al. Pregnancy outcome following prenatal exposure to triptan medications: a meta-analysis. Headache 2015;55(4): 490–501.

48. Marmura MJ, Siberstein SD, Schwedt TJ. The acute treatment of migraine in adults: the American Headache Society evidence assessment of migraine pharmacotherapies. Headache 2015;55(1):3–20.

Manganese Exposure and Neurologic Outcomes in Adult Populations

Kaitlin V. Martin, PhD, MPH[a],*, David Edmondson, PhD[b,c],
Kim M. Cecil, PhD[b,c,d], Cassandra Bezi, MPH[e],
Miriam Leahshea Vance[f], Dani McBride, BS[g],
Erin N. Haynes, DrPH, MS[h]

KEYWORDS

• Brain • Manganese • Cognition • Motor

KEY POINTS

• Chronic increased manganese (Mn) exposure is associated with cognitive and motor impairments in both occupational and community settings.
• Numerous biomarkers are used to ascertain Mn exposure.
• Neuroimaging is an innovate tool used as both a biomarker of Mn exposure and a biomarker of effect.
• Older adults are a novel population that can provide insight into the impacts of chronic Mn exposure and the role of Mn in the development and progression of neurodegenerative diseases.

INTRODUCTION

Manganese (Mn) plays a critical role in many physiologic processes, including protein and energy metabolism, cellular protection from damaging free radicals, bone mineralization, immune function, reproduction, digestion, and metabolic regulation.[1]

^a Department of Epidemiology, College of Public Health, University of Kentucky, 111 Washington Avenue Room 212C, Lexington, KY 40536, USA; ^b Department of Radiology, University of Cincinnati College of Medicine, Cincinnati, OH, USA; ^c Imaging Research Center, Cincinnati Children's Hospital Medical Center, 3333 Burnet Avenue, MLC 5033, Cincinnati, OH 45229, USA; ^d Department of Environmental Health, University of Cincinnati College of Medicine, Cincinnati, OH, USA; ^e Division of Infectious Diseases, Department of Pediatrics, Cincinnati Children's Hospital Medical Center, 3333 Burnet Avenue, MLC 7017, Cincinnati, OH 45229, USA; ^f Department of Epidemiology, College of Public Health, University of Kentucky, 111 Washington Avenue, Lexington, KY 40536, USA; ^g Department of Environmental Health, University of Cincinnati College of Medicine, Cincinnati, OH 45267, USA; ^h Department of Epidemiology, College of Public Health, University of Kentucky, 111 Washington Avenue Room 212G, Lexington, KY 40536, USA
* Corresponding author.
E-mail address: Kaitlin.vollet.martin@uky.edu

Neurol Clin 38 (2020) 913–936
https://doi.org/10.1016/j.ncl.2020.07.008
0733-8619/20/© 2020 Elsevier Inc. All rights reserved.

neurologic.theclinics.com

Although vital in trace amounts, Mn overexposure has been associated with neurodegeneration and neurotoxicity.[2] Chronic exposure to increased levels of Mn in occupational settings has resulted in a condition called manganism. Manganism is characterized by extrapyramidal symptoms, including bradykinesia, dystonia, gait instabilities, and speech impairments.[3] In 1837, Dr John Couper first reported neurologic features associated with Mn exposure when several employees of a Mn processing facility presented with extrapyramidal symptoms. During the twentieth century, research remained focused on occupational exposure to Mn with workplace studies in industries such as welding, mining, and the manufacturing of Mn-containing products. In recent decades, research has become more focused on investigating the impact of chronic low-level exposure to Mn within the general population to understand the subsequent cognitive and neuromotor effects. In 1999, Mergler and colleagues[2] were among the first to investigate the impact of low-level environmental exposure to Mn within a community setting. Subtle neurologic impairments were observed in relation to blood Mn levels. Current research builds on this concept by substantiating that lower-level environmental exposures are associated with subclinical neurologic effects.[4]

Abundant exposure to Mn occurs through diet,[5] with factors such as age, gender, and nutritional status affecting absorption rates, which range from 1% to 5%.[6] Although Mn is naturally present throughout the environment, anthropogenic sources such as industrial air pollution, agricultural fungicides, and gasoline additives contribute to the burden of excess environmental Mn. The inhalation of Mn is concerning because of greater absorption rates, especially within the brain.[5] Homeostatic regulation is efficient at stabilizing levels of ingested Mn; however, airborne Mn may bypass these mechanisms and directly enter the brain by crossing the blood-brain barrier through membrane transporter proteins, transferrin and transferrin receptors,[7] or via the olfactory nerve.[8]

Depending on the route of exposure, Mn absorption occurs via the gastrointestinal tract or lung with subsequent distribution throughout the body.[9] The highest levels of Mn are reported in various organs, including the liver, bone, kidneys, pancreas, adrenal gland, and the pituitary gland within the brain.[10] Typical levels of Mn in blood range from 4 to 15 μg/L.[5] Circulating Mn is typically bound to hemoglobin; thus, the main compartment for Mn is the erythrocytes.[11] The liver plays the primary role in the biological regulation of Mn by conjugating excess Mn to bile for excretion through the intestine.[9] As indicated by the neurologic impairments associated with Mn exposure, the brain is very vulnerable to Mn toxicity. Mn accumulates in the brain with an affinity toward the basal ganglia structures.[12] With a half-life estimated to be around 150 days, Mn has a slow clearance rate from the brain.[13,14] In addition, it is thought that the high energy requirement and longevity of neurons contributes to enhanced neurologic susceptibility to Mn.[9]

This article examines the recent literature investigating the neurologic impact of Mn exposure on adult populations. This article synthesizes study findings to create a better understanding of the current state of research and to provide suggestions for future research directions.

METHODS

This systematic review investigates the effect of Mn exposure on adult neurocognitive and neuromotor function. In 2016, a systematic review assessing Mn exposure and cognition across the lifespan was published.[4] Thus, to incorporate the findings from current research into the discussion regarding adult Mn exposure and neurocognition, the authors searched for studies that were published between January 2016 and November 2019 investigating Mn exposure and neurocognition. We identified studies that met our criteria though PubMed and Medline using the following search terms: (manganese) AND (neurocognition OR cognition OR neuro) AND (adults) AND (occupation OR occupational OR environment OR environ*) ("2016/01/01"[Date – Publication]: "2019/11/01"[Date – Publication]). Previously, a review was published to assess the literature regarding Mn exposure and neuromotor outcomes.[15] Therefore, we searched for studies that evaluated Mn exposure among adults and were published between November 2007 and November 2019. Studies that met our criteria were obtained using both PubMed and Medline and the following search terms: (manganese) AND (neurofunctional OR neuromotor OR motor OR neurobehavioral) AND (adults) AND (welders OR occupational OR occupational OR environ*) ("2007/07/01"[Date – Publication]: "2019/11/01"[Date – Publication]).

DISCUSSION
Exposure Biomarkers

There is a substantial amount of research characterizing Mn exposure through environmental matrices such as water,[16–18] soil,[16,18,19] and air.[16,20–36] Although these markers indicate levels of external exposure, they are not able to specify individual dose concentrations. In epidemiologic studies, personalized biomarkers of exposure strengthen study findings by capturing internal dose measurements and minimizing reporting bias. However, there is no concurrence on which biomarker of Mn exposure is ideal. **Table 1** provides an overview of several different biomarkers commonly used in the studies included in this article.

Blood Mn/iron ratio (MIR) was used as the biomarker for exposure in a study conducted in Guizhou, China.[27] The decline in fine motor movement was worsened by Mn exposure, and plasma MIR was inversely associated with fine motor skills. Viana and colleagues[44] in 2014 incorporated saliva measurements in a study of residents in Brazil living near a ferromanganese refinery to assess Mn exposure; however, no significant correlations were detected with saliva. Urine has been used as a Mn biomarker in many studies[16,18,19,28,29]; however, the future use of urine as a biomarker is not recommended. Toenails, fingernails, and hair are more frequently collected and analyzed for Mn content.[21,44–47] A Brazilian community study also collected scalp hair, axillary hair, and fingernail specimens, all of which were positively correlated with neuromotor function. Bone, a novel biomarker of Mn exposure, is an appealing biomarker of exposure because of the long-term storage of Mn. Rolle-McFarland and colleagues[45] in 2019 described associations between bone Mn levels and cognitive deficits, which may stem from underlying hippocampal and striatal impairments. Wells and colleagues[48] in 2018 found similar associations between increased hand bone Mn concentrations and reduced manual dexterity in an occupational cohort.

Many factors influence personal exposure levels, including ingestion or inhalation rates, age,[4] gender,[49] iron (Fe) status,[50] and nutritional status.[6] Although exposure may remain constant, variability in individual accumulation of Mn has also been noted. Mutations in Mn transporter and Fe metabolism genes are associated with variations in Mn accumulation,[51–54] thus predisposing an individual to Mn excess or depletion. An Italian study discovered that there was a higher prevalence of Parkinson disease (PD) in the areas surrounding a ferroalloy smelter.[19] Polymorphisms in ATP13A2 (PARK9), a PD-related gene, had a significant impact on the observed effects among the older participants.

Table 1
Biomarkers of manganese exposure

	Acute Exposures		Cumulative Exposures		
Blood	**Urine**	**Saliva**	**Hair**	**Nails**	**Bone**
Most widely used biomarker of Mn exposure[38]	Poor correlation between Mn exposure and Mn levels in urine[39]	Although levels are present at concentrations similar to blood, saliva is an alternative noninvasive biomarker for Mn exposure[39]	Quantifies longer-term cumulative exposures transpiring over several months[40]	Fingernails and toenails are noninvasive measures that represent aggregate exposures spanning from several months to approximately 1 y[37]	Approximately 40% of Mn is stored in bone[45]
Mn in blood has a short half-life of hours[10]	Past studies have not made significant observations using urine as a Mn biomarker[38]	Saliva Mn levels seem to linearly increase with exposure[39]	Exogenous contamination is a significant concern[40]	Mn concentrations quantified in nails have been associated with levels of Mn in the striatum and midbrain regions[41,42] of the brain	Estimated half-life of Mn in bone is 8 y[10]
Optimal for acute exposures[37] such as occupational settings	The future use of urine as a marker of Mn exposure is not recommended[30]	Use of saliva as a Mn biomarker is questionable[10,38,39]	Used as a noninvasive biomarker in many studies[40]		Bone Mn concentrations have been correlated with Mn levels in the brain, specifically the striatum, hippocampus, and choroid plexus[43]

Occupational Findings

With known increased exposure levels, the earliest adverse effects related to Mn exposure were first noted in occupational settings. Since the initial observations, regulatory measures have been established to govern exposure; however, a strong consensus on the proper exposure limits is lacking.[55] **Table 2** provides an overview of the occupational studies included in this review. A recent study of welders assessed Mn exposure through reported work history[56] and accumulated exposure to welding fumes.[57] Lower cognitive scores were associated with welding fume exposure. In China, a questionnaire was administered to welders to assess potential Mn exposure through queries such as duration of work and type of workplace.[35] Similarly, increased Mn exposure through welding histories was associated with negative health outcomes.

In a cohort study, welders compared with nonwelder referents had poorer performance on motor tests; however, there were no statistically significant associations indicating poorer test performance related to Mn exposure.[28] Similarly, Mn exposure assessed from personal monitoring was significantly associated with worse stability of handwriting among welders.[30] When measuring Mn dust at a ferromanganese alloy plant, initial and follow-up examinations on exposed workers showed a significant association between poorer motor performance and exposure.[58] In a cohort of welders, Mn cumulative exposure was strongly associated with the progression of limb bradykinesia and limb rigidity.[22] In another study, the duration of Mn exposure and Mn small respirable particulates were strongly associated with motor function.[59]

To assess the permanency of Mn-associated health outcomes among acutely exposed welders, a follow-up neuromotor examination was done 3.5 years after cessation of confined-space welding.[60] Symptoms including extrapyramidal, olfactory, and mood disturbances did not improve over time and may even have deteriorated, whereas cognitive function seemed to improve for the retired welders. To investigate even longer-term cessation of exposure to Mn, a study recruited welders who had been retired for an average of 18 years.[61] Results were similar among retired welders and referents.[61]

Community Findings

The studies of community exposure to Mn are described in **Table 3**. A study among people living near a ferromanganese refinery in Ohio and a demographically similar community examined the effects of long-term, low-level environmental Mn exposure on neuromotor function.[33] No association was found between blood Mn levels and Unified Parkinson's Disease Rating Scale (UPDRS) data or postural sway; however, adjusted models showed significant differences between the exposed and the referents, with heightened impairments observed among the exposed. Similar results were seen using the same study population, where blood Mn and cumulative exposure index did not predict any motor outcomes.[62] Another study conducted in the same region showed a significant association of airborne Mn with several neuromotor outcomes.[25] Increased tremor and motor symptoms, executive dysfunction, and tremor-dominant and non–tremor-dominant symptom clusters were identified in chronically exposed residents.[20]

Older populations are vulnerable to environmental exposures for multiple reasons. First, older adults have the opportunity for chronic exposure, particularly if they reside in a community with a Mn point source. Second, older generations were likely exposed to contaminants at greater levels than are present today because of changes in regulations and advances in control technology. Third, aging is a key risk factor for

Table 2
Epidemiologic studies investigating occupational exposure to manganese

Author	Location	Study Design	Participants Age at Motor Assessment	Source of Mn Exposure	Biomarker/ Environmental Measures	Covariates	Outcome Measure	Results
Bouchard et al,[58] 2007	Canada	Prospective cohort	Exposed n = 69 Referents n = 68 Mean age 58.1 y	Mn ferroalloy plant	Dust (mg Mn/m^3 years) n = 69	Age, education, alcohol, and smoking	Motor Scale of the Luria-Nebraska, finger tapping, Dynamometer, 9-hole Hand Steadiness Test	Exposed had poorer scores compared with referents both in the initial and follow-up examinations for the Luria-Nebraska test. Increasing levels of CEI were significantly associated with poorer scores on the Luria Motor Scale and the Hand Steadiness Test
Shin et al,[26] 2007	Korea	Cross-sectional study	350 workers Age not specified	Manufacturing factories	Air (mg/m^3) n = 121 Blood (µg/dL) n = 121 Duration of work (years) n = 121 CEV n = 121 PI n = 111	Age, alanine aminotransferase, and educational level	WHO-NCTB and computerized finger tapping	The proportion of workers with increased signals increased with all the Mn exposure variables. The PI was significantly associated with a correct score of pursuit aiming II tests and finger tapping of the dominant hand
Cowan et al,[27] 2009	Guizhou, China	Cross-sectional study	Smelters n = 26 18–56 y	Ferroalloy plant	Air (mg/m^3) Blood MIR n = 136 Plasma MIR n = 143 Mn concentration in erythrocytes n = 144	Age, years of education, sex, income, and years of employment	Groove-type steadiness tester, 9-hole tests, and Purdue Pegboard Coordination Test	Plasma MIR was significantly correlated with pegboard scores. Age-related decline in fine-movement coordination was observed among all study participants regardless of Mn exposure

Study	Location	Study design	Participants	Setting	Exposure measurement	Covariates adjusted	Tests	Findings
Chang et al,[24] 2009	Korea	Cross-sectional study	Welders n = 43, Controls n = 29, 40–57 y	Steel block factory	Air (mg/m³), Blood (µg/dL), n = 72, PI n = 73	Age, educational level, alcohol consumption, and smoking	Grooved pegboard, finger-tapping test, CATSYS, hand pronation/supination test	Grooved-pegboard and finger-tapping tests showed significant differences between the 2 groups. Blood Mn levels were shown to be significantly associated with grooved pegboard (dominant hand)
Chang et al,[32] 2010	Korea	Cross-sectional study	Welders n = 42, Controls n = 26, 40–57 y	Steel block factory	Air (mg/m³) n = 73 Blood (µg/dL) n = 73 Pallidal index n = 73	Age, educational level, alcohol consumption, and smoking	Grooved pegboard, finger-tapping test, CATSYS, hand pronation/supination test	Hand pronation/supination and finger-tapping tests were significantly lower among the welders than among the controls
Bowler et al,[60] 2011	California	Prospective cohort	Welders n = 26, 32–65 y	Mn-containing welding fumes	Blood (µg/L) n = 24	Age, ethnicity, duration of welding, type of welding, blood Pb, and smoking	UPDRS3 and the CATSYS Tremor system	Rigidity, dominant postural hand tremor, and body sway increased significantly at follow-up
Sen et al,[88] 2011	United States	Cross-sectional study	Welders n = 7, Controls n = 7, Mean age 48 y	Not specified	CEI (Mg Mn/m³) n = 7	Age	Grooved pegboard; MRI	The welders scored worse than the controls on the grooved-pegboard test for both dominant and nondominant hand
Laohaudomchok et al,[30] 2011	United States	Cross-sectional study	Welders n = 46, Mean age 37.4 y	Welding school	Air (µg/m³) n = 46	Age, race, education, income, dietary Mn, and BMI	Neuroskill device and finger tapping	Mn exposure over a work shift was significantly associated with worse stability of handwriting

(continued on next page)

Table 2
(continued)

Author	Location	Study Design	Participants Age at Motor Assessment	Source of Mn Exposure	Biomarker/ Environmental Measures	Covariates	Outcome Measure	Results
Kim et al,[33] 2011	Korea	Cross-sectional study	Welders n = 30 Controls n = 19 40–58 y	Factory	Air (μg/m³) n = 100 Blood (μg/L) n = 191	Age, educational level, smoking status, and alcohol consumption status	Finger-tapping tests and the grooved-pegboard test	Fractional anisotropy and radial diffusivity were significantly associated with grooved-pegboard (dominant and nondominant hand) and finger-tapping (dominant and nondominant hand) test outcomes
Racette et al,[56] 2012	United States	Prospective cohort	389 welders 40–58 y	Factories and shipyards	CEI (Mg Mn/m³) n = 886	Age at baseline, sex, race, tobacco smoking, alcohol consumption, and occupational pesticide exposure	UPDRS3	Exposure was most strongly associated with progression of upper limb bradykinesia, upper and lower limb rigidity
Wastensson et al,[61] 2012	Sweden	Cross-sectional study	Welders n = 17 Referents n = 21 Mean age 69 y	Shipyard	CEI (mA/m²) n = 17	Age and smoking habits	The Kløwe-Matthews static steadiness test, CATSYS, finger-tapping test, grooved-pegboard test, eurythmokinesimeter, diadochokinesimeter, and Jamar dynamometer	Former welders performed less well than referents in the grooved-pegboard test, and poorer performance was associated with CEI
Chang et al,[75] 2013	Korea	Cross-sectional study	Welders n = 40 Controls n = 26 40–58 y	Steel block factory	Air (mg/m³) Blood (μg/dL) n = 66	Age, educational level, alcohol consumption, and smoking	MRI, Grooved-pegboard, and finger-tapping test	Significant brain volume reductions were found in welders compared with controls, and these volume reductions are associated with motor deficits

Study	Location	Study design	Population	Setting	Exposure (n)	Adjustments	Tests	Results
Ellingsen et al,[28] 2014	Russia	Cross-sectional study	Welders n = 137, Referents n = 137, 19–70 y	Shipyard	Air (μg/m³) n = 130, Blood (μg/L) n = 123, Urine (μg/g) n = 126	Age, tobacco smoking, the concentration of carbohydrate-deficient transferrin in serum, self-reported mild head injury, shift work, duration of education, coffee consumption	Finger-tapping, foot-tapping, grooved-pegboard, dynamometer, CATSYS 2000, Kløve-Matthews Static Steadiness and Hand Pronation-Supination tests	Welders had poorer performance on motor tests compared with nonwelder referents
Park et al,[59] 2014	Quebec, Canada	Cross-sectional study	Referents n = 67, Alloy workers n = 68, Mean age 43.9 y	Silico-Mn and ferro-Mn production plant	CE (mg/m³) n = 68	Age and educational level	Luria-Nebraska Neuropsychological Battery-Motor Scale and Finger Tapping	The duration of Mn exposure and Mn as small respirable particulates is strongly associated with the Luria-Nebraska Motor Scale
Long et al,[29] 2014	Guangxi, China	Cross-sectional study	Smelters n = 9, Controls n = 23, Mean age 39.3 y	Mn-iron alloy factory	Air (mg/m³) n = 9, Blood (mg/L) n = 32, Urine (μg/L) n = 32	Age	Purdue pegboard motor testing	Increase in GABA level was significantly associated with the duration of exposure and significant inverse associations between GABA levels and all Purdue Pegboard Test scores in the smelter workers
Baker et al,[71] 2015	Washington	Prospective cohort	Welders n = 56, Mean age 28 y	Welding	Air (μg/m³) n = 56, Tl-weighted indices n = 17	Smoking status, alcohol drinker, prior self-reported loss of consciousness, self-reported respirator use, and age at baseline	Grooved pegboard (Lafayette Instrument Evaluation, West Lafayette, IN), UPDRS3	There were no associations between cumulative exposure and UPDRS3 score or grooved-pegboard time
Lewis et al,[69] 2016	Pennsylvania	Cross-sectional study	Welders n = 20, Controls n = 13, Mean age 47.1 y	Not specified	hW (hours) n = 20, yW (years) n = 20	Age, education level, BMI, and respirator use	Maximal voluntary contraction tasks, single-finger ramp tasks, quick force pulse production tasks, UPDRS, and the grooved-pegboard test	There also were no significant differences between welders and controls on the grooved-pegboard test

(continued on next page)

Table 2
(continued)

Author	Location	Study Design	Participants Age at Motor Assessment	Source of Mn Exposure	Biomarker/ Environmental Measures	Covariates	Outcome Measure	Results
Seo et al,[73] 2016	Korea	Cross-sectional study	Welders n = 53 Controls n = 44 40+ y	Factories for mild steel blocks and shipbuilding	Air (mg/m3) n = 53 Blood (µg/dL) n = 97	Age, education level, tobacco use, alcohol consumption, use of medication, medical history, subjective symptoms, job type (type of welding and duration), work history	fMRI, Wisconsin Card-sorting Task, Word-Color Test, Computerized Neuropsychological Test	Blood Mn level was significantly higher in welders than in controls. Reaction time for given tasks were not significantly different between groups even though welders took longer. Based on fMRI images, no specific regions had significant activity in welders while WCST was being completed
Al-Lozi et al,[57] 2017	United States	Cross-sectional study	Welders n = 82 Nonwelders n = 13 23–66 y	Welding	Exposure welding metrics (duration, intensity and total exposure)	Work history, cumulative Mn exposure, age, sex, race, ethnicity, medical history, history of head injury, previous exposures, alcohol/ tobacco use	Assess cognitive control in response inhibition, working memory, verbal fluency, letter-number sequencing, Two Black Letter Task, Go-N-Go, Simon Task, Cognitive Control Summary was scored for those completing all 5 tasks, WAIS3- verbal/matrix reasoning	Poorer performance in cognitive control tasks in relation to welding fume exposure. Welders had lower IQ and cognitive control scores
Zhang et al,[35] 2017	Qingdao City, China	Cross-sectional study	n = 505 19–54 y	Welding	Work history	Smoking habits, years of work, education level, age	Questionnaires assessing symptoms	Correlation between the highest level of symptom reports with highest level of air Mn measurements. Those with >15 y of welding reported high levels of tremor and motor disabilities

Study	Country	Study type	Population	Setting/Exposure	Exposure measure	Covariates	Outcome measures	Key findings
Bowler et al,[23] 2018	United States	Cross-sectional study	Welders n = 26, Controls n = 17, ≥18 y	Welding for semitruck manufacture	Air (mg/m³) n = 43, MRI n = 43	Age, education, ethnicity, alcohol consumption, smoking habits	Rey-O Copy Trial, Trials B Test, Trials A, Digit Symbol Coding, WAIS3, WHO-AVLT, verbal fluency	Welders scored lower than controls in verbal fluency, Parallel Lines Test, and Digit Symbol Coding. Welders had shorter T1 relaxation times
Lee et al,[36] 2018	Pennsylvania	Cross-sectional study	Welders n = 43, Controls n = 32, Age not stated	Welding	Blood (ng/mL) n = 75	Recent hours welding, lifetime exposure, cumulative exposure inhaled over lifetime	Grooved-pegboard test, UPDRS3, single-finger/multifinger pressing task, MRI	Results of Phonemic Fluency Test suggest that processes associated with phonemic fluency are among some of the earliest changes in welders with low Mn exposure
Ma et al,[31] 2018	United States	Cross-sectional study	Welders n = 39, Controls n = 22, Mean age 40 y	Mn fumes	Air (mg/m³) n = 39	Age	UPDRS3	High exposure to Mn showed a significant increase of thalamic GABA levels, as well as significantly worse performance in general motor function
Wells et al,[48] 2018	United States	Cross-sectional study	Workers n = 7, Comparison n = 12, 18-62 y	Trailer manufacturer	Bone Mn (μg/g) n = 19	Age and occupation	Purdue Pegboard Test	High MnBn was significantly associated with lower manual dexterity based on the Purdue pegboard assembly task
Criswell et al,[65] 2019	Midwest United States	Cross-sectional study	Mn-exposed welders n = 27, Other Mn-exposed workers n = 12, Nonexposed n = 29, 22-69 y	Welding worksites	CEI n = 68, PI n = 68	Sex; age; imaging scan date; current consumption of cigarettes, caffeine or alcohol	UPDRS3	Cumulative Mn exposure is associated with increased PI. PI was associated with clinical parkinsonism
Palzes et al,[46] 2019	Zarcero County, Costa Rica	Cross-sectional study	Organic farmers n = 26, Conventional farmers n = 22, 18+ y	Farmers from organic and conventional farms	Hair (μg/g) n = 33, Toenails (μg/g) n = 40	Sociodemographic characteristics, work history, medical history, computer literacy, age	Letter retrieving/working memory task, fNIR	Brain activity decreased with every 2-fold increase in nail and hair Mn concentration

(continued on next page)

Table 2
(continued)

Author	Location	Study Design	Participants Age at Motor Assessment	Source of Mn Exposure	Biomarker/ Environmental Measures	Covariates	Outcome Measure	Results
Rolle-McFarland et al,[45] 2019	Zunyi, China	Cross-sectional study	Ferroalloy smelters n = 30 Manufacturing workers n = 30 ≥18 y	Equipment manufacturing and installation company (control) and ferroalloy smelting facility	Bone (μg/g) n = 60 Fingernail (μg/g) n = 55 Blood (μg/L) n = 60	Age, education, drinking status, smoking status	Animal naming, fruit naming, WHO/UCLA Verbal Learning Test (AVLT), UPenn Smell Identification Test	MnBn and MnFn are associated with decreased performance in cognitive function but not smell MnB had no association with cognitive function

Abbreviations: AVLT, auditory verbal learning test; BMI, body mass index; CEI, Cumulative Exposure Index; CEV, cumulative exposure variable; CATSYS, Coordination Ability Test System; GABA, gamma-aminobutyric acid; Ferro-Mn, ferromanganese; fMRI, functional MRI; fNIR, functional near infrared; IQ, intelligence quotient; hW, hours spent welding in the 90 day period preceding MRI; MnBn, Bone Mn; MnB, Blood Mn; MnFn, Fingernail Mn; NCTB, Neurobehavioral Core Test Battery; PI, pallidal index; UCLA, University of California, Los Angeles; UPenn, University of Pennsylvania; WAIS, Wechsler Adult Intelligence Scale; WHO, World Health Organization; yW, cumulative lifetime years welding.

Data from Refs.[23,24,26–32,34–36,45,46,48,56,57,59–61,65,71,73–75,88,91]

Table 3
Epidemiologic studies investigating community-level manganese exposures

Author	Location	Study Design	Participants; Age at Motor Assessment	Source of Mn Exposure	Biomarker/ Environmental Measures	Covariates	Outcome Measure	Results
Kim et al,[33] 2011	Ohio	Cross-sectional study	Exposed n = 100 Reference n = 90 30–75 y	Ferro-Mn and silico-Mn smelter	Air (µg/m³) n = 100 Blood (µg/L) n = 190	Age, sex, ethnicity, smoking status, drinking status, educational level, household income, insurance status, serum ferritin, ALT, and GGT; BMI; medication history; blood lead, cadmium, and mercury	UPDRS and CATSYS 2000	UPDRS motor and postural sway scores were significantly higher in the exposed group than in the comparison group. No significant difference between the exposed and comparison groups was evident as to MnB
Bowler et al,[62] 2012	Ohio	Cross-sectional study	Exposed n = 100 Reference n = 91 30–75 y	Ferro-Mn smelter	CEI air (µg/m³) n = 100 Blood (µg/L) n = 190	Age, sex, education, diabetes, mental health medication, and health insurance status	Finger tapping, grooved pegboard, dynamometer, and UPDRS	MnB did not predict any motor outcomes either in the exposed or in the comparison group
Rentschler et al,[19] 2012	Italy	Cross-sectional study	255 adults 63–80 y	Ferroalloy smelters	Soil (ppm) Blood (µg/L) Urine (µg/L)	Age and gender	Luria-Nebraska Motor Battery, stylus and balance plate	For both adolescents and elderly, negative correlations between Mn in soil and motor coordination were shown

(continued on next page)

Table 3
(continued)

Author	Location	Study Design	Participants; Age at Motor Assessment	Source of Mn Exposure	Biomarker/ Environmental Measures	Covariates	Outcome Measure	Results
Lucchini et al,[16] 2014	Brescia, Italy	Cross-sectional study	Exposed n = 153 Reference n = 102 65–75 y	Ferroalloy plant	Air (ng/m³) n = 254 soil (ppm) n = 255 Blood (μg/L) n = 238 Urine (μg/L) n = 239	Age, gender, alcohol, smoke, and distance from the nearest ferro-Mn plant	Luria-Nebraska Neuro-psychological Battery	Air Mn was negatively associated with the motor coordination tests of the Luria-Nebraska Neuropsychological Battery
Viana et al,[44] 2014	Bahia, Brazil	Cross-sectional study	89 adults 15–55 y	Ferro-Mn refinery	Scalp hair (μg/g) n = 81 Fingernail (μg/g) n = 73 Axillary hair (μg/g) n = 18 Saliva (μg/g) n = 82	Age, gender, years of schooling, locale of residence, time in years of residence in the communities, drinking habits, and family income	Grooved-pegboard Test	MnH, MnFN, and MnAxH levels were positively correlated with motor function for the dominant hand
Bowler et al,[25] 2016	Ohio	Cross-sectional study	186 adults 30–75 y	Ferro-Mn smelter	Air (μg/m³) n = 186	Sex, employment status, household income	Finger tapping, hand dynamometer, grooved pegboard, and the CATSYS tremor system	Tremor and motor function were associated with higher exposure to airborne Mn

Study	Location	Design	N / Age	Exposure source	Biomarker/Media	Covariates	Assessment	Findings
Cabral Pinto et al,[18] 2018	Estarreja, Portugal	Cross-sectional study	N = 103 residents 55+ y	Industrial activity	Urine, Water, Soil	Years of residency, medical history, health status, work history, education, water used in irrigation and drinking, use of homegrown foods, daily habits	MMSE, MoCA, CDR Scale	Association between mild dementia and moderate dementia with high contents of Cr, Mn, Cd, and Se. Stream water was associated with dementia and high levels of Cr, Mn, Cd and Se in urine
Kornblith et al,[20] 2018	Ohio	Cross-sectional study	N = 182 30–75 y	Ferro-Mn smelter	Air (µg/m3) n = 182	Age, gender, employment, race, and years of residence	CATSYS, UPDRS	Increased tremor and motor symptoms and executive dysfunction were observed, and TD and NTD symptom clusters were identified

Abbreviations: ALT, alanine transaminase; CDR, Clinical Dementia Rating; GGT, gamma-glutamyl transferase; MMSE, Mini-Mental State Examination; MnAxH, Auxiliary Hair Mn; MoCA, Montreal Cognitive Assessment; NTD, non-tremor dominant; TD, tremor dominant.

neurologic decline and the development of neurodegenerative disorders. Studying older populations provides an insight into the potential health issues that may burden future generations if exposure patterns are not altered. An Italian study recruited older adults living near a ferroalloy plant to represent people with lifelong exposure to environmental Mn.[16] The researchers observed a negative correlation between airborne Mn and coordination, with women showing greater motor dysfunction than men. Using the same cohort, Rentschler and colleagues,[19] in 2012 described a negative association between soil Mn and motor coordination, again with women showing greater motor dysfunction.[19]

Although personal biomarkers are generally preferred, some studies justify applying environmental measures to indicate Mn exposure. In a study of environmentally exposed adults,[20,63] Mn exposure was estimated based on the US Environmental Protection Agency's AERMOD (atmospheric dispersion modeling) dispersion models. Researchers aimed to determine whether subtypes of Mn neurotoxicity were similar to those observed in PD.[20] Among those exposed to low levels of Mn, subtle cognitive impairment was observed; however, there was no indication of motor dysfunction. Findings indicate that PD and Mn-induced motor disorders have distinct pathophysiology patterns.

Neuroimaging

MRI is useful as a biomarker of exposure because of its ability to show Mn accumulation in the brain. Because of its paramagnetic properties, Mn is a longitudinal relaxation time (T1) contrast agent, which means that, when water is excited with radiofrequency pulses within the MRI scanner, the manner in which the signal decays is influenced by accumulated Mn. For T1-weighted images, regions of the brain with Mn accumulation show higher signal than other regions. One method to assess Mn accumulation is with the pallidal index (PI). This metric takes the ratio of signal intensity in 2 anatomic locations of a T1-weighted image, usually the globus pallidus and frontal white matter. PI seems to be higher in exposed groups versus controls[64] and shows a dose-response relationship with blood Mn and recent air-exposure Mn,[26,64] as well as workers' cumulative Mn exposure.[65] Shin and Aschner[66] found a significant relationship between PI and motor dysfunction, as measured by pursuit aiming tests and finger tapping, respectively.

Another method for assessing Mn accumulation in the brain is by directly measuring T1. Because Mn accumulation leads to shorter T1 values, the inverse of the T1, R1 (R1 = 1/T1), is commonly used. Researchers have found that the relationship between Mn exposure and Mn accumulation in the brain is not straightforward. For 1 cohort of welders, R1 increased after 300 hours of work in the past 90 days, suggestive of a Mn exposure threshold below which there are no significant increases in R1.[36,67] In another cohort of welders, R1 increased significantly only for those exposed to air exposure greater than $0.1 \ mg/m^3$.[68] In addition, R1 was sensitive to changes in Mn exposure and changed proportionately with fluctuating levels of Mn exposure.[69] However, changes in R1 in relation to short-term Mn exposure are influenced by the person's lifetime cumulative exposure,[70] suggesting that lifetime exposure may have a longer-lasting effect on Mn retention in the brain. Some studies associated T1 with impaired cognitive performance. Shorter T1 was related to lower performance on verbal fluency, verbal learning, memory, and preservation tests.[23] Verbal dysfunction, which is not commonly tested, may be an early symptom of Mn exposure. In addition, T1 changes have been detected when there is low Mn exposure and before neurologic changes are clinically evident.[71]

MRI technology can also be used to measure neurochemicals in vivo with magnetic resonance spectroscopy (MRS). MRS can measure many chemicals in the millimolar range, including gamma-aminobutyric acid (GABA), the major inhibitory neurotransmitter in the central nervous system. Because of its high abundance in the basal ganglia, GABA has been targeted as a potential biomarker for motor dysfunction with Mn exposure. Consequently, thalamic GABA levels have been found to be higher in workers in smelters[29,72] and welders,[31,70] where it also correlated with Mn exposure as measured at 12-month and -month intervals. In a study of welders by Ma and colleagues[31] (2018), highly exposed welders had higher thalamic GABA levels as well as higher UPDRS3 scores compared with less exposed welders and controls. Although thalamic GABA also correlated with R1 in the substantia nigra and frontal cortex, thalamic GABA did not correlate with UPDRS3 scores. Thalamic GABA changes proportionately with increasing or decreasing Mn exposure in the workplace; however, UPDRS3 scores seem to remain static.[70]

To measure cognitive processes during tasks, functional MRI (fMRI) is a useful biomarker of effect. fMRI is based on the principle that the brain uses more energy in regions of the brain that are used during particular tasks, which results in measurable increased blood flow (seen as blood oxygen level–dependent contrast) in regions of increased cognitive use. To test the effect of Mn on memory, Chang and colleagues[32] (2010) used a commonly used paradigm, the N-back task, where participants are asked to remember pertinent items from N trials previously presented. Chang and colleagues[32] used a 2-back task and found welders have increased brain activity in working memory networks compared with controls. Using the Wisconsin Card-sorting Task (WCST), Seo and colleagues[73] (2016) found that welders had lower activation compared with controls in the areas of the brain related to executive function, such as the prefrontal cortex, under conditions of higher cognitive demand. However, although air Mn exposure was measured in both of these studies, there was large variability within each cohort and air Mn exposure was not taken into account in any of the reported analyses.

In addition, brain structure can be assessed using diffusion tensor imaging (DTI) and voxel-based morphometry (VBM). DTI measures the integrity of white matter by determining how free water can diffuse within a given location. The greater water diffusion is restricted within fibers, the higher its fractional anisotropy (FA), and vice versa. Higher FA corresponds with increased fiber organization. In general, FA has been found to be lower in the corpus collosum,[34] frontal white matter,[34] and basal ganglia[36,74] in welders. Specifically, lower FA was found in the basal ganglia of welders with 30 years or more of experience welding,[36] suggesting that long-term exposure to Mn might have a degradational effect on neuronal integrity beyond normal aging. Lower FA was also related to fine motor dysfunction, as measured by synergy indices.[74]

Using VBM, Chang and colleagues[75] (2013) found decreased brain volume in the globus pallidus and cerebellar regions in welders, which correlated with cognitive performance and grooved-pegboard performance. However, this is the only study to have been performed with significant results in morphometry, which is confounded because of the difficulty in segmenting the basal ganglia because of high signal intensity caused by Mn exposure.

Manganese and Neurodegenerative Diseases

Evidence suggests that, because of accumulation in the brain, neurotoxic metals may play a role in neurodegenerative diseases.[76] Exposure to toxic levels of Mn results in manganism, a neurodegenerative condition, and is implicated in the etiopathogenesis of several prevalent neurodegenerative diseases, including PD and Alzheimer disease

(AD).[77] Because of numerous links between Mn and PD-like symptoms, Mn exposure may be involved with PD development; however, inconsistent results have been reported.[78] A meta-analysis was conducted in 2018 and results suggest that increased Mn concentrations may be a potential risk factor for PD.[79] Multiple assessments may be used to observe the prevalence of parkinsonian symptoms, such as the UPDRS, pegboard tasks, and various motor tasks.[22,36,56] Lee and colleagues[36] observed significantly lower stability in welders compared with controls; however, UPDRS scores were similar. There was an association between cumulative Mn exposure and UPDRS scores in a cohort of US welders.[22] Findings suggest that there are associations between neurodegenerative patterns in Mn toxicity and parkinsonian features along with further potential associations with movement disorder symptoms.[20] Mn seems to accelerate the transmission of misfolded alpha-synuclein, a protein that, when misfolded, clumps and becomes toxic to neurons and has thus been linked to PD.[80] However, contrary to PD, Mn-induced movement disorders likely result from the reduced ability to release dopamine.[78,81,82]

Because of the age distribution among workers, many occupationally based studies do not include senior participants. However, when investigating cognitive decline, older adults may be among the most vulnerable populations to consider when studying the neurotoxic impacts of Mn exposure. More than 35 million people worldwide have dementia and the incidence rate is expected to increase over the next few decades.[83] Dementia is a condition that encompasses significant impairments in memory, thinking abilities, social skills, and behavior.[83] AD, the most common form of dementia, has suggestive causal links with preceding Mn exposure. Pinto and colleagues[18] examined a group of older participants living in close proximity to Estarreja Chemical Complex (ECC), a source of environmental contamination in Portugal. The investigators described an association between mild and moderate dementia and high concentrations of several metals, including Mn. Previous research has proposed that Mn may be a contributing factor in the pathogenesis of AD by disrupting amyloid-β (Aβ) peptide degradation.[84] In a sample of Portuguese residents, Pinto and colleagues[18] observed associations between high concentrations of Mn measured in water and moderate levels of dementia. In mouse models, the intraperitoneal injection of a Mn chelator was effective at reducing Mn levels within the brain, decreasing Aβ peptides, and restoring cognitive function,[84] thereby providing a potential avenue to explore with regard to human intervention. However, opposing observations have been made as well. A meta-analysis conducted by Du and colleagues[85] described low serum Mn levels among people with mild cognitive impairment and AD. Further investigation into the potential relationship between Mn and AD is of great public health and socioeconomic interest.

Summary

Overall, the research included in this review contributes novel and valuable information to the existing literature and provides directions for future research. Innovative biomarkers, including those from advanced neuroimaging, were incorporated into many studies to assess both Mn exposure and neurologic outcomes. Studies examining the effects of occupational exposures to Mn continue to show adverse neurologic outcomes. With participants from communities located near Mn point sources, usually industrial facilities, studies in these populations show variability in the observed effects, which reflects the complexities of Mn exposure measurement, individual absorption, and impairment assessment. Unique populations, specifically those incorporating older adults, were used to study the impact of lifelong Mn exposure and provide insight into what the future may hold for younger exposed populations.

Limitations

The literature is saturated with studies investigating occupational Mn exposure, and, as a result, studies involving women are lacking. Although gender influences the development and progression of AD[86] and PD,[87] hormonal uniqueness is hypothesized to affect the pharmacokinetics of Mn as well.[49] Therefore, gender-based selection bias limits the ability to generalize from many studies. Regarding occupational research, there is possible bias from the healthy worker effect because sicker workers may no longer be actively employed.[58] Inaccurate work history and the lack of a reliable biomarker may contribute to recall bias and exposure misclassification among participants.[22,24,26,30,32,33] In addition, sample size constraints pose a challenge to many epidemiologic studies.[27,30,44–46,60,73,74,88] It is known that coexposures may influence the neurotoxicity of Mn; therefore, possible confounding may be present because of failure to consider concomitant exposures such as tobacco smoke[89] and lead.[90] In addition, because of the cross-sectional nature of many of the reviewed studies, temporality is not feasible to definitively establish and future studies would benefit from using a longitudinal design.

Future Directions

- Elucidating the optimal biomarker of Mn exposure
- Leveraging novel methods, such as neuroimaging, to directly measure Mn exposure and characterize effects
- Considering individual variability with regard to both Mn accumulation and neurotoxicity
- Understanding the role of Mn in neurodegenerative diseases and ultimately developing intervention methods

CLINICS CARE POINTS

- Environmental exposures should be considered when assessing neurodevelopmental deficits and neurodegenerative diseases.
- Those with increased susceptibility to Mn accumulation (ie. individuals with liver diseases, patients receiving parenteral nutrition) should be carefully monitored for Mn associated effects.
- Efforts to mitigate elevated environmental Mn exposure, especially in vulnerable populations, should be taken.

DISCLOSURE

The authors have nothing to disclose.

REFERENCES

1. Aschner M. Manganese: brain transport and emerging research needs. Environ Health Perspect 2000;108(Suppl 3):429–32.
2. Mergler D, Baldwin M, Belanger S, et al. Manganese neurotoxicity, a continuum of dysfunction: results from a community based study. Neurotoxicology 1999; 20(2–3):327–42.
3. Rodier J. Manganese poisoning in Moroccan miners. Br J Ind Med 1955;12(1): 21–35.
4. Vollet K, Haynes EN, Dietrich KN. Manganese exposure and cognition across the lifespan: contemporary review and argument for biphasic dose-response health effects. Curr Environ Health Rep 2016;3(4):392–404.

5. Agency for Toxic Substances and Disease Registry. Toxicological profile for manganese 2019. Available at: https://www.atsdr.cdc.gov/toxprofiles/tp.asp?id=102&tid=23. Accessed July 29, 2019.

6. Aschner JL, Aschner M. Nutritional aspects of manganese homeostasis. Mol Aspects Med 2005;26(4–5):353–62.

7. Peres TV, Schettinger MR, Chen P, et al. Manganese-induced neurotoxicity: a review of its behavioral consequences and neuroprotective strategies. BMC Pharmacol Toxicol 2016;17(1):57.

8. Crossgrove J, Zheng W. Manganese toxicity upon overexposure. NMR Biomed 2004;17(8):544–53.

9. Chen P, Bornhorst J, Aschner M. Manganese metabolism in humans. Front Biosci (Landmark Ed) 2018;23:1655–79.

10. O'Neal SL, Zheng W. Manganese Toxicity Upon Overexposure: a Decade in Review. Curr Environ Health Rep 2015;2(3):315–28.

11. Montes S, Riojas-Rodriguez H, Sabido-Pedraza E, et al. Biomarkers of manganese exposure in a population living close to a mine and mineral processing plant in Mexico. Environ Res 2008;106(1):89–95.

12. Bouabid S, Tinakoua A, Lakhdar-Ghazal N, et al. Manganese neurotoxicity: behavioral disorders associated with dysfunctions in the basal ganglia and neurochemical transmission. J Neurochem 2016;136(4):677–91.

13. Takeda A. Manganese action in brain function. Brain Res Brain Res Rev 2003; 41(1):79–87.

14. Leggett RW. A biokinetic model for manganese. Sci Total Environ 2011;409(20): 4179–86.

15. Zoni S, Albini E, Lucchini R. Neuropsychological testing for the assessment of manganese neurotoxicity: a review and a proposal. Am J Ind Med 2007;50(11): 812–30.

16. Lucchini RG, Guazzetti S, Zoni S, et al. Neurofunctional dopaminergic impairment in elderly after lifetime exposure to manganese. Neurotoxicology 2014;45: 309–17.

17. Lucchini RG, Aschner M, Landrigan PJ, et al. Neurotoxicity of manganese: Indications for future research and public health intervention from the Manganese 2016 conference. Neurotoxicology 2018;64:1–4.

18. Cabral Pinto MMS, Marinho-Reis AP, Almeida A, et al. Human predisposition to cognitive impairment and its relation with environmental exposure to potentially toxic elements. Environ Geochem Health 2018;40(5):1767–84.

19. Rentschler G, Covolo L, Haddad AA, et al. ATP13A2 (PARK9) polymorphisms influence the neurotoxic effects of manganese. Neurotoxicology 2012;33(4): 697–702.

20. Kornblith ES, Casey SL, Lobdell DT, et al. Environmental exposure to manganese in air: Tremor, motor and cognitive symptom profiles. Neurotoxicology 2018;64: 152–8.

21. Hassani H, Golbabaei F, Shirkhanloo H, et al. Relations of biomarkers of manganese exposure and neuropsychological effects among welders and ferroalloy smelters. Ind Health 2016;54(1):79–86.

22. Racette BA, Searles Nielsen S, Criswell SR, et al. Dose-dependent progression of parkinsonism in manganese-exposed welders. Neurology 2017;88(4):344–51.

23. Bowler RM, Yeh CL, Adams SW, et al. Association of MRI T1 relaxation time with neuropsychological test performance in manganese- exposed welders. Neurotoxicology 2018;64:19–29.

24. Chang Y, Kim Y, Woo ST, et al. High signal intensity on magnetic resonance imaging is a better predictor of neurobehavioral performances than blood manganese in asymptomatic welders. Neurotoxicology 2009;30(4):555–63.
25. Bowler RM, Beseler CL, Gocheva VV, et al. Environmental exposure to manganese in air: Associations with tremor and motor function. Sci Total Environ 2016;541:646–54.
26. Shin YC, Kim E, Cheong HK, et al. High signal intensity on magnetic resonance imaging as a predictor of neurobehavioral performance of workers exposed to manganese. Neurotoxicology 2007;28(2):257–62.
27. Cowan DM, Fan Q, Zou Y, et al. Manganese exposure among smelting workers: blood manganese-iron ratio as a novel tool for manganese exposure assessment. Biomarkers 2009;14(1):3–16.
28. Ellingsen DG, Kusraeva Z, Bast-Pettersen R, et al. The interaction between manganese exposure and alcohol on neurobehavioral outcomes in welders. Neurotoxicol Teratol 2014;41:8–15.
29. Long Z, Li XR, Xu J, et al. Thalamic GABA predicts fine motor performance in manganese-exposed smelter workers. PLoS One 2014;9(2):e88220.
30. Laohaudomchok W, Lin X, Herrick RF, et al. Neuropsychological effects of low-level manganese exposure in welders. Neurotoxicology 2011;32(2):171–9.
31. Ma RE, Ward EJ, Yeh CL, et al. Thalamic GABA levels and occupational manganese neurotoxicity: Association with exposure levels and brain MRI. Neurotoxicology 2018;64:30–42.
32. Chang Y, Lee JJ, Seo JH, et al. Altered working memory process in the manganese-exposed brain. Neuroimage 2010;53(4):1279–85.
33. Kim Y, Bowler RM, Abdelouahab N, et al. Motor function in adults of an Ohio community with environmental manganese exposure. Neurotoxicology 2011;32(5):606–14.
34. Kim Y, Jeong KS, Song HJ, et al. Altered white matter microstructural integrity revealed by voxel-wise analysis of diffusion tensor imaging in welders with manganese exposure. Neurotoxicology 2011;32(1):100–9.
35. Zhang H, Xu C, Wang H, et al. Health effects of manganese exposures for welders in Qingdao City, China. Int J Occup Med Environ Health 2017;30(2):241–7.
36. Lee EY, Flynn MR, Lewis MM, et al. Welding-related brain and functional changes in welders with chronic and low-level exposure. Neurotoxicology 2018;64:50–9.
37. Laohaudomchok W, Lin X, Herrick RF, et al. Toenail, blood, and urine as biomarkers of manganese exposure. J Occup Environ Med 2011;53(5):506–10.
38. Zheng W, Fu SX, Dydak U, et al. Biomarkers of manganese intoxication. Neurotoxicology 2011;32(1):1–8.
39. Wang D, Du X, Zheng WJTI. Alteration of saliva and serum concentrations of manganese, copper, zinc, cadmium and lead among career welders. Toxicol Lett 2008;176(1):40–7.
40. Coetzee DJ, McGovern PM, Rao R, et al. Measuring the impact of manganese exposure on children's neurodevelopment: advances and research gaps in biomarker-based approaches. Environ Health 2016;15(1):91.
41. Sriram K, Lin GX, Jefferson AM, et al. Manganese accumulation in nail clippings as a biomarker of welding fume exposure and neurotoxicity. Toxicology 2012;291(1–3):73–82.
42. Liu Y, Byrne P, Wang H, et al. A compact DD neutron generator–based NAA system to quantify manganese (Mn) in bone in vivo. Physiol Meas 2014;35(9):1899.

43. O'Neal SL, Hong L, Fu S, et al. Manganese accumulation in bone following chronic exposure in rats: steady-state concentration and half-life in bone. Toxicol Lett 2014;229(1):93–100.

44. Viana GF, de Carvalho CF, Nunes LS, et al. Noninvasive biomarkers of manganese exposure and neuropsychological effects in environmentally exposed adults in Brazil. Toxicol Lett 2014;231(2):169–78.

45. Rolle-McFarland D, Liu Y, Mostafaei F, et al. The association of bone, fingernail and blood manganese with cognitive and olfactory function in Chinese workers. Sci Total Environ 2019;666:1003–10.

46. Palzes VA, Sagiv SK, Baker JM, et al. Manganese exposure and working memory-related brain activity in smallholder farmworkers in Costa Rica: Results from a pilot study. Environ Res 2019;173:539–48.

47. Ward EJ, Edmondson DA, Nour MM, et al. Toenail manganese: a sensitive and specific biomarker of exposure to manganese in career welders. Ann Work Expo Health 2017;62(1):101–11.

48. Wells EM, Liu Y, Rolle-McFarland D, et al. In vivo measurement of bone manganese and association with manual dexterity: A pilot study. Environ Res 2018; 160:35–8.

49. Finley JW, Johnson PE, Johnson LK. Sex affects manganese absorption and retention by humans from a diet adequate in manganese. Am J Clin Nutr 1994; 60(6):949–55.

50. Finley JW. Manganese absorption and retention by young women is associated with serum ferritin concentration. Am J Clin Nutr 1999;70(1):37–43.

51. Haynes EN, Heckel P, Ryan P, et al. Environmental manganese exposure in residents living near a ferromanganese refinery in Southeast Ohio: a pilot study. Neurotoxicology 2010;31(5):468–74.

52. Thompson K, Molina RM, Donaghey T, et al. Olfactory uptake of manganese requires DMT1 and is enhanced by anemia. FASEB J 2007;21(1):223–30.

53. Claus Henn B, Kim J, Wessling-Resnick M, et al. Associations of iron metabolism genes with blood manganese levels: a population-based study with validation data from animal models. Environ Health 2011;10:97.

54. Anagianni S, Tuschl K. Genetic disorders of manganese metabolism. Curr Neurol Neurosci Rep 2019;19(6):33.

55. Deveau M, Maier A, Krewski D. Application of a framework for the selection of an appropriate occupational exposure limit for manganese. Neurotoxicology 2017; 58:249–56.

56. Racette BA, Criswell SR, Lundin JI, et al. Increased risk of parkinsonism associated with welding exposure. Neurotoxicology 2012;33(5):1356–61.

57. Al-Lozi A, Nielsen SS, Hershey T, et al. Cognitive control dysfunction in workers exposed to manganese-containing welding fume. Am J Ind Med 2017;60(2): 181–8.

58. Bouchard M, Mergler D, Baldwin M, et al. Neurobehavioral functioning after cessation of manganese exposure: a follow-up after 14 years. Am J Ind Med 2007;50(11):831–40.

59. Park RM, Bouchard MF, Baldwin M, et al. Respiratory manganese particle size, time-course and neurobehavioral outcomes in workers at a manganese alloy production plant. Neurotoxicology 2014;45:276–84.

60. Bowler RM, Gocheva V, Harris M, et al. Prospective study on neurotoxic effects in manganese-exposed bridge construction welders. Neurotoxicology 2011;32(5): 596–605.

61. Wastensson G, Sallsten G, Bast-Pettersen R, et al. Neuromotor function in ship welders after cessation of manganese exposure. Int Arch Occup Environ Health 2012;85(6):703–13.

62. Bowler RM, Harris M, Gocheva V, et al. Anxiety affecting parkinsonian outcome and motor efficiency in adults of an Ohio community with environmental airborne manganese exposure. Int J Hyg Environ Health 2012;215(3):393–405.

63. Bowler RM, Kornblith ES, Gocheva VV, et al. Environmental exposure to manganese in air: Associations with cognitive functions. Neurotoxicology 2015;49: 139–48.

64. Li SJ, Jiang L, Fu X, et al. Pallidal index as biomarker of manganese brain accumulation and associated with manganese levels in blood: a meta-analysis. PLoS One 2014;9(4):e93900.

65. Criswell SR, Nielsen SS, Warden MN, et al. MRI signal intensity and parkinsonism in manganese-exposed workers. J Occup Environ Med 2019;61(8):641–5.

66. Soldin OP, Aschner M. Effects of manganese on thyroid hormone homeostasis: potential links. Neurotoxicology 2007;28(5):951–6.

67. Lee EY, Flynn MR, Du G, et al. T1 relaxation rate (R1) indicates nonlinear Mn accumulation in brain tissue of welders with low-level exposure. Toxicol Sci 2015;146(2):281–9.

68. Pesch B, Dydak U, Lotz A, et al. Association of exposure to manganese and iron with relaxation rates R1 and R2*- magnetic resonance imaging results from the WELDOX II study. Neurotoxicology 2018;64:68–77.

69. Lewis MM, Flynn MR, Lee EY, et al. Longitudinal T1 relaxation rate (R1) captures changes in short-term Mn exposure in welders. Neurotoxicology 2016;57:39–44.

70. Edmondson DA, Ma RE, Yeh CL, et al. Reversibility of neuroimaging markers influenced by lifetime occupational manganese exposure. Toxicol Sci 2019; 172(1):181–90.

71. Baker MG, Criswell SR, Racette BA, et al. Neurological outcomes associated with low-level manganese exposure in an inception cohort of asymptomatic welding trainees. Scand J Work Environ Health 2015;41(1):94–101.

72. Dydak U, Jiang YM, Long LL, et al. In vivo measurement of brain GABA concentrations by magnetic resonance spectroscopy in smelters occupationally exposed to manganese. Environ Health Perspect 2011;119(2):219–24.

73. Seo J, Chang Y, Jang KE, et al. Altered executive function in the welders: A functional magnetic resonance imaging study. Neurotoxicol Teratol 2016;56:26–34.

74. Lewis MM, Lee EY, Jo HJ, et al. Synergy as a new and sensitive marker of basal ganglia dysfunction: A study of asymptomatic welders. Neurotoxicology 2016;56: 76–85.

75. Chang Y, Jin SU, Kim Y, et al. Decreased brain volumes in manganese-exposed welders. Neurotoxicology 2013;37:182–9.

76. Chen P, Miah MR, Aschner M. Metals and neurodegeneration. F1000Res 2016;5: 366. https://doi.org/10.12688/f1000research.7431.1.

77. Bowman AB, Kwakye GF, Herrero Hernandez E, et al. Role of manganese in neurodegenerative diseases. J Trace Elem Med Biol 2011;25(4):191–203.

78. Guilarte TR. Manganese and Parkinson's disease: a critical review and new findings. Environ Health Perspect 2010;118(8):1071–80.

79. Du K, Liu MY, Pan YZ, et al. Association of circulating manganese levels with Parkinson's disease: A meta-analysis. Neurosci Lett 2018;665:92–8.

80. Harischandra DS, Ghaisas S, Zenitsky G, et al. Manganese-induced neurotoxicity: new insights into the triad of protein misfolding, mitochondrial impairment, and neuroinflammation. Front Neurosci 2019;13:654.

81. Guilarte TR. Manganese neurotoxicity: new perspectives from behavioral, neuro-imaging, and neuropathological studies in humans and non-human primates. Front Aging Neurosci 2013;5:23.

82. Guilarte TR, Gonzales KK. Manganese-induced parkinsonism is not idiopathic parkinson's disease: environmental and genetic evidence. Toxicol Sci 2015; 146(2):204–12.

83. Organization; WH. Dementia. 2019. Available at: https://www.who.int/news-room/fact-sheets/detail/dementia. Accessed October, 10, 2019.

84. Tong Y, Yang H, Tian X, et al. High manganese, a risk for Alzheimer's disease: high manganese induces amyloid-beta related cognitive impairment. J Alzheimers Dis 2014;42(3):865–78.

85. Du K, Liu M, Pan Y, et al. Association of serum manganese levels with alzheimer's disease and mild cognitive impairment: a systematic review and meta-analysis. Nutrients 2017;9(3):231.

86. Mielke MM, Vemuri P, Rocca WA. Clinical epidemiology of Alzheimer's disease: assessing sex and gender differences. Clin Epidemiol 2014;6:37–48.

87. Haaxma CA, Bloem BR, Borm GF, et al. Gender differences in Parkinson's disease. J Neurol Neurosurg Psychiatry 2007;78(8):819–24.

88. Sen S, Flynn MR, Du G, et al. Manganese accumulation in the olfactory bulbs and other brain regions of "asymptomatic" welders. Toxicol Sci 2011;121(1):160–7.

89. Pappas RS, Gray N, Gonzalez-Jimenez N, et al. Triple Quad-ICP-MS measurement of toxic metals in mainstream cigarette smoke from spectrum research cigarettes. J Anal Toxicol 2016;40(1):43–8.

90. Neal AP, Guilarte TR. Mechanisms of lead and manganese neurotoxicity. Toxicol Res (Camb) 2013;2(2):99–114.

91. Bouchard M, Laforest F, Vandelac L, et al. Hair manganese and hyperactive behaviors: pilot study of school-age children exposed through tap water. Environ Health Perspect 2007;115(1):122–7.

Neurologic Toxicities Associated with Tumor Necrosis Factor Inhibitors and Calcineurin Inhibitors

Christopher L. Coe, MD[a], Sarah N. Horst, MD, MPH[b],
Manhal J. Izzy, MD[c],*

KEYWORDS

- Calcineurin inhibitors • TNF inhibitors • Demyelination • Tremor • PRES
- Transplantation • Rheumatology • Inflammatory bowel disease

KEY POINTS

- Neurotoxic side effects of calcineurin inhibitors range from common and bothersome to rare and serious.
- Tremor and headache are common side effects of calcineurin inhibitors; seizure and severe encephalopathy are much rarer.
- If calcineurin inhibitor toxicity is suspected, a drug trough level should be checked; depending on severity, dose-reduction or medication change should be considered.
- Tumor necrosis factor (TNF) inhibitors are generally well tolerated but may increase the risk of central and peripheral demyelinating disorders.
- If TNF inhibitor demyelination is suspected, usual care for the provoked disorder should be sought, the drug withdrawn, and the class avoided in the future.

CALCINEURIN INHIBITORS
Introduction to the Calcineurin Inhibitors

The calcineurin inhibitors (CNIs) include cyclosporine and tacrolimus. Cyclosporine is a 1203-Da peptide that was discovered from a fungus in the early 1970s in Switzerland. It was unique in that it exhibited immunosuppressive effects without

[a] Department of Medicine, Section of Hospital Medicine, Vanderbilt University Medical Center, 1161 21st Avenue South, Nashville, TN 37232, USA; [b] Division of Gastroenterology, Hepatology and Nutrition, Vanderbilt University Medical Center, 1211 21st Avenue South, Medical Arts Building, Suite 220, Nashville, TN 37232, USA; [c] Division of Gastroenterology, Hepatology and Nutrition, Vanderbilt University Medical Center, Transplant Hepatology, 1660 The Vanderbilt Clinic, Nashville, TN 37232, USA
* Corresponding author.
E-mail address: manhal.izzy@vumc.org
Twitter: @ccoemd (C.L.C.); @HorstIBDDoc (S.N.H.); @manhalizzy (M.J.I.)

Neurol Clin 38 (2020) 937–951
https://doi.org/10.1016/j.ncl.2020.07.009
0733-8619/20/© 2020 Elsevier Inc. All rights reserved.

neurologic.theclinics.com

cytotoxicity.[1] A decade later, a search for fungal derivatives with similar immunosup-pressive effects in a Japanese laboratory led to the discovery of tacrolimus.[2] These drugs have become important parts of the pharmacologic armamentarium against autoimmune disease and rejection of transplanted grafts.

The CNIs exert their immunosuppressive effect by inhibiting T-lymphocyte prolifer-ation and activation.[3,4] They interact with 2 intracellular proteins of the immunophilin class: cyclosporine binds cyclophilin and tacrolimus binds FK-binding protein.[3] The drug-immunophilin compound inactivates calcineurin, which typically dephosphory-lates cytosolic transcription factors, such as nuclear factor of activated T cells, leading to production of critical immunoregulatory proteins, including interleukin-2, inter-leukin-4, CD40, and tumor necrosis factor-α (TNF-α).[5] Deactivation of calcineurin leads to impaired release of these molecules and mediates the immunosuppressive effect of CNIs.[5,6]

Epidemiology and Clinical Impact of Calcineurin Inhibitor–Induced Neurotoxicity

Tremor is among the most common neurotoxicity in patients treated with tacrolimus and cyclosporine. It is seen in up to 56% and 46% of patients, respectively, although studies differ widely.[7] A retrospective review of 386 liver transplant patients treated with postoperative intravenous cyclosporine revealed that all patients with cyclosporine-related neurotoxicity exhibited tremor, identifying this symptom as an important indicator of toxicity.[8] Tremor is more common in tacrolimus than in cyclo-sporine.[7,9] CNI-related tremor is classically fine and involves the upper extremities, especially upon extention.[10,11]

Headache is also commonly reported. Large multicenter comparisons between tacrolimus and cyclosporine place the incidence of headache to be between 44% to 64% and 38% to 60%, respectively, and show increased incidence in tacrolimus-treated patients.[7,12] The headache associated with calcineurin inhibition is typically migrainous, occipital, and frequent, tending to occur at least weekly.[13] In a 2005 review of symptoms after solid organ transplantation, 38% of 74 transplant pa-tients reported new headache after treatment with cyclosporine or tacrolimus, and 23% reported worsening of pretransplant headache symptoms.[13]

Paresthesia and peripheral neuropathy have also been reported. Incidence rates vary, but may be as high as 40% for tacrolimus and 30% for cyclosporine.[7] Palmar and plantar burning have been reported as well.[14]

Neuropsychiatric activation ranging from agitation and insomnia to psychosis is a frequently cited complication of calcineurin inhibition.[12,15] A small review of 13 pa-tients with cyclosporine-associated neurotoxicity noted that 11 had "flushing, headache, and insomnia secondary to mind racing." The same paper noted that 8 patients had symptoms including "agitation and anxiety."[16] In a larger review, Pirsch and colleagues[12] reported that 32% of patients treated with cyclosporine and 30% of patients treated with tacrolimus complained of insomnia. Anxiety was noted in 14% and 8%, respectively. The difference in incidence between cyclosporine and tacrolimus was not significant. In a 545-patient trial in liver trans-plants, psychosis was identified in about 5% of cyclosporine- and tacrolimus-treated patients.[17]

Major neurologic complications have also been reported. The reported incidence of posttransplant seizure, regardless of immunosuppression, varies widely (2%–24% based on 1 review).[11] A study that followed approximately 800 transplant patients treated with tacrolimus revealed that the incidence of seizure was less than 1%.[18] Although generalized seizures are typical for CNI-related seizures,[8,10] focal seizures have also been described.[18]

A collection of severe symptoms are described in case reports, including visual changes and cortical blindness,[19,20] dysarthria and akinetic mutism with swallowing difficulties,[21,22] extrapyramidal or Parkinsonian symptoms,[23] severe psychomotor depression, stupor, or coma,[24,25] and delusions and psychosis.[26] Although often mentioned in previous reviews,[10,15,27] these symptoms are inconsistently detailed in larger studies, and reliable epidemiologic data remain lacking.

Encephalopathy associated with treatment with cyclosporine or tacrolimus is often accompanied by transient white matter changes consistent with posterior reversible encephalopathy syndrome (PRES). Since the syndrome's identification as a clinical entity by Hinchey and colleagues[28] in 1996, calcineurin inhibition, along with acute hypertension, has been identified as a potential cause of PRES. A large retrospective review of more than 4000 solid organ transplants found that PRES occurred in 0.5% of patients treated with cyclosporine or tacrolimus.[29] Although cyclosporine has been shown to increase blood pressure more than tacrolimus,[30] available data suggest that tacrolimus is more likely to precipitate PRES.[31] A 2015 review of multiple case reports of CNI-associated PRES noted that more than 50% of CNI-treated patients with seizures or encephalopathy had radiographic findings associated with PRES.[32] The incidence of PRES may be higher when CNIs are used after stem cell transplant.[33]

The long-term neurologic sequelae of immunosuppression with CNIs have not been well studied. Recently, however, data have emerged revealing that patients treated with long-term calcineurin inhibition have impaired visuospatial ability and impaired global cognitive function when compared with controls.[34] The study was small (20 controls treated with CNI-free immunosuppression after liver transplant and 35 patients treated with CNI), and further conformational data are needed.

Mechanisms of Neurotoxicity

Calcineurin is enriched in the central nervous system (CNS) and is thought to be the only calcium-activated phosphatase in the brain.[14,35] Both cyclosporine (1203 Da) and tacrolimus (804 Da) are large molecules and are not expected to permeate the blood-brain barrier (BBB) quickly.[4,14] Furthermore, both cyclosporine[36] and tacrolimus[37] are substrates of the drug efflux pump p-glycoprotein, which limits penetration into the CNS.

Data from in vitro studies show that cyclosporine and tacrolimus may increase permeability of the BBB, possibly by decreasing the expression of p-glycoprotein.[38] The vasoconstrictive properties of CNIs may also increase BBB permeability.[38,39] The BBB in patients treated with cyclosporine and tacrolimus is further compromised by a plethora of comorbid conditions, including hypertension (a known effect of CNIs), infection (not uncommon in immunosuppressed patients), or the attendant metabolic derangements involved in recent organ failure or ongoing inflammatory conditions (**Fig. 1**).

Altered magnesium handling has also been implicated in seizure and encephalopathy, although with conflicting evidence.[27] CNI-treated patients tend to be more hypomagnesemic than controls.[40] Tacrolimus causes more hypomagnesemia than cyclosporine, which may in part explain its more severe neurotoxic profile.[9,41]

Once within the CNS, the toxic effects of cyclosporine and tacrolimus are likely mediated by calcineurin inhibition.[14,27] It has been shown that cyclosporine decreases brain concentrations of gamma-aminobutyric acid (GABA), a critical neurotransmitter that decreases neuroexcitation.[42] In addition, N-methyl-D-aspartate (NMDA) plays a role in seizure,[43] and calcineurin has been shown to modulate the sensitivity of NMDA receptors.[44]

There are conflicting data regarding the mechanism of CNI-induced headache, but nitrous oxide (NO) may be involved. NO is thought to play an important role in the

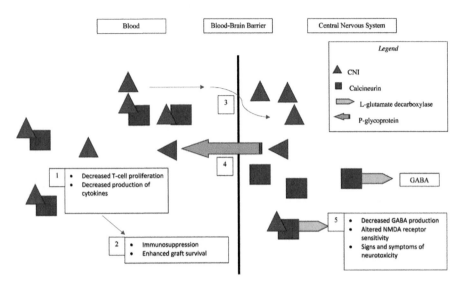

Fig. 1. Simplified schema of the mechanism of action and mechanism of neurotoxicity of the CNIs. (1) CNIs bind and inhibit calcineurin, leading to decreased T-cell proliferation and decreased production of cytokines. (2) This leads to immunosuppression and increased graft survival. (3) The BBB makes access to the CNS difficult, but CNI-induced vasoconstriction and metabolic derangements present in patients receiving CNIs may increase permeability. (4) The efflux pump p-glycoprotein works to decrease CNI concentration in the CNS, but CNIs themselves may decrease its expression. (5) Within the CNS, calcineurin inhibition leads to the neurotoxic effects presented in this article. One mechanism may be decreased GABA production via inhibition of L-glutamate decarboxylase.

cause of cephalgia.[45] In vitro, cultured human brain endothelial cells exposed to cyclosporine and tacrolimus have been shown to produce significantly more NO than controls not exposed to CNIs.[13] Interestingly, this is at odds with previous data that show that calcineurin is needed to activate NO synthase.[46]

There are emerging neuroradiologic data using MRI that reveal structural changes in the brains of CNI-treated transplant recipients. In a recently published study, Goede and colleagues[47] followed patients who were initially treated with standard CNI doses post–liver transplant but were then transitioned to CNI-free, low-, standard-, or high-dose CNI regimens. Compared with controls, brain MRIs of those treated with low-dose and CNI-free regimens showed more cerebral free water, decreased neuronal transmission, and decreased spatial organization of nerve fibers. The median time since liver transplant was 10 years in this study. The investigators hypothesize that the patients switched to low-dose or CNI-free regimens were switched because of toxicity, and that the changes seen on MRI may be due to CNI toxicity. Other investigators have found increased microangiopathic brain lesions in CNI-treated transplant patients, raising vascular changes as a possible neurotoxic mechanism.[34]

Although many studies have focused on the toxic role that CNIs may play in the CNS, peripheral neuropathy remains an important neurotoxic effect that warrants consideration. A 2013 study showed that peripheral nerves of kidney transplant recipients treated with CNIs had changes in multiple parameters, including the depolarization threshold.[48] The investigators propose that the mechanism is mediated by calcineurin's role in modulating Na/K ATPase activity.

Risk Factors for Neurotoxicity

As noted above, available data suggest that treatment with tacrolimus is more likely to lead to neurotoxicity than treatment with cyclosporine. Cyclosporine comes as a standard formulation (Sandimmune, Gengraf) or a lipid emulsion (Neoral); although some have argued that patients treated with the microemulsion may be less likely to develop toxicities,[10] this has not been demonstrated by available data.[49]

The setting in which calcineurin inhibition is prescribed can confer risk for development of neurotoxicity. In liver transplant, older recipient age, pretransplant model for end-stage liver disease score, and pretransplant and posttransplant sodium levels were identified as risk factors for CNI neurotoxicity.[25,50,51] The several days to months immediately after transplant may be particularly high risk for significant CNI-related neurotoxicity.[31,52]

Yamauchi and colleagues[53] showed that distinct polymorphisms in the MDR1 gene, which encodes p-glycoprotein, can confer increased risk of tacrolimus-induced developing neurotoxicity. This test is not available for clinical use.

Although high blood levels of tacrolimus are associated with tacrolimus-induced neurotoxicity,[53] drug levels do not appear to correlate well with the incidence of PRES.[29,54] Measured drug levels are often reported as troughs, but peak levels may be more useful in determining risks of neurotoxicity.[55] Indeed, dosing with intravenous formulations, which leads to rapid peak levels, appears to confer a greater risk of neurotoxicity.[27]

Management

Any CNI-treated patient who presents with neurologic symptoms suspicious for CNI-induced neurotoxicity should be assessed by a transplant physician as well as a transplant pharmacist. Dose reduction is recommended and is often effective, based on the outcome of case reports.[52] Although supported by limited data, some investigators suggest a tacrolimus trough concentration between 5 and 8 ng/mL to reduce the risk of neurotoxicity.[56] If the patient is receiving tacrolimus, symptoms are likely to improve if switched to cyclosporine.[57] If there is suboptimal clinical response to medication adjustment, consultation by a neurologist should be sought.

In addition to CNI regimen-related changes, several interventions have been proposed to manage neurotoxicity in this patient population. It has been noted that CNI-related tremor responds well to β-blockade.[11] When treating seizure, magnesium may be an important adjunct to the anticonvulsive prescription.[27,40] Electroencephalography should be considered to assess for focal status epilepticus. Neuroimaging should be pursued in patients with convulsions or encephalopathy to rule out structural or infectious causes of symptoms, and to assess for the presence of PRES. The diagnosis of PRES is best made with MRI; gadolinium enhancement is not necessary.[58] If PRES is confirmed, blood pressure should be strictly controlled, and, with the guidance of a multidisciplinary transplant team, the offending immunosuppressant should be discontinued.[54]

Clinics Care Points

- CNIs are associated with multiple neurotoxicities.
- Common neurotoxic effects include tremor, headache, and neuropathy.
- Rarer and serious neurotoxic events include seizure, PRES, and encephalopathy.
- Tacrolimus is more neurotoxic than cyclosporine.

- In addition to usual treatment of the provoked event, management includes dose-reduction, switching between CNIs, or using a CNI-sparing regimen.

TUMOR NECROSIS FACTOR-α INHIBITORS
Introduction to the Tumor Necrosis Factor-α Inhibitors

The anti-TNFs include adalimumab, etanercept, infliximab, certolizumab, and golimumab. Biosimilar formulations of these parent compounds have recently entered the market. Biosimilars are biologic compounds that are similar enough to their parent compound as to have no meaningful pharmacologic difference.[59]

Anti-TNF medications exert their therapeutic effect by inhibiting TNF-α, a cytokine that has a central role in inflammation and immunity.[60] TNF-α mediates downstream immunoregulatory and proinflammatory effects after binding 1 of 2 TNF receptors (TNFr1 and TNFr2), which are present peripherally and in the CNS.[61,62] Anti-TNFs have important roles in the treatment of autoimmune conditions, such as inflammatory arthropathies, psoriasis, and inflammatory bowel disease (IBD), which includes Crohn disease (CD) and ulcerative colitis (UC). Side effects are rare. They include infections, infusion or injection reactions, and neurotoxicity, particularly a possible link to demyelinating conditions.

Epidemiology and Clinical Impact of Anti–tumor Necrosis Factor–Associated Neurotoxicity

Mohan and colleagues[63] first raised the possibility of a link between anti-TNFs and demyelinating disorders in 2001 when they identified 19 patients with inflammatory arthritis treated with etanercept (17) and infliximab (2) who presented with visual symptoms, paresthesias, and confusion. Neuroimaging was consistent with demyelinating disease. Symptoms improved after discontinuation of anti-TNF therapy. Because of these concerns and subsequent case reports, the most recent Food and Drug Administration (FDA) prescription guides for all 5 anti-TNF inhibitors include a warning regarding multiple sclerosis (MS), optic neuritis, transverse myelitis, Guillain-Barre, seizure, and demyelinating peripheral neuropathies.[64–68]

Neurotoxicities, namely central (MS[63,69,70]) and peripheral (Guillain-Barre and Miller-Fischer syndrome,[71,72] chronic inflammatory demyelinating peripheral neuropathy,[73] and, more rarely, mononeuropathy simplex, mononeuropathy multiplex, and multifocal motor neuropathy[74,75]) demyelinating disorders, have been detailed in case reports. In a large safety analysis of adalimumab for CD that evaluated multiple clinical trials, the incidence of demyelinating disorders was calculated to be less than 0.1 event per 100 patient-years.[76] A retrospective study that followed 500 patients treated with infliximab for CD identified only 1 patient who developed an MS-like syndrome.[77] Smaller studies evaluating the safety of certolizumab (n = 60) and golimumab (n = 115) in CD identified only 1 neurotoxic event (peripheral neuropathy) in a patient treated with golimumab.[78,79] Overall, the risk of demyelinating disease is estimated at less than 1 event per 1000 patients during anti-TNF treatment.[80] In a review of 75 cases of patients treated with anti-TNFs who developed a demyelinating disorder, the mean time to onset was 17 months from initiation of anti-TNF therapy. The range was 1 month to 6 years.[61] Peripheral demyelinating neuropathies are even rarer.[81]

There are similarly low incidences of neurologic toxicity when assessing the rheumatologic literature. A large (10,050 patients over 12,506 patient-years) safety analysis of patients with rheumatoid arthritis (RA) treated with adalimumab identified only 10 patients who developed demyelinating disease and calculated a rate of 0.08 demyelinating events per 100 patient-years.[82] Some large studies evaluating safety of anti-TNFs in rheumatologic diseases do not identify any instances of demyelinating conditions.[83,84]

Other neurologic complications have been noted as well, although are even rarer. Deepak and colleagues[85] searched the FDA Adverse Events Reporting System for neurologic complications of anti-TNFs. They noted reports of encephalopathy, facial palsy, and transverse myelitis. Seizures during anti-TNF have also been noted but are exceedingly rare, and a causal link has not been definitively established.[86,87]

Causation or Disease Association?

Data support an association between MS and other autoimmune conditions, such as IBD and psoriasis, regardless of drug exposure. Nielsen and colleagues[88] showed that among patients with MS, the relative risk of developing CD is about 2. Another study by Kimura and colleagues[89] established a relative risk of developing MS in the IBD population of 3.7. A large 2005 cohort study that compared incidence rates of MS, optic neuritis, and other demyelinating diseases in 20,000 patients with IBD to more than 80,000 controls established an incidence rate ratio of 1.54 for CD and 2.63 for UC.[90] This association has been further supported by a large metaanalysis by Dobson and Giovannoni,[91] who reported a significantly increased risk of CD and UC in patients with MS, with an overall odds ratio of 1.4 and 2.2, respectively. Similarly, Egeberg and colleagues[92] demonstrated that patients with psoriasis have an increased risk of developing MS. Importantly, they controlled for confounders, including exposure to anti-TNFs.

Patients with IBD also have a higher baseline risk of peripheral nerve disease, regardless of anti-TNF exposure. In a retrospective study of 638 IBD patients, nearly 1% also carried a diagnosis of Guillain-Barre syndrome.[93] Another study reported that 19% of 21 patients with IBD complained of tingling or numbness in the hands or feet. Notably, objective measurements of motor and sensory conduction velocities were normal in these patients.[94]

Although a large case-controlled analysis of RA patients showed a trend toward increased incidences of demyelinating disorders in those treated with anti-TNFs, this trend did not meet statistical significance.[95] A similar longitudinal case-control study that included 22,310 patients with CD on various treatment regimens failed to definitively show that anti-TNF therapy increased the risk of MS significantly above baseline. Interestingly, when the investigators included optic neuritis in their analysis, the association with anti-TNF therapy was significant.[96]

Other data do support a causal relationship between anti-TNF exposure and development of demyelinating conditions. The anti-TNF lenercept was evaluated as a possible treatment for MS in a double-blind, placebo-controlled study. This study was terminated early after patients in the lenercept arm experienced more frequent MS exacerbations.[97] Furthermore, in a systemic review of 122 cases of TNF-associated demyelination, the mean age of onset of demyelination was 45.7 years, older than expected for MS generally, suggesting of a causal role for anti-TNF exposure.[61]

Possible Mechanisms of Neurotoxicity

It is notable that higher levels of TNF-α are found in the sera of MS patients before a flare and in MS-associated cerebral plaques.[98] Anti-TNFs are not expected to penetrate the BBB and would not be able to neutralize TNF-α within the CNS. In decreasing systemic TNF-α concentrations, the relative concentration of TNF-α in the CNS would increase, and it has been proposed that this may lead to upregulation of central TNF-α receptors, leading to inflammation.[99]

Interestingly, TNF-α been shown to suppress T-cell proliferation and cytokine production in certain murine models.[100] It has been suggested that anti-TNF treatment may thus lead to increased survival of peripheral myelin-specific T cells, which can then move within the CNS and attack nerve sheaths.[99]

Management and Prognosis

Given the rarity of anti-TNF–associated neurotoxicities, there are no guidelines for their management beyond the standard care and withdrawal of the anti-TNF. Anti-TNFs should be avoided in patients with a history of MS if feasible.[61] Sometimes, usual

Table 1
Highlighted neurotoxicities of calcineurin inhibitors and antitumor necrosis factors, their frequency, and notes on management

	Neurotoxicities	Frequency	Management[a]
Calcineurin inhibitors Cyclosporine (Gengraf) Tacrolimus (Prograf)	Tremor	May affect >50% of patients, tacrolimus > cyclosporine[7,12]	Consider β-blockade[11]
	Headache	Up to 38% may experience new headache after drug initiation; 23% may have worsening of existing headache symptoms[13]	Standard treatment. Note that verapamil may increase cyclosporine levels and worsen headache[10]
	Paraesthesia	30%-40% of patients tacrolimus > cyclosporine[7,12]	Limited data
	Seizure	Likely around 1%, although some studies with incidence as high as 20%[11,18]	Standard treatment; also consider magnesium administration. Note that phenytoin, carbamazepine, and phenobarbital will decrease cyclosporine levels[27]
	PRES	Around 0.5%, tacrolimus > cyclosporine[29]	Standard treatment, including strict blood pressure control. The offending immunosupressant should be discontinued with the guidance of a multidiscplinary transplant team
Anti-TNFs Adalimumab (Humira) Certolizumab (Cimzia) Etanercept (Enbrel) Golimumab (Simponi) Infliximab (Remicade)	Central demyelinating disorders and peripheral demyelinating disorders	Very rare; incidence rates have been calculated to be as low as 0.1 event per 100 patient-years. Peripheral disorders may be even rarer[76,81]	Consider avoiding this class in patients with personal history of demyelination. Consider cessation of drug

[a] For all symptoms, dose reduction, switching to the other CNI, or using a CNI-free regimen should be considered in collaboration with a multidisciplinary transplant team.

treatment of demyelinating neuropathies is required, such as intravenous immuno-globulin, corticosteroids, and plasma exchange.[61,81]

Prognoses are generally, although not universally, favorable. For example, in a report of infliximab-associated central demyelination, symptoms improved after discontinuation of infliximab.[70] A report of adalimumab-associated Guillain-Barre syndrome also showed improvement at 8 months after drug discontinuation.[71] However, in a case of etanercept-associated MS, new lesions developed even after discontinuation of the anti-TNF, and high-dose steroids were required to induce remission.[69] In a case series presented by Lozeron and colleagues,[81] of 5 patients with anti-TNF–associated peripheral neuropathy, 2 had complete recovery after discontinuation and intravenous immune globulin administration, 2 were left with minor symptoms, and 1 continued to have disabling symptoms. In a larger series of 15 patients with anti-TNF–associated neurotoxicities who were assessed at a follow-up interval between 6 weeks and 7 months, 10 had at least partial resolution of their symptoms.[63]

Clinics Care Points

- Patients treated with anti-TNFs may be at higher risk of developing central or peripheral demyelinating disorders.

- Management includes withdrawal of the anti-TNF and usual care for the demyelinating disorder, which may include intravenous immunoglobulin, plasma exchange, or high-dose steroids.

- Prognosis is typically, but not always, favorable.

- Anti-TNFs should be avoided if possible in patients with a history of demyelination.

SUMMARY

In conclusion, neurotoxicity from CNIs is common and ranges from tremor to encephalopathy, whereas anti-TNF neurotoxicity is rare and mainly manifests as demyelinating disease (**Table 1**). Outcomes are variable, but most reports suggest resolution or improvement with cessation of the offending medication. Switching to a different class is needed in case of anti-TNF–related demyelinating disease, whereas switching to an alternative of the same class may sometimes suffice in case of CNI-related neurotoxicity. Recognition of the risk factors for these toxicities is essential for decreasing their incidence in this patient population.

DISCLOSURE

M.J. Izzy and C.L. Coe report no commercial or financial conflicts of interest. S.N. Horst has been a consultant to Janssen. S.N. Horst has also been a consultant for Gilead.

REFERENCES

1. Borel JF, Feurer C, Gubler HU, et al. Biological effects of cyclosporin A: a new antilymphocytic agent. Agents Actions 1976;6(4):468–75.
2. Kino T, Hatanaka H, Miyata S, et al. FK-506, a novel immunosuppressant isolated from a streptomyces. II. Immunosuppressive effect of FK-506 in vitro. J Antibiot (Tokyo) 1987;40(9):1256–65.

3. Azzi JR, Sayegh MH, Mallat SG. Calcineurin inhibitors: 40 years later, can't live without. J Immunol 2013;191(12):5785–91.

4. Kapturczak MH, Meier-Kriesche HU, Kaplan B. Pharmacology of calcineurin antagonists. Transplant Proc 2004;36(2 Suppl):25S–32S.

5. Rao A, Luo C, Hogan PG. Transcription factors of the NFAT family: regulation and function. Annu Rev Immunol 1997;15:707–47.

6. Bunjes D, Hardt C, Rollinghoff M, et al. Cyclosporin A mediates immunosuppression of primary cytotoxic T cell responses by impairing the release of interleukin 1 and interleukin 2. Eur J Immunol 1981;11(8):657–61.

7. U.S. Multicenter FK506 Liver Study Group. A comparison of tacrolimus (FK 506) and cyclosporine for immunosuppression in liver transplantation. N Engl J Med 1994;331(17):1110–5.

8. Wijdicks EF, Wiesner RH, Krom RA. Neurotoxicity in liver transplant recipients with cyclosporine immunosuppression. Neurology 1995;45(11):1962–4.

9. Margreiter R. European Tacrolimus vs Ciclosporin Microemulsion Renal Transplantation Study G. Efficacy and safety of tacrolimus compared with ciclosporin microemulsion in renal transplantation: a randomised multicentre study. Lancet 2002;359(9308):741–6.

10. Wijdicks EF. Neurotoxicity of immunosuppressive drugs. Liver Transpl 2001; 7(11):937–42.

11. Senzolo M, Ferronato C, Burra P. Neurologic complications after solid organ transplantation. Transpl Int 2009;22(3):269–78.

12. Pirsch JD, Miller J, Deierhoi MH, et al. A comparison of tacrolimus (FK506) and cyclosporine for immunosuppression after cadaveric renal transplantation. FK506 Kidney Transplant Study Group. Transplantation 1997;63(7):977–83.

13. Ferrari U, Empl M, Kim KS, et al. Calcineurin inhibitor-induced headache: clinical characteristics and possible mechanisms. Headache 2005;45(3):211–4.

14. Tan T, Robinson P. Mechanisms of calcineurin inhibitor-induced neurotoxicity. Transplant Rev 2006;20:49–60.

15. Gijtenbeek JM, van den Bent MJ, Vecht CJ. Cyclosporine neurotoxicity: a review. J Neurol 1999;246(5):339–46.

16. de Groen PC, Aksamit AJ, Rakela J, et al. Central nervous system toxicity after liver transplantation. The role of cyclosporine and cholesterol. N Engl J Med 1987;317(14):861–6.

17. Neuhaus P, McMaster P, Calne R, et al. Neurological complications in the European multicentre study of FK 506 and cyclosporin in primary liver transplantation. Transpl Int 1994;7(Suppl 1):S27–31.

18. Eidelman BH, Abu-Elmagd K, Wilson J, et al. Neurologic complications of FK 506. Transplant Proc 1991;23(6):3175–8.

19. Kapoor KG, Mirza SN, Gonzales JA, et al. Visual loss associated with tacrolimus: case report and review of the literature. Cutan Ocul Toxicol 2010;29(2):137–9.

20. Knower MT, Pethke SD, Valentine VG. Reversible cortical blindness after lung transplantation. South Med J 2003;96(6):606–12.

21. Najera JE, Alousi A, De Lima M, et al. Akinetic mutism-a serious complication to tacrolimus-based GVHD prophylaxis. Bone Marrow Transplant 2013;48(1): 157–8.

22. Bronster DJ, Gurkan A, Buchsbaum MS, et al. Tacrolimus-associated mutism after orthotopic liver transplantation. Transplantation 2000;70(6):979–82.

23. Gmitterova K, Minar M, Zigrai M, et al. Tacrolimus-induced parkinsonism in a patient after liver transplantation - case report. BMC Neurol 2018;18(1):44.

24. Beresford TP. Neuropsychiatric complications of liver and other solid organ transplantation. Liver Transpl 2001;7(11 Suppl 1):S36–45.
25. DiMartini A, Fontes P, Dew MA, et al. Age, model for end-stage liver disease score, and organ functioning predict posttransplant tacrolimus neurotoxicity. Liver Transpl 2008;14(6):815–22.
26. Krishna N, Chiappelli J, Fischer BA, et al. Tacrolimus-induced paranoid delusions and fugue-like state. Gen Hosp Psychiatry 2013;35(3):327.e5-6.
27. Bechstein WO. Neurotoxicity of calcineurin inhibitors: impact and clinical management. Transpl Int 2000;13(5):313–26.
28. Hinchey J, Chaves C, Appignani B, et al. A reversible posterior leukoencephalopathy syndrome. N Engl J Med 1996;334(8):494–500.
29. Bartynski WS, Tan HP, Boardman JF, et al. Posterior reversible encephalopathy syndrome after solid organ transplantation. AJNR Am J Neuroradiol 2008;29(5):924–30.
30. Lucey MR, Abdelmalek MF, Gagliardi R, et al. A comparison of tacrolimus and cyclosporine in liver transplantation: effects on renal function and cardiovascular risk status. Am J Transplant 2005;5(5):1111–9.
31. Cruz RJ Jr, DiMartini A, Akhavanheidari M, et al. Posterior reversible encephalopathy syndrome in liver transplant patients: clinical presentation, risk factors and initial management. Am J Transplant 2012;12(8):2228–36.
32. Song T, Rao Z, Tan Q, et al. Calcineurin inhibitors associated posterior reversible encephalopathy syndrome in solid organ transplantation: report of 2 cases and literature review. Medicine (Baltimore) 2016;95(14):e3173.
33. Kapoor R, Simalti A, Kumar R, et al. PRES in pediatric HSCT: a single-center experience. J Pediatr Hematol Oncol 2018;40(6):433–7.
34. Pflugrad H, Schrader AK, Tryc AB, et al. Longterm calcineurin inhibitor therapy and brain function in patients after liver transplantation. Liver Transpl 2018;24(1):56–66.
35. Mansuy IM. Calcineurin in memory and bidirectional plasticity. Biochem Biophys Res Commun 2003;311(4):1195–208.
36. Shirai A, Naito M, Tatsuta T, et al. Transport of cyclosporin A across the brain capillary endothelial cell monolayer by P-glycoprotein. Biochim Biophys Acta 1994;1222(3):400–4.
37. Yokogawa K, Takahashi M, Tamai I, et al. P-glycoprotein-dependent disposition kinetics of tacrolimus: studies in mdr1a knockout mice. Pharm Res 1999;16(8):1213–8.
38. Kochi S, Takanaga H, Matsuo H, et al. Effect of cyclosporin A or tacrolimus on the function of blood-brain barrier cells. Eur J Pharmacol 1999;372(3):287–95.
39. Kochi S, Takanaga H, Matsuo H, et al. Induction of apoptosis in mouse brain capillary endothelial cells by cyclosporin A and tacrolimus. Life Sci 2000;66(23):2255–60.
40. Ledeganck KJ, De Winter BY, Van den Driessche A, et al. Magnesium loss in cyclosporine-treated patients is related to renal epidermal growth factor down-regulation. Nephrol Dial Transplant 2014;29(5):1097–102.
41. Aisa Y, Mori T, Nakazato T, et al. Effects of immunosuppressive agents on magnesium metabolism early after allogeneic hematopoietic stem cell transplantation. Transplantation 2005;80(8):1046–50.
42. Shuto H, Kataoka Y, Fujisaki K, et al. Inhibition of GABA system involved in cyclosporine-induced convulsions. Life Sci 1999;65(9):879–87.
43. Kapur J. Role of NMDA receptors in the pathophysiology and treatment of status epilepticus. Epilepsia Open 2018;3(Suppl 2):165–8.

44. Krupp JJ, Vissel B, Thomas CG, et al. Calcineurin acts via the C-terminus of NR2A to modulate desensitization of NMDA receptors. Neuropharmacology 2002;42(5):593–602.

45. Olesen J. The role of nitric oxide (NO) in migraine, tension-type headache and cluster headache. Pharmacol Ther 2008;120(2):157–71.

46. Dawson TM, Steiner JP, Dawson VL, et al. Immunosuppressant FK506 enhances phosphorylation of nitric oxide synthase and protects against glutamate neurotoxicity. Proc Natl Acad Sci U S A 1993;90(21):9808–12.

47. Goede LL, Pflugrad H, Schmitz B, et al. Quantitative magnetic resonance imaging indicates brain tissue alterations in patients after liver transplantation. PLoS One 2019;14(9):e0222934.

48. Arnold R, Pussell BA, Pianta TJ, et al. Association between calcineurin inhibitor treatment and peripheral nerve dysfunction in renal transplant recipients. Am J Transplant 2013;13(9):2426–32.

49. Cole E, Keown P, Landsberg D, et al. Safety and tolerability of cyclosporine and cyclosporine microemulsion during 18 months of follow-up in stable renal transplant recipients: a report of the Canadian Neoral Renal Study Group. Transplantation 1998;65(4):505–10.

50. Lue A, Martinez E, Navarro M, et al. Donor age predicts calcineurin inhibitor induced neurotoxicity after liver transplantation. Transplantation 2019;103(8): e211–5.

51. Balderramo D, Prieto J, Cardenas A, et al. Hepatic encephalopathy and post-transplant hyponatremia predict early calcineurin inhibitor-induced neurotoxicity after liver transplantation. Transpl Int 2011;24(8):812–9.

52. Mueller AR, Platz KP, Bechstein WO, et al. Neurotoxicity after orthotopic liver transplantation. A comparison between cyclosporine and FK506. Transplantation 1994;58(2):155–70.

53. Yamauchi A, Ieiri I, Kataoka Y, et al. Neurotoxicity induced by tacrolimus after liver transplantation: relation to genetic polymorphisms of the ABCB1 (MDR1) gene. Transplantation 2002;74(4):571–2.

54. Fischer M, Schmutzhard E. Posterior reversible encephalopathy syndrome. J Neurol 2017;264(8):1608–16.

55. Wijdicks EF, Wiesner RH, Dahlke LJ, et al. FK506-induced neurotoxicity in liver transplantation. Ann Neurol 1994;35(4):498–501.

56. Varghese J, Reddy MS, Venugopal K, et al. Tacrolimus-related adverse effects in liver transplant recipients: its association with trough concentrations. Indian J Gastroenterol 2014;33(3):219–25.

57. Emre S, Genyk Y, Schluger LK, et al. Treatment of tacrolimus-related adverse effects by conversion to cyclosporine in liver transplant recipients. Transpl Int 2000;13(1):73–8.

58. Karia SJ, Rykken JB, McKinney ZJ, et al. Utility and significance of gadolinium-based contrast enhancement in posterior reversible encephalopathy syndrome. AJNR Am J Neuroradiol 2016;37(3):415–22.

59. Biosimilar and interchangable products. U.S Food and Drug Administration. 2017. Available at: https://www.fda.gov/drugs/biosimilars/biosimilar-and-interchangeable-products. Accessed November 15, 2019.

60. Carswell EA, Old LJ, Kassel RL, et al. An endotoxin-induced serum factor that causes necrosis of tumors. Proc Natl Acad Sci U S A 1975;72(9):3666–70.

61. Kemanetzoglou E, Andreadou E. CNS demyelination with TNF-alpha blockers. Curr Neurol Neurosci Rep 2017;17(4):36.

62. Probert L. TNF and its receptors in the CNS: the essential, the desirable and the deleterious effects. Neuroscience 2015;302:2–22.

63. Mohan N, Edwards ET, Cupps TR, et al. Demyelination occurring during anti-tumor necrosis factor alpha therapy for inflammatory arthritides. Arthritis Rheum 2001;44(12):2862–9.

64. AMGEN. Enbrel: full prescribing information. US Food and Drug Administration. 2018. Available at: https://www.accessdata.fda.gov/scripts/cder/safetylabelingchanges/index.cfm?event=searchdetail.page&DrugNameID=540. Accessed November 15, 2019.

65. AbbVie. Humira: full prescribing information. US Food and Drug Administration. 2018. Available at: https://www.accessdata.fda.gov/drugsatfda_docs/label/2018/125057s410lbl.pdf. Accessed November 15, 2019.

66. Janssen. Remicade: full prescribing information. US Food and Drug Administration. 2017. Available at: https://www.accessdata.fda.gov/drugsatfda_docs/label/2018/103772s5385lbl.pdf. Accessed November 15, 2019.

67. UCB. Cimzia: full prescribing information. US Food and Drug Administration. 2019. Available at: https://www.fda.gov/media/73404/download. Accessed November 15, 2019.

68. Janssen. Simponi: full prescribing information. US Food and Drug Administration. 2018. Available at: https://www.accessdata.fda.gov/drugsatfda_docs/label/2019/125289s146lbl.pdf. Accessed November 15, 2019.

69. Sicotte NL, Voskuhl RR. Onset of multiple sclerosis associated with anti-TNF therapy. Neurology 2001;57(10):1885–8.

70. Thomas CW Jr, Weinshenker BG, Sandborn WJ. Demyelination during anti-tumor necrosis factor alpha therapy with infliximab for Crohn's disease. Inflamm Bowel Dis 2004;10(1):28–31.

71. Cancado GG, Vilela EG. Guillain-Barre syndrome during adalimumab therapy for Crohn s disease: coincidence or consequence? Scand J Gastroenterol 2017;52(4):473–6.

72. Shin IS, Baer AN, Kwon HJ, et al. Guillain-Barre and Miller Fisher syndromes occurring with tumor necrosis factor alpha antagonist therapy. Arthritis Rheum 2006;54(5):1429–34.

73. Kamel AY, Concepcion O, Schlachterman A, et al. Chronic inflammatory demyelinating polyneuropathy following anti-TNF-alpha therapy with infliximab for Crohn's disease. ACG Case Rep J 2016;3(3):187–9.

74. Stubgen JP. Tumor necrosis factor-alpha antagonists and neuropathy. Muscle Nerve 2008;37(3):281–92.

75. Richette P, Dieude P, Damiano J, et al. Sensory neuropathy revealing necrotizing vasculitis during infliximab therapy for rheumatoid arthritis. J Rheumatol 2004;31(10):2079–81.

76. Colombel JF, Sandborn WJ, Reinisch W, et al. Long-term safety of adalimumab in clinical trials in adult patients with Crohn's disease or ulcerative colitis. Aliment Pharmacol Ther 2018;47(2):219–28.

77. Colombel JF, Loftus EV Jr, Tremaine WJ, et al. The safety profile of infliximab in patients with Crohn's disease: the Mayo clinic experience in 500 patients. Gastroenterology 2004;126(1):19–31.

78. Vavricka SR, Schoepfer AM, Bansky G, et al. Efficacy and safety of certolizumab pegol in an unselected Crohn's disease population: 26-week data of the FACTS II survey. Inflamm Bowel Dis 2011;17(7):1530–9.

79. Martineau C, Flourie B, Wils P, et al. Efficacy and safety of golimumab in Crohn's disease: a French National Retrospective Study. Aliment Pharmacol Ther 2017; 46(11–12):1077–84.

80. Moris G. Inflammatory bowel disease: an increased risk factor for neurologic complications. World J Gastroenterol 2014;20(5):1228–37.

81. Lozeron P, Denier C, Lacroix C, et al. Long-term course of demyelinating neuropathies occurring during tumor necrosis factor-alpha-blocker therapy. Arch Neurol 2009;66(4):490–7.

82. Schiff MH, Burmester GR, Kent JD, et al. Safety analyses of adalimumab (HUMIRA) in global clinical trials and US postmarketing surveillance of patients with rheumatoid arthritis. Ann Rheum Dis 2006;65(7):889–94.

83. Bykerk VP, Cush J, Winthrop K, et al. Update on the safety profile of certolizumab pegol in rheumatoid arthritis: an integrated analysis from clinical trials. Ann Rheum Dis 2015;74(1):96–103.

84. Yoo DH, Prodanovic N, Jaworski J, et al. Efficacy and safety of CT-P13 (biosimilar infliximab) in patients with rheumatoid arthritis: comparison between switching from reference infliximab to CT-P13 and continuing CT-P13 in the PLANETRA extension study. Ann Rheum Dis 2017;76(2):355–63.

85. Deepak P, Stobaugh DJ, Sherid M, et al. Neurological events with tumour necrosis factor alpha inhibitors reported to the Food and Drug Administration Adverse Event Reporting System. Aliment Pharmacol Ther 2013;38(4):388–96.

86. Desai SB, Furst DE. Problems encountered during anti-tumour necrosis factor therapy. Best Pract Res Clin Rheumatol 2006;20(4):757–90.

87. Singh S, Kumar N, Loftus EV Jr, et al. Neurologic complications in patients with inflammatory bowel disease: increasing relevance in the era of biologics. Inflamm Bowel Dis 2013;19(4):864–72.

88. Nielsen NM, Frisch M, Rostgaard K, et al. Autoimmune diseases in patients with multiple sclerosis and their first-degree relatives: a nationwide cohort study in Denmark. Mult Scler 2008;14(6):823–9.

89. Kimura K, Hunter SF, Thollander MS, et al. Concurrence of inflammatory bowel disease and multiple sclerosis. Mayo Clin Proc 2000;75(8):802–6.

90. Gupta G, Gelfand JM, Lewis JD. Increased risk for demyelinating diseases in patients with inflammatory bowel disease. Gastroenterology 2005;129(3): 819–26.

91. Dobson R, Giovannoni G. Autoimmune disease in people with multiple sclerosis and their relatives: a systematic review and meta-analysis. J Neurol 2013; 260(5):1272–85.

92. Egeberg A, Mallbris L, Gislason GH, et al. Risk of multiple sclerosis in patients with psoriasis: a Danish Nationwide Cohort Study. J Invest Dermatol 2016; 136(1):93–8.

93. Lossos A, River Y, Eliakim A, et al. Neurologic aspects of inflammatory bowel disease. Neurology 1995;45(3 Pt 1):416–21.

94. Stahlberg D, Barany F, Einarsson K, et al. Neurophysiologic studies of patients with Crohn's disease on long-term treatment with metronidazole. Scand J Gastroenterol 1991;26(2):219–24.

95. Bernatsky S, Renoux C, Suissa S. Demyelinating events in rheumatoid arthritis after drug exposures. Ann Rheum Dis 2010;69(9):1691–3.

96. Marehbian J, Arrighi HM, Hass S, et al. Adverse events associated with common therapy regimens for moderate-to-severe Crohn's disease. Am J Gastroenterol 2009;104(10):2524–33.

97. TNF neutralization in MS: results of a randomized, placebo-controlled multicenter study. The Lenercept Multiple Sclerosis Study Group and The University of British Columbia MS/MRI Analysis Group. Neurology 1999;53(3):457–65.

98. Hofman FM, Hinton DR, Johnson K, et al. Tumor necrosis factor identified in multiple sclerosis brain. J Exp Med 1989;170(2):607–12.

99. Robinson WH, Genovese MC, Moreland LW. Demyelinating and neurologic events reported in association with tumor necrosis factor alpha antagonism: by what mechanisms could tumor necrosis factor alpha antagonists improve rheumatoid arthritis but exacerbate multiple sclerosis? Arthritis Rheum 2001; 44(9):1977–83.

100. Cope AP, Liblau RS, Yang XD, et al. Chronic tumor necrosis factor alters T cell responses by attenuating T cell receptor signaling. J Exp Med 1997;185(9): 1573–84.

A Concise Review of Neurologic Complications Associated with Chimeric Antigen Receptor T-cell Immunotherapy

Michael W. Ruff, MD[a,b], Elizabeth L. Siegler, PhD[a,c], Saad S. Kenderian, MD[a,c,d,e],*

KEYWORDS

- Neurotoxicity • Chimeric antigen receptor • CAR-T • Tisagenlecleucel
- Axicabtagene ciloleucel

KEY POINTS

- Chimeric antigen receptor–engineered T (CAR-T) cell–associated neurotoxicity, also referred to as immune effector cell–associated neurotoxicity syndrome (ICANS), is mild and reversible in most cases but may be severe and rarely is fatal.
- The pathogenesis of ICANS is similar to but distinct from cytokine release syndrome (CRS) and involves blood-brain barrier permeability, endothelial cell dysfunction, and excitotoxicity.
- Proposed risk factors for ICANS include but are not limited to an abnormal baseline brain magnetic resonance imaging or preexisting neurologic comorbidities. The CAR-T cell product itself has a significant influence on ICANS incidence and severity.
- In general, patients with more severe CRS are more likely to experience a higher-grade ICANS.
- Deeper understanding of the mechanisms driving ICANS has led to improved mitigation strategies and novel preventative treatments.

INTRODUCTION

Chimeric antigen receptor–engineered T (CAR-T) cells combine the antigen recognition capacity of an antibody with the effector functions of a T cell. A patient's T cells

[a] T Cell Engineering, Mayo Clinic, 200 First Street Southwest, Rochester, MN 55905, USA; [b] Department of Neurology, Mayo Clinic, 200 First Street Southwest, Rochester, MN 55905, USA; [c] Division of Hematology, Mayo Clinic, 200 First Street Southwest, Rochester, MN 55905, USA; [d] Department of Molecular Medicine, Mayo Clinic, 200 First Street Southwest, Rochester, MN 55905, USA; [e] Department of Immunology, Mayo Clinic, 200 First Street Southwest, Rochester, MN 55905, USA
* Corresponding author. Division of Hematology, Mayo Clinic, 200 First Street Southwest, Rochester, MN 55905.
E-mail address: Kenderian.saad@mayo.edu

Neurol Clin 38 (2020) 953–963
https://doi.org/10.1016/j.ncl.2020.08.001
0733-8619/20/© 2020 Elsevier Inc. All rights reserved.

are extracted and genetically modified to express a synthetic cell surface receptor consisting of the single-chain variable fragment (scFv) of an antibody coupled to a transmembrane domain and intracellular T-cell receptor–derived signaling domains. The chimeric antigen receptor (CAR) renders the CAR-T cell major histocompatibility complex independent. When CAR-T cells encounter target cells expressing the appropriate cell surface antigen, signaling through the CAR induces CAR-T cell proliferation, cytokine secretion, and target cell lysis.

First-generation CAR-T cells consist of the scFv coupled to a transmembrane domain and the intracellular CD3ζ domain derived from the T-cell receptor. These CAR-T cells, however, did not persist or demonstrate antitumor efficacy in vivo. Second-generation CAR-T cells incorporate a costimulatory domain, such as CD28 or 4-1BB, into the CAR construct and have demonstrated greatly improved persistence and antitumor activity in vivo. Third-generation CAR-T cells contain multiple costimulatory domains, but a clear advantage over second-generation CAR-T cells remains to be seen. The 2 current Food and Drug Administration (FDA)-approved CAR-T products are second generation and both target CD19 but differ in their costimulatory domains: the Kite/Gilead Yescarta, El Segundo, CA, USA (axicabtagene ciloleucel) utilizes CD28, whereas the Novartis Kymriah, Morris Plains, NJ, USA (tisagenlecleucel) utilizes 4-1BB. Preclinical studies have shown that the choice of costimulatory domain has a large impact on CAR-T cell metabolism and function.[1,2] More direct clinical comparisons are needed to further examine the differences between CD28 and 4-1BB CAR-T cells.

TOXICITIES AFTER CHIMERIC ANTIGEN RECEPTOR–ENGINEERED T-CELL THERAPY

CD19-targeting CAR-T cells have been wildly successful in treating some hematologic malignancies; however, CAR-T therapy is associated with severe adverse effects, such as cytokine release syndrome (CRS), as well as a bizarre, idiosyncratic, largely reversible encephalopathy, termed immune effector cell–associated neurotoxicity syndrome (ICANS), summarized in **Table 1**. This syndrome may accompany CRS or occur independently.[3–5] CRS and ICANS are the most common CAR-T–associated toxicities. Rapid expansion of CD19-directed CAR-T cells often results in systemic inflammatory CRS, which commonly occurs after CAR-T infusion. Although it is an undesirable toxicity, CRS appears to be associated with favorable response to CAR-T therapy, likely due to the expansion and activation of CAR-T cells. The first symptom of CRS is fever, which may be followed by more dire clinical manifestations, including systemic capillary leak, respiratory insufficiency, hyperferritinemia, hemophagocytic lymphohistiocytosis/macrophage activation syndrome, coagulopathy, and multiorgan failure. CRS-related fatalities have been reported, especially in patients with concurrent infections. CRS is present to some degree in 74% to 100% of patients undergoing CD19-directed CAR-T therapy. CRS typically appears within the first week after infusion and can progress in the ensuing 1 weeks to 2 weeks. Earlier onset of prolonged fever is associated with more severe CRS. Symptoms predictably and rapidly improve on the administration of tocilizumab, a monoclonal antibody against interleukin (IL)-6 receptor.[6–8]

CLINICAL MANIFESTATIONS OF IMMUNE EFFECTOR CELL–ASSOCIATED NEUROTOXICITY SYNDROME

ICANS presentation is variable and manifests with encephalopathy and focal neurologic deficits, in particular aphasia and seizures. In a majority of cases reported in the literature as well as in the author's experience, there is complete resolution of

Table 1
Pathophysiology of immune effector cell–associated neurotoxicity syndrome

Clinical Symptoms	Laboratory Markers	Risk Factors	Pathologic Findings	Potential Mechanisms
Encephalopathy Headache Obtundation Somnolence Aphasia Tremor Coma Seizures	Elevated cytokine levels (including IL-6, IL-10, IL-12, IL-15, IFN-γ, TNF-α, granzyme B, GM-CSF, MCP-1, IP-10) Elevated CRP	ALL Higher disease burden Higher CAR-T cell dose Higher peak CAR-T expansion CD28-costimulated CAR-T products Preexisting conditions (including prior severe CRS and abnormal baseline brain MRI)	Ischemic and hemorrhagic stroke Subarachnoid hemorrhages Severe white matter, cerebral, and dorsal pontine edema Blood-brain barrier breakdown Microglial activation Astrocyte injury Macrophage and T-cell infiltration	Activated CAR-T cells stimulate myeloid and endothelia cells Systemic inflammation drives blood-brain barrier dysfunction and astrocyte/neuron injury Microglial activation leads to elevated NDMA agonists

low-grade ICANS. Fatal manifestations of ICANS include intracerebral hemorrhage and malignant cerebral edema. The estimated incidence of fatal ICANS is less than 5% from all acute lymphoblastic leukemia (ALL) and diffuse large B-cell lymphoma CAR-T experience. ICANS may be seen with other CD19-targeting strategies, including bispecific antibodies as well as with CD20-targeting and CD22-targeting CAR-T cells.[9] ICANS has not been seen in other solid tumors or in glioblastoma treated with CAR-T therapy to date.

Subsequent descriptions of ICANS, specifically by Rubin and colleagues,[10] detail that clinical characteristics associated with ICANS most frequently are encephalopathy followed by headache, tremor, aphasia, and somnolence. Focal weakness was much less common, occurring in 11 of the cohort of 100 consecutive patients. They reported 1 ICANS-associated death in their patient cohort, 2 CRS-associated deaths, and 2 deaths associated with disease progression. The ICANS was described as an encephalopathy with a state of waxing and waning inattentiveness with or without confusion, disorientation, impulsivity, and emotional lability. Somnolence or a depressed level of arousal was noted in 21 cases, ranging from mild somnolence to significant lethargy, with difficulty arousing the patient. Agitated delirium associated with impulsivity and aggression was observed in 15 cases. Four patients were described as abulic.

Mild ICANS has been described as encephalopathy: disorientation to time and place, impaired attention, or impaired short-term memory with preserved alertness. In many cases, frontal release signs (eg, palmomental, grasp, and snout reflexes) are present. Additionally, headaches also were frequent manifestations of mild ICANS and were described as tension or pressure-type headaches over the occiput, occasionally migrainous, and rarely thunderclap. Tremor was noted in some patients, described as heightened physiologic tremor, asterixis, and myoclonus. These symptoms, which can wax and wane, appear to worsen during fever.

The distinction between mild and severe ICANS is that of focal neurologic deficits, most frequently aphasia. The symptoms typically occur in a stepwise gradation and disappear in reverse order during recovery. Severe ICANS is manifested most frequently by expressive aphasia. The order of events typically includes somnolence and impaired attention, followed by anomia and paraphasic errors, progressing over hours to global aphasia, myoclonus, coma, and seizures. There are a multitude of manifestations, however, including apraxia, automatisms, autonomic instability, sensorimotor neuropathy, allodynia, and perseverative behaviors. In most patients, the neurologic symptoms are self-limiting and resolve within 1 week. There have been fatal cases, however, described in the literature.[11]

ICANS onset typically begins within 7 days of CAR-T administration and is associated with prior CRS symptoms, although there are cases of later-onset ICANS. In general, patients with more severe CRS are more likely to experience higher-grade ICANS, although there are cases of grade 3 and grade 4 ICANS accompanying relatively minor grade 1 CRS.[12] ICANS rarely has been observed in the absence of any CRS and, if reported, usually is mild and subjective (grade 1); however, there may be late, abrupt onset of ICANS after CRS has subsided.

CLINICAL RISK FACTORS AND LABORATORY MARKERS OF IMMUNE EFFECTOR CELL–ASSOCIATED NEUROTOXICITY SYNDROME

Clinical risk factors associated with an increased risk of ICANS include the disease type and burden as well as CAR-T treatment specifics. ICANS is more common in ALL than lymphoma and appears to be negligible in multiple myeloma and solid tumors to date. Higher disease burden, in particular, the percent of marrow disease in

ALL, has been associated with increased risk of ICANS. Higher CAR-T cell dose and higher peak CAR-T expansion in the blood have been associated with ICANS.

The particular CAR-T product used in treatment also may increase the risk of ICANS. A CD28-costimulated CD19-directed CAR-T product from (Juno Therapeutics/Celgene, Seattle, WA, USA) was abandoned due to cerebral edema resulting in 5 patient deaths during the ROCKET clinical trial.[11] Yescarta contains the CD28 costimulatory domain and is associated with higher incidence and severity of ICANS (ICANS of any grade in 87% of patients and severe ($\geq$ grade 3) in 31% of patients), whereas Kymriah is 4-1BB–costimulated and is associated with lower incidence and severity of ICANS (ICANS of any grade in 58% of patients and severe in 18% of patients). Newer CAR-T products may have a reduced risk of ICANS development, such as the (Celgene/Bristol-Myers Squibb, Summit, NJ, USA) lisocabtagene maraleucel, which displayed less frequent incidences of ICANS compared with those observed in pivotal trials of Kymriah or Yescarta.[3,9,13–16]

Prior severe CRS, preexisting neurologic comorbidities (eg, neuropathy), and an abnormal brain magnetic resonance imaging (MRI) at baseline—demonstrating, for example, optic atrophy—have been associated with a greater risk of ICANS. Additionally, there has been an association between ICANS and fludarabine conditioning regimens. Elevated levels of IL-6, C-reactive protein (CRP), interferon gamma, IL-15, granulocyte-macrophage colony-stimulating factor (GM-CSF), gingival crevicular fluid, IL-5, IL-10, IL-12, IP-10, monocyte chemoattractant protein (MCP)-1, IL-1A, granzyme B, and tumor necrosis factor (TNF)-α as well as central nervous system (CNS)-specific production of IL-6, IL-8, MCP-1, and interferon gamma-inducible protein (IP)-10 and elevated cerebrospinal fluid (CSF) protein have been associated with ICANS and evidence of blood-brain barrier breakdowns.[17]

Surprisingly, CNS disease and white blood cell or CAR-T cell counts in the CSF are not clearly associated with ICANS. There is a paucity of clinical data, however, in patients with CNS disease, because many CAR-T clinical trials have excluded patients with (1) active or previous CNS involvement; (2) a history of CNS disorders, such as seizures, stroke, hemorrhage, dementia, and cerebellar diseases; or (3) autoimmune diseases with CNS involvement. Recently, however, there have been reports of successful off-treatment of patients with CNS metastases of lymphoma with both FDA-approved CAR-T products.[18,19]

PATHOLOGIC FINDINGS OF IMMUNE EFFECTOR CELL–ASSOCIATED NEUROTOXICITY SYNDROME AFTER CHIMERIC ANTIGEN RECEPTOR–ENGINEERED T-CELL THERAPY

In 2018, Santomasso and colleagues[9] described characteristic radiographic findings associated with ICANS in patients treated with CAR-T therapy. MRI findings associated with ICANS include T2/fluid-attenuated inversion recovery (FLAIR) signal hyperintensity present in the thalami, periventricular white matter, external capsule, extreme capsule, claustrum, and dorsal pons. Some of these elements are similar to the radiographic findings seen in extrapontine myelinolysis and to findings seen on occasion in Wernicke encephalopathy. Radiographic abnormalities present during severe ICANS resolve along with symptomatic improvement.[9] Splenial lesions with restricted diffusion have been described. In addition to the fairly unique radiographic findings seen with ICANS, there also have been reports of ischemic and hemorrhagic stroke as well as nonaneurysmal convexity subarachnoid hemorrhages in patients with severe ICANS.[12] In the ROCKET clinical trial, which subsequently was halted due to ICANS-related deaths, there was evidence of severe white matter and dorsal pontine edema; blood-brain barrier breakdown with contrast extravasation into the deep nuclei, including the thalamus; and restricted diffusion with subsequent laminar necrosis. Rubin and colleagues published findings of hypometabolism with focal electroencephalogram slowing in patients with neurologic toxicity, noting rhythmic and periodic electrical activity. There were alterations in the velocities of transcranial Doppler ultrasound in patients with focal neurologic deficits, thereby implicating dysfunctional cerebrovascular autoregulation in ICANS pathophysiology.

At autopsy in fatal ICANS cases, fulminant cerebral edema with evidence of microglial activation, astrocytic injury, and expansion of the Virchow-Robin spaces were noted. In other cases, loss of cerebrovascular integrity, manifesting as multifocal hemorrhage, was observed.[13] A patient with a prior history of optic atrophy, fludarabine lymphodepletion, and follicular lymphoma developed progressive encephalopathy with neurologic deterioration that resulted in death. Postmortem examination of the brain demonstrated diffuse gliosis with severe, widespread neuronal loss and degeneration of white matter associated with an inflammatory process that involved a dense macrophage infiltration of white matter, numerous microglial cells, and moderate $CD8^+$ T-cell infiltrate. There was no evidence of herpes-like virus 1 or 2, cytomegalovirus, zoster virus, JC virus, adenovirus, or Epstein-Barr virus.[4]

A 21-year-old patient had a sudden relapse of pre–B-cell ALL and died from fulminant cerebral edema after CAR-T cell infusion. Upon postmortem examination of the brain, there was note of activated microglial expansion of perivascular spaces and clasmatodendrosis, which is a beading of glial fibrillary acid protein associated with astrocytic injury. Infrequent T cells were identified in the brain parenchyma, and there was no evidence of ALL cells or CAR-T cells. The findings were nonspecific and consistent with fulminant cerebral edema. This raised the possibility, however, of astrocytic and blood-brain barrier functioning as a potential etiology of fatal CAR-T–associated ICANS in this patient.[20]

MANAGEMENT OF IMMUNE EFFECTOR CELL–ASSOCIATED NEUROTOXICITY SYNDROME

Current management protocols differ between institutions. In many institutions, however, the assistance of neurology specialists is required from day 1 of hospitalization. ICANS is largely treated with corticosteroids, such as dexamethasone and methylprednisolone, as well as antiepileptics and CSF diversion, although there is concern that corticosteroids may have a negative impact on the therapeutic functions of CAR-T cells.[21–23] ICANS frequently is treated with an anticonvulsant medication, levetiracetam (500 mg twice a day), with dose escalation with increasing encephalopathy due to the concern for excitotoxicity resulting in seizure provocation.

Recent preclinical studies have demonstrated that blocking the inflammatory cytokine IL-1 may prevent or ameliorate ICANS.[24,25] IL-1 is a key driver of CRS and is secreted by activated macrophages, which also appear play a large role in ICANS development. Several clinical trials have been initiated to test the IL-1 inhibitor, anakinra, as a protective agent against ICANS during CAR-T therapy (NCT03430011, NCT04359784, NCT04150913, NCT04148430, and NCT04205838). Another novel approach involves using defibrotide to protect endothelial cells from activation and subsequent blood-brain barrier disruption; a clinical trial has been initiated to test this therapy for the prevention of ICANS as well (NCT03954106). Current treatment strategies for ICANS are summarized in **Table 2**.

CASE PRESENTATION

A 26-year-old man with refractory large B-cell lymphoma with predominantly mediastinal disease underwent a Yescarta infusion and tolerated this without issue. On day 1

Table 2
Immune effector cell–associated neurotoxicity syndrome treatment strategies

Treatment Strategy	Therapeutic Agent	Rationale	Stage	References
Antiseizure medication	Levetiracetam	Excitotoxicity and cerebral edema increases seizure risk; treats symptoms	Clinical	Santomasso et al,[9] 2018; Gust et al,[14] 2019
Corticosteroids	Dexamethasone, methylprednisolone	Steroids dampen overactive immune response and mitigate cerebral edema by effect on cerebrovasculature; treats underlying cause	Clinical	Neelapu et al,[3] 2017 Davila et al,[23] 2014 Kalos et al,[21] 2011
Osmotic agents	Mannitol, hypertonic saline	Osmotic agents reduce cerebral edema; treats symptoms	Clinical	Neelapu et al,[28] 2018
CSF	Shunt	Severe ICANS can lead to progressive cerebral edema and increased intracranial pressure; treats symptoms	Clinical	Gust et al,[14] 2019
IL-1 inhibition	Anakinra	IL-1 elevated during ICANS, produced by activated myeloid cells; treats underlying cause	Preclinical, clinical trial initiated	Norelli et al,[24] 2018 Giavridis et al,[25] 2018 NCT03430011, NCT04359784, NCT04150913, NCT04148430, NCT04205838
Endothelial cell protection	Defibrotide	Endothelial cell activation leads to blood-brain barrier breakdown; treats underlying cause	Clinical trial initiated	NCT03954106

postinfusion, the patient became febrile to 39.1°C and tachycardic with a heart rate of 132 beats per minute. His blood pressure and oxygenation saturation remained normal. On days 1 to 3, the patient remained febrile without hypotension, hypoxia, or organ dysfunction and was nonencephalopathic. By the afternoon of day 3, the patient developed urinary retention and had a Foley urinary catheter placed with good urine output. Subsequent desaturation required a 2-L nasal cannula. It also was noted on the afternoon of day 3 that the patient developed a mild tremor. By 7:00 AM of the fourth day postinfusion, the patient had a tremor as well as expressive and receptive aphasia without dysarthria. He attempted to read sentences but had fluent and anomic aphasia. The patient subsequently was transferred to the intensive care unit, where tocilizumab and dexamethasone were administered. By 12:00 PM of day 4, the patient had global aphasia and a worsening neurologic examination. He was intubated for airway protection and given 1 g of methylprednisolone. Lumbar puncture was performed and demonstrated an elevated opening pressure of 44-cm water. He was given mannitol as well as a bolus of hypertonic saline (23%) and subsequently underwent emergent external ventricular drain placement with a resulting intracranial pressure of 3 mm Hg. The patient was sedated on propofol. CSF analysis demonstrated a white blood cells of 13 white blood cells per cubic mm with 16% polymorphonuclear cells, 52% lymphocytes, and 31% monocytes, with an elevated protein of 585 g/dL and a glucose of 100 g/dL. The patient received tocilizumab every 8 hours for 3 doses, with resolution of fever after 1 dose. He received dexamethasone, 10 mg intravenously, as well as methylprednisolone, 1 g daily for 3 days, and intravenous mannitol with a taper.

The patient's symptoms improved, and he was able to be extubated on day 6. On day 7, the patient underwent MRI, which demonstrated T2/FLAIR signal hyperintensity within the thalami, extreme capsule, the posterior right lateral ventricular horn, white and posterior pons, and periventricular white matter. The external ventricular drain was able to be removed on day 8. He was transferred back to the hospital floor on day 9 and discharged on day 11 without recurrence or prolonged sequelae of his neurologic deficits. He was evaluated 1 month postdischarge by a neurologist, who documented a normal neurologic examination.

POTENTIAL MECHANISMS OF IMMUNE EFFECTOR CELL–ASSOCIATED NEUROTOXICITY SYNDROME

One proposed common pathway of CRS and subsequent ICANS is as follows: activated CAR-T cells release effector cytokines that, in turn, activate endothelial cells and antigen-presenting cells and macrophages. These cells produce IL-6, driving the onset of CRS. Robust systemic cytokine production results in cytokine-mediated endothelial activation, which results in altered cerebrovascular regulation and blood-brain barrier dysfunction as well as vascular dysfunction, astrocytic injury, and, in extreme cases, neuronal injury. Additionally, thrombocytopenia and coagulopathy may lead to intracerebral hemorrhage. Also, microglial activation with CNS-specific production of cytokines leads to elevated glutamate and quinolinic acid (an N-methyl-D-aspartate [NMDA] agonist) in the CSF. The production of these NMDA agonists results in cytotoxicity manifesting in seizures and motor phenomenon, such as tremulousness. Additionally, CAR-T cells are able to penetrate the blood-brain barrier. In a recently published animal study, rhesus macaque monkeys with CAR-T–associated ICANS were found to have elevated proinflammatory cytokines in the CSF and high levels of CAR-T and endogenous T cells in both the gray matter and white matter of the brain parenchyma as well as in the CSF.[26] These factors likely contribute to increased blood-brain barrier permeability and the passive passage of cytokines into the CNS. Pericytes and endothelial cells thus are exposed to effector cytokines or IL-6, further driving ICANS.[8]

CRS and ICANS both involve excessive IL-6 production by myeloid cells, pericytes, and endothelial cells, leading to endothelial activation and dysregulation. As such, CRS may trigger the development of ICANS, which can continue to develop independently. Paradoxically, blocking IL-6 receptors actually may worsen ICANS.[8,27,28] Tocilizumab blocks the IL-6 receptor but is a monoclonal antibody that cannot cross the blood-brain barrier; therefore, the systemic sink for IL-6 is eliminated, and tocilizumab may exacerbate ICANS. Increased understanding of the mechanisms behind CRS and ICANS will lead to improved treatment protocols as well as novel treatment strategies.

SUMMARY

In conclusion, ICANS is mild and reversible in most cases. The pathogenesis of this disorder is similar but distinct from CRS and involves blood-brain barrier permeability, endothelial cell dysfunction, and excitotoxicity. Preexisting neurologic comorbidities are associated with clinically significant ICANS, among many other risk factors associated with this occurrence. Additionally, the CAR-T cell product itself seems to have a significant influence on ICANS incidence and severity. Ongoing developments and strategies to mitigate the occurrence of this serious adverse effect hopefully will render ICANS an artifact of the pioneering days of CAR-T therapy, which continues to hold tremendous promise across multiple disease domains.

CLINICALS CARE POINTS

- ICANS presentation is variable and manifests with encephalopathy and focal neurologic deficits, in particular aphasia and seizures.
- In the majority of reported cases, there is complete resolution of low-grade ICANS.
- History of neurologic disease, high tumor burden, early CRS, abnormal MRI brain are all proposed risk factors for ICANS.
- Management of ICANS includes the use of corticosteroids such as dexamethasone and methylprednisolonde, anti-epileptics and CSF diversion.
- Treatments under investigation include Anakinra and Defibrotide.
- Tocilizumab is not used to treat ICANS.

DISCLOSURE

S.S. Kenderian is an inventor on patents in the field of CAR immunotherapy that are licensed to Novartis (through an agreement between Mayo Clinic, University of Pennsylvania, and Novartis), Humanigen (through Mayo Clinic), and Mettaforge (through Mayo Clinic). S.S. Kenderian receives research funding from Kite, Gilead, Juno, Celgene, Novartis, Humanigen, MorphoSys, Tolero, Sunesis, and Lentigen. S.S. Kenderian has participated in advisory boards with Humanigen, Kite, and Juno.

REFERENCES

1. Long AH, Haso WM, Shern JF, et al. 4-1BB costimulation ameliorates T cell exhaustion induced by tonic signaling of chimeric antigen receptors. Nat Med 2015;21(6):581–90.

2. Kawalekar OU, O' Connor RS, Fraietta JA, et al. Distinct Signaling of Coreceptors Regulates Specific Metabolism Pathways and Impacts Memory Development in CAR T Cells. Immunity 2016;44(2):380–90.

3. Neelapu SS, Locke FL, Bartlett NL, et al. Axicabtagene Ciloleucel CAR T-Cell Therapy in Refractory Large B-Cell Lymphoma. N Engl J Med 2017;377(26): 2531–44.

4. Schuster SJ, Svoboda J, Chong EA, et al. Chimeric Antigen Receptor T Cells in Refractory B-Cell Lymphomas. N Engl J Med 2017;377(26):2545–54.

5. Turtle CJ, Hay KA, Hanafi LA, et al. Durable Molecular Remissions in Chronic Lymphocytic Leukemia Treated With CD19-Specific Chimeric Antigen Receptor-Modified T Cells After Failure of Ibrutinib. J Clin Oncol 2017;35(26):3010–20.

6. Grupp SA, Kalos M, Barrett D, et al. Chimeric antigen receptor-modified T cells for acute lymphoid leukemia. N Engl J Med 2013;368(16):1509–18.

7. Maude SL, Barrett D, Teachey DT, et al. Managing cytokine release syndrome associated with novel T cell-engaging therapies. Cancer J 2014;20(2):119–22.

8. Titov A, Petukhov A, Staliarova A, et al. The biological basis and clinical symptoms of CAR-T therapy-associated toxicites. Cell Death Dis 2018; 9(9):897.

9. Santomasso BD, Park JH, Salloum D, et al. Clinical and biological correlates of neurotoxicity associated with CAR T-cell \ tients with B-cell Acute Lymphoblastic Leukemia. Cancer Discov 2018;8(8):958–71.

10. Rubin DB, Danish HH, Ali AB, et al. Neurological toxicities associated with chimeric antigen receptor T-cell therapy. Brain 2019;142(5):1334–48.

11. Gilbert MJ. Severe neurotoxicity in the phase 2 trial of JCAR015 in adult B-ALL (ROCKET Study): analyses of patient, protocol and product attributes. SITC Annual Meeting, National Harbor, MD: November 8-12, 2017. 102.

12. Lee DW, Santomasso BD, Locke FL, et al. ASTCT Consensus Grading for Cytokine Release Syndrome and Neurologic Toxicity Associated with Immune Effector Cells. Biol Blood Marrow Transplant 2019;25(4):625–38.

13. Gust J, Hay KA, Hanafi LA, et al. Endothelial activation and blood-brain barrier disruption in neurotoxicity after adoptive immunotherapy with CD19 CAR-T cells. Cancer Discov 2017;7(12):1404–19.

14. Gust J, Finney OC, Li D, et al. Glial injury in neurotoxicity after pediatric CD19-directed chimeric antigen receptor T cell therapy. Ann Neurol 2019; 86(1):42–54.

15. Kochenderfer JN, Somerville RPT, Lu T, et al. Lymphoma remissions caused by anti-cd19 chimeric antigen receptor T cells are associated with high serum interleukin-15 levels. J Clin Oncol 2017;35(16):1803–13.

16. Park JH, Rivière I, Gonen M, et al. Long-term follow-up of CD19 CAR therapy in acute lymphoblastic leukemia. N Engl J Med 2018;378(5):449–59.

17. Hunter BD, Jacobson CA. CAR T-cell associated neurotoxicity: mechanisms, clinicopathologic correlates, and future directions. J Natl Cancer Inst 2019;111(7): 646–54.

18. Novo M, Ruff MW, Skrabek PJ, et al. Axicabtagene ciloleucel chimeric antigen receptor T cell therapy in lymphoma with secondary central nervous system involvement. Mayo Clin Proc 2019;94(11):2361–4.

19. Frigault MJ, Dietrich J, Martinez-Lage M, et al. Tisagenlecleucel CAR T-cell therapy in secondary CNS lymphoma. Blood 2019;134(11):860–6.

20. Torre M, Solomon IH, Sutherland CL, et al. Neuropathology of a case with fatal CAR T-cell-associated cerebral edema. J Neuropathol Exp Neurol 2018;77(10): 877–82.

21. Kalos M, Levine BL, Porter DL, et al. T cells with chimeric antigen receptors have potent antitumor effects and can establish memory in patients with advanced leukemia. Sci Transl Med 2011;3(95):95ra73.

22. Maude SL, Frey N, Shaw PA, et al. Chimeric antigen receptor T cells for sustained remissions in leukemia. N Engl J Med 2014;371(16):1507–17.

23. Davila ML, Riviere I, Wang X, et al. Efficacy and toxicity management of 19-28z CAR T cell therapy in B cell acute lymphoblastic leukemia. Sci Transl Med 2014;6(224):224ra25.

24. Norelli M, Camisa B, Barbiera G, et al. Monocyte-derived IL-1 and IL-6 are differentially required for cytokine-release syndrome and neurotoxicity due to CAR T cells. Nat Med 2018;24(6):739–48.

25. Giavridis T, van der Stegen SJC, Eyquem J, et al. CAR T cell-induced cytokine release syndrome is mediated by macrophages and abated by IL-1 blockade. Nat Med 2018;24(6):731–8.

26. Taraseviciute A, Tkachev V, Ponce R, et al. Chimeric antigen receptor T cell-mediated neurotoxicity in nonhuman primates. Cancer Discov 2018;8(6):750–63.

27. Lee DW, Gardner R, Porter DL, et al. Current concepts in the diagnosis and management of cytokine release syndrome. Blood 2014;124(2):188–95.

28. Neelapu SS, Tummala S, Kebriaei P, et al. Chimeric antigen receptor T-cell therapy - assessment and management of toxicities. Nat Rev Clin Oncol 2018;15(1): 47–62.

Neurotoxicity and Chemoreception
A Systematic Review of Neurotoxicity Effects on Smell and Taste

Madeline C. Aulisio, MPH[a], Amanda C. Glueck, PhD[b],
Michael R. Dobbs, MD, MHCM[c], Sandro Pasagic, BSN[b],
Dong Y. Han, PsyD, CELM[b,d,e,*]

KEYWORDS

- Neurotoxicity - Chemoreception - Smell - Taste - Olfaction - Gustation - Anosmia
- Ageusia

KEY POINTS

- Olfactory and gustatory dysfunctions owing to neurotoxicity can severely impact quality of life and requires greater attention.
- This review provides evidence that neurotoxic exposures via manganese dust, pesticides, toxic composites, such as debris from the World Trade Center disaster, and certain types of medications can produce deficits in olfaction and gustation.
- Continued research is needed to further explore these preliminary associations.

INTRODUCTION

The senses of smell and taste, although separate, are intimately linked. Both rely on chemoreceptors to transmit information about the surrounding environment to the brain and cooperate with each other extensively. Therefore, olfactory dysfunction, a significant public health problem that affects as many as 13.9% to 31.7% of older adults in the United States, can significantly impact quality of life, because humans use their sense of smell, and in turn taste, for a variety of activities.[1–3] For instance,

[a] Department of Health Management and Policy, University of Kentucky College of Public Health, 138 Leader Avenue, Lexington, KY 40506, USA; [b] Department of Neurology, University of Kentucky College of Medicine, 740 South Limestone Street, Lexington, KY 40536, USA; [c] Department of Neurology, University of Texas Rio Grande Valley School of Medicine, 1201 West University Drive, Edinburg, TX 78539, USA; [d] Department of Neurosurgery, University of Kentucky College of Medicine, Lexington, KY, USA; [e] Department of Physical Medicine and Rehabilitation, University of Kentucky College of Medicine, Lexington, KY, USA
* Corresponding author. Department of Neurology, University of Kentucky College of Medicine, 740 South Limestone Street, Lexington, KY 40536.
E-mail address: d.han@uky.edu

Neurol Clin 38 (2020) 965–981
https://doi.org/10.1016/j.ncl.2020.08.002
0733-8619/20/© 2020 Elsevier Inc. All rights reserved.

smell and taste play an important role in the development of dietary preferences and evaluation of foods for toxins. Human sexual arousal is partially mediated through the subconscious detection of the scent of pheromones and sex hormones.[4–7] The detection of environmental hazards, such as gas leaks, burning substances, and putrefaction, acts as early warning signs of danger to humans. The sensation of pleasure and a person's general well-being are all also impacted by olfactory and gustatory function.[8]

The nose and upper-respiratory tract are integral to olfaction by serving as the gatekeepers of the respiratory system, warming and humidifying air and trapping and expelling foreign particulate matter while facilitating the sense of smell and chemical somatosensation.[9,10] However, these abilities come at a cost. The first cranial nerve (CN I) comprises olfactory neurons. Its position in the roof of the nasal cavity exposes it to the outside environment, facilitating its activities but also making it susceptible to exposure to toxins and injurious materials, such as air pollution.[8] In addition to damage to the olfactory nerve, these exposures can also produce inflammation of the nasal epithelium and systemic introduction of chemicals that have bypassed the filtration process in the liver.[11]

The oral cavity and primarily the tongue within it are integral to taste, housing the chemical receptors responsible for the sensation. These chemical receptors or taste buds distinguish between 5 basic tastes (sweet, sour, salty, bitter, and umami) via their interactions with the molecules and ions within food.[12] Several CNs play an important role in transmitting sensory information pertaining to taste. Taste sensations from the anterior two-thirds of the tongue are transmitted by CN VII (the facial nerve), whereas CN IX (the glossopharyngeal nerve) carries information from the posterior one-third of the tongue. A branch of CN X (the vagus nerve) transmits sensory information from the back of the mouth. Finally, CN V (the trigeminal nerve) relays information about food texture and heat from spices.[12–14]

Both olfactory and gustatory systems are integrated in the brain for the perception of flavor.[15] Orthonasal and retronasal olfactory processing begins at the external nares and from the back of the mouth through the nasopharynx to stimulate the olfactory system. In addition, with the stimulation of the primary taste cortex, and all additional precursory stimuli processes, flavor perception involves nearly all of the human senses.[15] Among said perceptual processes, olfaction, not gustation, is the primary contributor for flavor perception. These systems are also linked to systems for learning, memory, emotion, and even language.[15] Physical damage to any of the aforementioned structures, the production of inflammation, or the introduction of chemicals can have the cumulative effect of causing deficits of varying degrees to smell, taste, and the overall flavor perception.

Despite the multitude of activities of daily living impacted by smell and taste, deficits within the two remain relatively understudied. In addition, these deficits are infrequently discussed in the context of neurotoxicity. Environmental exposures facilitate much of the damage sustained by those with olfactory and gustatory dysfunction; however, a gap exists in the literature with regards to a comprehensive review of neurotoxic agents known to cause deficits in smell and taste. Therefore, the goal of this systematic review was to evaluate the preexisting evidence linking potentially neurotoxic environmental exposures to deficits in taste and/or smell.

METHODS

The PRISMA (Preferred Reporting Items for Systematic Reviews and Meta-Analyses) guided this review, and a search of the CINAHL, Cochrane Library, PsychInfo, PsychNet, and PubMed databases was conducted using search terms: "toxin(s)," "toxicity," "neurotoxin(s)," "neurotoxicity," "smell," "taste," "olfaction," "olfactory," "gustation," "gustatory," "dysosmia," "anosmia," "parosmia," "dysgeusia," "ageusia," and "parageusia" for studies published within the last 10 years up to February 1, 2019. Three authors independently assessed eligibility of articles to reduce risk of bias. Studies reported on several different types of toxic exposures; however, this review defines neurotoxicity as an alteration of the normal activity of the nervous system following exposure to natural or synthetic toxic substances in accordance with the National Institute of Neurological Disorders and Stroke.[16] Only studies available in English and published in a refereed scholarly journal were considered for this review.

The assessment criteria of Van Tulder and colleagues[17] were modified and used to operationalize what constituted strong, moderate, limited, or conflicting evidence. Evidence linking a potential toxic exposure to deficits in smell and taste was considered "strong" if multiple studies with higher-quality methods, such as randomized controlled trials, reported the association. Evidence was considered "moderately strong" if multiple lower-quality studies, such as observational or cohort studies, or 1 high-quality study reported the association. Evidence was considered "limited" if 1 lower-quality study reported the association between a potential toxin and deficits in smell and taste. Finally, inconsistent evidence among multiple studies of varying quality comprised "conflicting" evidence of an association between a potential neurotoxin and smell and taste deficits.

RESULTS

After deleting duplicate results, 20 studies were identified with 17 deemed suitable for inclusion (**Fig. 1**). Included studies were read in full, and their characteristics and results are displayed in **Table 1**. Data on study design, sample size, exposure, outcome measures, and main results were extracted. Several of the studies described possible correlations between potentially neurotoxic substances and olfactory deficits not previously discussed in the literature.

The remaining studies were further categorized into 3 main causes of smell and taste dysfunction: manganese, chemical exposure, and medications. Of note, the search of the literature used for this systematic review predominantly produced articles relating to smell. Articles pertaining to taste were rare, a surprising finding given the close link between smell and taste dysfunction.

Manganese

Occupational and environmental exposures to potentially neurotoxic chemicals comprise a significant portion of all exposures that cause olfactory deficits, and smell and/or taste deficits owing to exposure to manganese feature prominently in the literature. Manganese is a versatile element that is vital for humans in small doses. It is also a crucial component of several industries, such as mining, dry-cell battery production, and the production of steel and metal alloys. Although OSHA has specified an acceptable exposure limit to manganese, inhalation of larger quantities of manganese dust can produce a constellation of neurologic symptoms, such as postural instability, hallucinations, and emotional lability owing to the fact that manganese is readily transported from olfactory epithelium to the olfactory bulb and deeper into the brain.[18–20]

Neurotoxicity owing to inhalation of manganese dust in an occupational setting was examined in the prospective, longitudinal study by Bowler and colleagues[18] examining olfactory changes in 25 welders working in poorly ventilated work conditions. Repeated measures were used to compare olfactory performance at baseline, while welders were actively working on a bridge reconstruction project that exposed

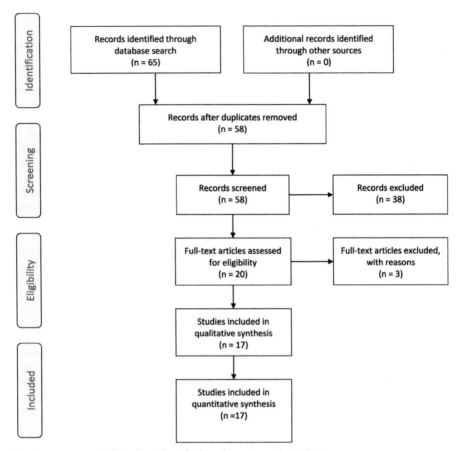

Fig. 1. Assessment of studies identified in the systematic review.

them to manganese and then again 3.5 years later (follow-up) after the completion of the project. Follow-up testing showed that that serum manganese levels decreased from 10 μg/L at baseline to 8.4 μg/L at follow-up. Administration of the University of Pennsylvania Smell Identification Test (UPSIT) demonstrated 68% of participants had a normal sense of smell or mild microsmia at follow-up compared with 56% at baseline. Forty-four percent of participants had originally presented with more severe microsmia or anosmia at baseline compared with 32% at follow-up. However, scores remained depressed, attributed to exposure to the manganese fumes encountered while welding. There was no significant statistical difference in the mean UPSIT scores at baseline and follow-up, indicating that olfaction did not improve significantly after cessation of welding, even after adjusting for age.[18]

Sen and colleagues[19] also explored the association between occupational manganese exposure and deficits in olfaction among a cohort of welders. The UPSIT was among a battery of tests administered to 7 welders with preexisting neurologic deficits and 6 age- and gender-matched controls. Findings included the accumulation of manganese in the olfactory bulb and other regions of the welders' brains, producing other deficits, such as difficulties with fine motor skills.[19] However, no significant difference in scores on the olfactory test was detected between the 2 groups. The investigators

Table 1
Characteristics and results of the studies included the systematic review

Author, Year	Study Design	Number of Patients	Neurotoxin	Result and Discussion
Adams et al,[2] 2016	Cross-sectional, secondary analysis of NSHAP data	1832	NO_2	Older adults who had higher yearly average NO_2 exposure levels had a significant 33% increase in the odds of olfactory impairment as measured by Sniffin' Sticks testing
Aïdli et al,[28] 2009	Case study	1	Pyrazinamide	Burning smell with onset 15 min after ingestion of drug did not recur after pyrazinamide was withdrawn
Ajmani et al,[9] 2016	Cross-sectional, secondary analysis of NSHAP data	2221	Fine particulate matter ($PM_{2.5}$)	Participants with greater exposure levels tended to face greater odds of having olfactory dysfunction. Significant interaction effects were also observed in variables of age, region, and employment status. Surprisingly, exposure to $PM_{2.5}$ air pollution had a stronger effect for younger participants compared with older adults
Altman et al,[26] 2011	Posttest only, quasiexperimental	198 (99 controls)	WTC debris	Exposed participants scored significantly lower on the UPSIT, and a relationship between age and olfactory function was also found. However, only 3% of exposed participants had anosmia and 15% had severe microsmia
Bello and Dumancas,[23] 2017	Cross-sectional (no control group)	839	2,4-DCP	A statistically significant association between olfactory impairment as measured by the 8-item NHANES PST and exposure to 2,4-DCP as measured by urinary levels was found

(continued on next page)

Table 1
(continued)

Author, Year	Study Design	Number of Patients	Neurotoxin	Result and Discussion
Bowler et al,[18] 2011	Pretest and posttest, quasiexperimental design (no control group)	26	Manganese (Mn)	UPSIT scores did not significantly improve from baseline to follow-up, even after adjusting for age. This was attributed to exposure to Mn fume exposure
Casjens et al,[20] 2017	Posttest only, observational cohort study	1385 (354 exposed)	Mn	Having ever worked as a welder was associated with better olfaction compared with participants in other "blue-collar" occupations. However, those in a "blue-collar" profession who had been exposed to Mn fumes had poorer olfaction testing results with Sniffin' Sticks kit than those who had worked in "white-collar" professions
Dalton et al,[10] 2010	Posttest only, quasiexperimental	196 (94 controls)	WTC debris	Significantly more participants in the exposed group had odor detection thresholds below the normal range, and 75% of the exposed group had irritant detection thresholds below the normal range. Although more members of the WTC-exposed group had extremely low scores, there were no significant differences between groups with regards to the prevalence of odor identification test scores below the normal range
Guarneros et al,[21] 2013	Posttest only, quasiexperimental cohort study	60 (30 controls)	Mn	Unexposed participants significantly outperformed exposed participants on Sniffin' Sticks measures of odor threshold detection, discrimination, and identification

Study	Design	Sample size	Exposure	Findings
Hisamitsu et al,[25] 2011	Observational, noncomparative (no control group)	41	Formaldehyde	32% of participants with preexisting allergic rhinitis experienced olfactory abnormalities during and immediately after exposure. 15% of participants with no history of allergic rhinitis experienced olfactory dysfunction, but only during the course itself. All symptoms resolved within 12 mo of completion of the course
Koizumi et al,[32] 2015	Case study	1	Crizotinib	Initial taste deficits deteriorated to all food having a bitter taste, leading to appetite loss. Alectinib was substituted for crizotinib, and dysgeusia improved after 2 wk cessation
Leyrer et al,[31] 2014	Pretest and posttest, prospective observational cohort study	20	Brain radiotherapy	25% of participants reported no dysgeusia and 60% reported no dysosmia following completion of radiotherapy. However, 55% reported increased dysgeusia and 35% reported an increase in dysosmia compared with their baseline scores before receiving radiotherapy
Quandt et al,[24] 2016	Posttest only, observational cohort study	551 (247 controls)	Pesticides	Proxy for exposure to pesticides (farmworker status) was not associated with odor identification ability as measured by Sniffin' Sticks test. Farmworker status was found to significantly impact odor threshold measurements
Riga et al,[29] 2015	Pretest and posttest, quasiexperimental design (no control group)	44	Chemotherapy regimen of oxaliplatin and antimetabolites, taxanes and platinum analogues, or taxanes and anthracyclines	All chemotherapy regimen groups demonstrated a significant decrease in composite threshold, detection, and identification scores from the Sniffin' Sticks testing kits with older age groups generally scoring worse

(continued on next page)

Table 1
(continued)

Author, Year	Study Design	Number of Patients	Neurotoxin	Result and Discussion
Sen et al,[19] 2011	Posttest only, quasiexperimental cohort study	13 (6 controls)	Mn	Mn was found to accumulate in the olfactory bulb and produce deficits in other areas, but no significant difference in performance on the UPSIT between a cohort of 7 welders, and 6 age- and gender-matched controls was found
Triebig et al,[22] 2016	Case crossover design with randomized exposure	52	ε-Caprolactam	Results appeared to demonstrate improvement in olfactory performance after exposure to ε-caprolactam, indicating no ε-caprolactam-induced impairment in olfaction
Zabernigg et al,[4] 2010	Longitudinal, prospective cohort study	197	One of 7 chemotherapy regimens	69.9% reported alterations in taste and smell during at least 1 assessment time, and 14.6% reported them at all assessment times. 21.6% of reported cases were mild deficits, and 17.6% of cases were moderate to severe. These findings were more than twice the levels of mild and moderate to severe deficits found in a reference sample taken from the general population

acknowledge that these findings may be attributed to the small sample size of this study.

Casjens and colleagues[20] continued work on the potential impact of manganese exposure on olfaction among welders with their secondary analysis of data from 1385 participants in the Heinz Nixdorf Recall Study (HNRS). During the second follow-up study of the HNRS, participants were asked to identify 12 odors (orange, leather, cinnamon, peppermint, banana, lemon, licorice, coffee, clove, pineapple, rose, and fish) presented individually via felt-tip Sniffin' Sticks odor pens. After being presented with an odor pen, participants identified the odor present through a 4-item multiple choice question. Participants who correctly identified 10 or more odors were considered normosmic, hyposmic if they identified between 7 and 9 odors correctly, and anosmic if they identified fewer than 7 odors correctly. Exposure to manganese was assessed with questionnaires about occupational history ("blue-collar" vs "white-collar" profession) and specific exposure to fumes from hot metals or other types of particulate matter that may contain manganese (regular welding, occasional welding, or other occupation that exposes one to manganese). Results revealed having worked as a welder was associated with better olfaction compared with participants in other "blue-collar" trade occupations (the reference group) that do not expose workers to manganese, such as foreman or technician. However, those who had worked in a "blue-collar" profession and had been exposed to manganese fumes (ie, welders) had poorer olfaction than those who had worked in "white-collar" professions as evidenced by identification of fewer Sniffin' Sticks odor pens.[20] The investigators note that significantly fewer welders reported ever having smoked than workers in "blue-collar" occupations, potentially impacting their olfaction. A relationship with age was also apparent within the data, with normosmic men being younger than hyposmic or anosmic men. Although no relationship between former exposure to manganese and olfactory impairment was found, these findings are potentially confounded by other variables, such as the higher rates of smoking among those with less manganese exposure.

Finally, the study by Guarneros and colleagues[21] also used the Sniffin' Sticks test to compare the olfaction of participants exposed to manganese because of their residence being located within 1 km or closer to a manganese processing plant (exposed participants). These residents were then compared with individuals matched in terms of age, sex, and education living 50 km or more away from the closest manganese source of exposure (unexposed participants). Olfaction was assessed with measures of odor threshold (ability to detect an odorant), odor discrimination (ability to distinguish between odorants), and odor identification (ability to name an odorant selecting from options within a checklist). For the purposes of this study, threshold testing assessed participants' ability to detect 2-phenyl ethanol (a roselike odor) when presented with 16 different dilutions. Discrimination testing assessed participants' ability to detect the different odorant in a triplet of odor pens. Finally, identification testing used the Sniffin' Sticks odor pens to measure participant ability to identify 13 common odorants. Unexposed participants significantly outperformed participants exposed to manganese on all measures. Furthermore, strong negative associations between performance and hair analysis manganese levels were noted in exposed participants.[21]

Collectively, these studies suggest that manganese can accumulate in regions of the brain and produce negative effects, such as deficits with fine motor skills, but provide conflicting evidence per the Van Tulder criteria that exposure to manganese dust can facilitate neurotoxic effects in the form of deficits in olfaction.[17] Although all studies controlled for some crucial confounders, such as smoking, other notable limitations are present. For example, only Bowler and colleagues[18] used a biomarker and reported manganese serum levels, considered a more accurate measure of exposure than estimation based on distance a study participant lives from an environmental exposure site. It is therefore impossible to determine at what level of manganese build-up in the body that deficits arise. Additional research is needed to more accurately characterize at what level manganese exposure can produce olfactory deficits and whether these deficits can resolve themselves after cessation of exposure.

Chemical exposure

The literature of neurotoxicity-induced deficits also explores potential associations between other common occupational chemical exposures and deficits in smell and taste. Triebig and colleagues[22] examined the neurotoxic potential of ε-caprolactam, an industrial chemical used for the production of plastic fibers, such as nylon. Although it has been previously characterized as having low toxicity to humans, local irritation following exposure to higher concentrations of aerosolized or vaporized ε-caprolactam such as ~12 ppm (56 mg/m^3) has been noted. Using a cross-over design with randomized conditions, 52 healthy adults were exposed to ε-caprolactam at levels of 0.05, 0.5, and 5.0 mg/m^3 for 6 hours over 4 days. Both volunteers and researchers were blinded to whether the exposure or control condition (0.0 mg/m^3) was being administered. Olfactory function pertaining to threshold, discrimination, and identification (TDI) was tested with the Sniffin' Sticks and summed into a composite score. Threshold measurements revealed a significant decrease in odor threshold after exposure to 0.05 mg/m^3 ε-caprolactam when compared with preexposure measurements.[22] Nonsignificant increases in odor threshold scores after exposure to 0.5 mg/m^3, 5.0 mg/m^3, and the control condition were also observed, indicating a reduced ability to detect an odor. However, there were no significant differences in threshold between the control air condition and the 5.0 mg/m^3 condition. In addition, composite TDI scores taken before the first and following the last day's exposure were compared, showing no significant difference between the 2 measurements. The TDI for the measurement taken after the last day's exposure to the 0.05 mg/m^3 ε-caprolactam concentration was significantly higher than the TDI score associated with the control air condition. Results from this study appeared to demonstrate improvement in olfactory performance after exposure to low concentrations of ε-caprolactam, indicating no ε-caprolactam-induced impairment in olfaction.[22]

Bello and Dumancas[23] explored exposure to another common chemical, 2,4-dichlorophenol (2,4-DCP), a known pollutant belonging to a class of chemicals found in commonly used products, such as pesticides, fungicides, and plastics.[23] Eight hundred thirty-nine middle-aged and older adults who had participated in the National Health and Nutrition Examination Survey (NHANES) were assessed using the NHANES Pocket Smell Test (PST), an 8-item "scratch-and-sniff" test with good agreement with the UPSIT. Participants were asked to identify 4 food-related odors (chocolate, grape, onion, and strawberry) and 4 nonfood-related odors (smoke, natural gas, leather, soap). Correctly identifying 6 to 8 odors classified participants as normosmic. Participants who correctly identified 4 to 5 odors were considered hyposmic, and those who correctly identified 3 or fewer were classified as anosmic. Exposure to 2,4-DCP was measured via urinalysis. After adjusting for covariates of age, gender, sex, race/ethnicity, poverty:income ratio, educational attainment, smoking status, alcohol consumption, body mass index (kg/m^2), and physical activity, a statistically significant association between olfactory impairment as measured by the PST and 2,4-DCP in urine levels was found. However, the investigators acknowledge that the study included numerous limitations. First, the PST, although quick and easy to implement, has lower sensitivity compared with the more comprehensive UPSIT. In addition, the PST only assessed odor identification and could not produce data pertaining to odor discrimination and odor threshold/sensitivity, which are other components of olfaction that are crucial for determining the presence of olfactory deficits. Finally, as this study is a cross-sectional analysis of NHANES data, the investigators are unable to infer a causal relationship between exposure to 2,4-DCP and olfactory impairment.[23]

In addition to 2,4-DCP, pesticides comprise another class of chemicals to which many people are frequently exposed. Quandt and colleagues[24] compared a sample of 304 current farmworkers and 247 non-farmworkers to measure olfactory performance, as measured by odor identification and odor threshold testing with Sniffin' Sticks, following significant pesticide exposure. Older age (but not farmworkers status, sex, or smoking status) was found to impact odor identification with those younger than 30 years of age having 1.93 times the odds of correctly identifying at least 13 out of 14 odors correctly than those who were 35 to 44 years of age and 2.7 times the odds than those who were 45 and older.[21] The association with age also held for odor threshold testing. Significant relationships were found between olfactory dysfunction and farmworker status and sex. Pesticide-exposed farmworkers had significantly poorer performance on the odor threshold measurements than non-farmworkers. In addition, odor threshold testing scores were also significantly worse for older participants and men.[24] No association with odor threshold was reported for those participants classified as smokers.

The previous articles have primarily described exposures associated with many types of "blue-collar" occupations; however, potential olfaction impairment can also occur in other professions and environments. Hisamitsu and colleagues[25] observed the effects of exposure to formaldehyde among a group of 41 medical students in a cadaver dissection course. A Nagashima jet nebulizing olfaction test was used to measure olfactory cognition threshold. Odor detection threshold and odor cognition threshold were assessed as the minimum concentration at which a student could smell any of 5 types of bromine and was able to recognize the odor, respectively. Thirty-two percent of participants with preexisting allergies experienced increased olfactory threshold during and immediately after completion of the dissection course. Fifteen percent of participants with no history of allergies experienced olfactory dysfunction, but only during the course itself. The study also demonstrated that formaldehyde may induce a temporary increase in nasal mucus production. Students who had originally demonstrated increased olfactory threshold were retested either 6 or 12 months after the initial study. Impaired olfaction was noted to have improved within 6 months of completion of the course and completely resolved within 12 months of completion of the course.[25]

Many of these same chemicals (in addition to inhalable nanoparticles and other toxins) also caused olfactory dysfunction following widespread exposure to them during the 2001 World Trade Center (WTC) disaster. Dalton and colleagues[10] compared the olfactory function of 102 individuals who were either survivors or involved in other activities at the WTC site, such as rescue, demolition, and cleanup, with an unexposed age-, sex-, and job title-matched control group from Philadelphia, Pennsylvania. Olfactory function was measured in a 3-part sensory evaluation: a test for odor detection of phenyl ethyl alcohol, a 20-item odor identification test, and threshold testing for detection of irritant n-butanol. Results demonstrated that significantly more participants in the WTC-exposed group had odor detection thresholds below the normal range, and 75% of the WTC-exposed group had irritant detection thresholds below the normal range. Although more members of the WTC-exposed group had extremely low scores, there were no significant differences between groups with regards to the prevalence of odor identification test scores below the normal range.[10]

Surprised by the findings of Dalton and colleagues,[10] Altman and colleagues[26] administered the UPSIT to 99 WTC-exposed persons and 99 controls matched on age, sex, and smoking history. As expected, WTC-exposed study participants scored significantly lower than control group participants on the UPSIT with regards to the ability to identify odors, and a relationship between age and olfactory function was also found. Although the relationships between WTC exposure, age, and olfaction were expected, less expected were the findings that only 3% of WTC-exposed participants had anosmia and 15% had severe microsmia, as indicated by the UPSIT scores.[26] Given that WTC-exposed persons were likely subjected to numerous chemicals and toxins,[27] such as polychlorinated biphenyls, volatile organic compounds, gypsum, glass fiber particles, and asbestos that typically induce deficits of smell and taste, the presence of more severe olfactory deficits was hypothesized.

Adams and colleagues[2] examined a more prolonged exposure to airborne pollutants in an analysis of National Social Life, Health, and Aging Project (NSHAP) data from 1832 participants aged 57 to 85 years, who lived within 60 km of a US Environmental Protection Agency (EPA) Aerometric Information Retrieval System (AIRS) ambient air monitoring site. Exposure to nitrogen dioxide (NO_2), a pervasive air pollutant generated by fossil fuel combustion, was assessed with hourly measurements obtained from the EPA AIRS ambient monitoring site closest to the participant's home. Odor identification abilities were assessed using Sniffin' Sticks odor pens. For the purposes of this study, respondents who correctly identified 4 or 5 odors were classified as normosmic, and those who identified 3 or fewer odors were classified as having olfactory dysfunction. As expected, older adults who were exposed to higher yearly average NO_2 exposure levels had a significant 33% increase in the odds of olfactory impairment after controlling for age, gender, race/ethnicity, and education. Additional analyses controlling for cognitive status, presence of comorbidities, smoking, and season of assessment and examining participants living 40 km away from a monitoring site found a similar relationship. These olfactory changes were produced at levels well below the acceptable EPA threshold of 53 ppb of NO_2.[2] However, it should be noted that this analysis may have been limited by a lack of a control group and its cross-sectional design, complicating inferences of a causal relationship between NO_2 experience and olfactory dysfunction.

Ajmani and colleagues[9] conducted another, cross-sectional analysis of NSHAP data to assess odor identification abilities for 2221 older respondents living in urban areas with an exposure to fine particulate matter with a diameter less than 2.5 ($PM_{2.5}$). $PM_{2.5}$ exposure was estimated at 1, 3, 6, 9, and 12 months for participants based on their home address and the date of their assessment. Participants were categorized into age groups of 57 to 64 years, 65 to 74 years, and 75 to 85 years. Olfactory function in the form of odor identification ability was assessed with Sniffin' Sticks test kits. Participants who identified 4 or 5 odors correctly were categorized as normosmic. Participants who identified 3 or fewer odors correctly were categorized as having olfactory dysfunction. Twenty-three percent of the study population was classified as having olfactory dysfunction. Of note, estimates of exposure were generated by demographic details. For example, participants had lived at their respective address for an average of 20.8 years, with a yearly average exposure to $PM_{2.5}$ of 13.9 ± 4.3 µg/m³. However, variation based on geographic location and season was observed. Participants who were exposed to higher $PM_{2.5}$ levels had increased odds of having olfactory dysfunction. Significant interaction effects were also observed in variables of age, region, and employment status (potentially because of occupational exposures that depended on age of retirement). Surprisingly, exposure to $PM_{2.5}$ air pollution had a stronger effect for younger participants (57–64 years old) compared with older adults.[9] However, this could potentially be explained by their longer duration of employment, giving them a longer exposure to the pollution.

Cumulatively, these studies demonstrate that many types of chemical exposures have the potential to produce neurotoxicity and cause deficits in smell and taste. However, further refinement of this conclusion is limited, per the Van Tulder criteria, by the relative lack of coverage in the literature of each of these individual chemical exposures.[17] Given the unavoidable nature of some of the chemical exposures for many populations, each of the aforementioned chemicals deserves additional study using more rigorous methods.

Medications

In addition to occupational and environmental exposure, olfactory and gustatory deficits are potential side effects of many medications or medication interactions with cardiovascular drugs, such as angiotensin-converting enzyme inhibitors, drugs used in anesthesia, and radiation therapy, and drugs used in the treatment of cancer being the most frequently implicated.[4,28–31] Aïdli and colleagues[28] described a case study of reversible dysosmia related to a regimen of antituberculous medication pyrazinamide. A 53-year-old woman reported a daily experience of the sensation of a burning smell with onset 15 minutes after ingestion of the drug. The smell would last for about 5 hours and then spontaneously resolve each day. The sensation did not recur after pyrazinamide was withdrawn but could be reliably reproduced with the reintroduction of the pyrazinamide. It is suspected that this result was due to the interaction between pyrazinamide and the patient's other medications; however, the ability to draw conclusions is limited by this case study with a sample size of one.[28]

Zabernigg and colleagues[4] assessed the prevalence of smell and taste abnormalities because of exposure to a chemotherapy regimen in a group of patients with pancreatic cancer (most patients were being treated with gemcitabine or a combination of gemcitabine and capecitabine), colorectal cancer (most were treated with the FOLFOX regimen 5-fluorouracil, leucovorin, and oxaliplatin or irinotecan monotherapy), or lung cancer (most were treated with vinorelbine plus a platinum agent or gemcitabine). Their longitudinal study using repeated measures with a short questionnaire ("Have you had problems with your sense of taste?"; "Did food and drink taste different from usual?") found that 69.9% of a sample of 197 patients assessed a total of 1024 times reported alterations in smell and taste during at least 1 assessment time and 14.6% of those patients reported them at all assessment times. These data indicate that 21.6% of reported cases were mild deficits and 17.6% of cases were moderate to severe and increased over the duration of the treatment.[4] In comparison, a reference sample taken from the general population demonstrated 4.5% of patients reporting mild deficits and 6.8% reporting moderate deficits. These findings are limited, however, by the brief nature of the questionnaire used to evaluate the participants and potential bias from the "leading" structure of the questions.

Riga and colleagues[29] also examined potential deficits in olfaction related to chemotherapy. Using the Sniffin' Sticks tests of odor threshold, odor discrimination, and odor identification, 44 patients undergoing chemotherapy were assessed for changes in olfaction. Patients belonged to one of 3 treatment groups: those undergoing therapy with oxaliplatin and antimetabolites (5-fluorouracil/capecitabine, or gemcitabine), those receiving taxanes and platinum-containing regimens (carboplatin or cisplatin), or those receiving taxanes and anthracyclines (doxorubicin or liposomal doxorubicin). Additional distinctions were made between age groups (39–50, 51–62, and 63–73 years). Ten patients were determined to have microsmia at baseline because of smoking history and older age. At follow-up at the end of chemotherapy, 42 of 44 patients were determined to be microsmic or anosmic. All chemotherapy groups demonstrated a significant decrease in composite TDI scores with older age groups scoring worse than younger age groups.[29] Odor threshold scores displayed a similar trend, and significant differences were found for all age groups with the exception of 39 to 50 years. All age groups experienced significant decreases in odor discrimination and odor identification scores.[29]

Leyrer and colleagues[31] examined reports of deficits for 20 patients with gliomas treated with brain irradiation in a prospective observational trial. Using questionnaires assessing smell and taste disturbances, taste complaints were assessed on a scale of 0 to 14 and smell complaints were assessed on a scale of 0 to 9 (higher scores indicating more significant deficits). Evaluations of dysgeusia and dysosmia were performed over the entire course of treatment. Twenty-five percent of participants reported no dysgeusia, and 60% reported no dysosmia following completion of radiotherapy. Fifty-five percent reported increased dysgeusia, and 35% reported an increase in dysosmia compared with their baseline scores before receiving radiotherapy. The mechanisms for dysgeusia and dysosmia in patients receiving brain irradiation are still unknown. However, scatter radiation may affect salivary glands and tissues in the nasopharynx, and dysfunction appears to be more common when the radiation-treated tumor is in the temporal lobe near the thalamus, the structure of the brain considered to be a central relay station for sensory information.[30,31] Alternatively, radiation may depopulate olfactory stem cells within the brain.[31]

Finally, Koizumi and colleagues[32] described a 54-year-old woman's case of severe dysgeusia after 5 days of crizotinib for the treatment of ALK-positive non–small cell lung cancer. Taste deficits began with reduced ability to detect salt and spicy flavors and progressed to inability to detect sweet, salty, or sour. Her condition deteriorated to a more severe toxicity whereby all food had a bitter taste, and she experienced loss of appetite. Alectinib was substituted for crizotinib, and dysgeusia improved after 2 weeks of crizotinib cessation. Readministration of crizotinib was not attempted because of the severity of symptoms.[32]

Taken together, these studies provide strong evidence that many classes of medication, particularly those that are chemotherapy agents, can produce neurotoxicity and cause deficits in smell and taste. Although physicians and patients depend on these therapies to extend lives or provide a cure, these symptoms can have a drastic impact on nutrition and quality of life. Therefore, these side effects deserve further investigation and empirical consideration. However, as demonstrated above, each of these singular case studies can only provide limited evidence based on the Van Tulder criteria that their unique exposure type is associated with deficits in smell and taste.[17]

DISCUSSION

Overall, neurotoxic exposures in the form of exposure to manganese dust; common chemicals such as pesticides and toxic composites, such as debris from the WTC disaster; and certain types of medications appear to have the ability to produce or contribute to deficits in olfaction and gustation. Such findings contribute to clinical management planning, especially in the context of quality-of-life management, and to policy planning for public awareness of these risks. However, most neurotoxins discussed in this review had limited coverage in the literature (as few as 1 article in many instances), revealing limited evidence to support the association and highlighting the necessity for expanded research in these topics. This situation may be further compli-cated by the potential presence of publication bias in the literature, further hindering efforts to draw more firm conclusions.

Although the findings of this review make an important contribution to the literature by considering the possible relationships between several potential neurotoxic agents and deficits in smell and taste, several limitations are also present that require consid-eration. The populations under study were often older and those within the studies of manganese were predominantly men, affecting generalizability of any conclusions to younger populations and particularly to women who typically demonstrate gender dif-ferences in human olfaction.[33] In addition, most of the studies were observational/case studies. The use of double-blinded experiments would have lent greater credi-bility to their findings per the Van Tulder criteria.[17] Furthermore, evaluation criteria (such as questionnaires) were often subjective, potentially introducing bias. Continued research in associations between potentially neurotoxic agents and deficits in smell and taste will lend weight to these preliminary associations, leading to important up-dates for clinical management, exposure limits, and workplace safety policies.

CLINICS CARE POINTS

- Chemoreceptive symptoms are often overlooked in clinical care, but are demon-strably notable to quality of life for patients.
- Olfactory and gustatory symptoms can aid in prodromal and syndromal differen-tials in toxic exposure.
- Olfactory and gustatory symptoms carry diagnostic value in addressing neuro-toxic exposure.
- Failure to address chemoreceptive symptoms after neurotoxic exposure may contribute to post-exposure affect disorder.

DISCLOSURE

The authors have no commercial or financial conflicts of interest to disclose.

REFERENCES

1. Ajmani GS, Suh HH, Pinto JM. Effects of ambient air pollution exposure on olfac-tion: a review. Environ Health Perspect 2016;124(11):1683–93.
2. Adams DR, Ajmani GS, Pun VC, et al. Nitrogen dioxide pollution exposure is associated with olfactory dysfunction in older US adults. Int Forum Allergy Rhinol 2016;6(12):1245–52.
3. Schubert CR, Cruickshanks KJ, Klein BE, et al. Olfactory impairment in older adults: five-year incidence and risk factors. Laryngoscope 2011;121:873–8.
4. Zabernigg A, Gamper E-M, Giesinger JM, et al. Taste alterations in cancer pa-tients receiving chemotherapy: a neglected side effect? Oncologist 2010;15: 913–20.
5. Mennella JA, Jagnow CP, Beauchamp GK. Prenatal and postnatal flavor learning by human infants. Pediatrics 2001;107(6):E88.
6. Tan R, Goldman MS. Exposure to male sexual scents (androstenone) influences women's drinking. Exp Clin Psychopharmacol 2017;25(6):456–65.
7. Wyart C, Webster WW, Chen JH, et al. Smelling a single component of male sweat alters levels of cortisol in women. J Neurosci 2007;27(6):1261–5.
8. Pinto JM. Olfaction. Proc Am Thorac Soc 2011;8:46–52.

9. Ajmani GS, Suh HH, Wroblewski KE, et al. Fine particulate matter exposure and olfactory dysfunction among urban-dwelling older US adults. Environ Res 2016; 151:797–803.

10. Dalton PH, Opiekun RE, Gould M, et al. Chemosensory loss: functional consequences of the World Trade Center disaster. Environ Health Perspect 2010; 118(9):1251–6.

11. Smith DD, Prezant DJ. Acute inhalation injury. In: Antosia R, Cahill JD, editors. Handbook of bioterrorism and disaster medicine. 2006 edition. New York: Springer Science; 2006. p. 227–34.

12. Chaudhari N, Roper SD. The cell biology of taste. J Cell Biol 2010;190(3):285.

13. Whitehead MC, Ganchrow JR, Ganchrow D, et al. Organization of geniculate and trigeminal ganglion cells innervating single fungiform taste papillae: a study with tetramethylrhodamine dextran amine labeling. Neuroscience 1999;93:931–41.

14. Small DM, Prescott J. Odor/taste integration and the perception of flavor. Exp Brain Res 2005;166:345–57.

15. Shepherd GM. Smell images and the flavour system in the human brain. Nature 2006;444(7117):316–21.

16. National Institute of Neurological Disorders and Stroke. Neurotoxicity. In: National Institute of Neurological Disorders and Stroke. 2018. Available at: https://www.ninds.nih.gov/Disorders/All-Disorders/Neurotoxicity-Information-Page. Accessed February 22, 2019.

17. Van Tulder M, Furlan A, Bombardier C, et al. Editorial Board of the Cochrane Collaboration Back Review Group. Updated method guidelines for systematic reviews in the Cochrane back review group. Spine 2003;28(12):1290–9.

18. Bowler RM, Gocheva V, Harris M, et al. Prospective study on neurotoxic effects in manganese-exposed bridge construction welders. Neurotoxicology 2011;32: 596–605.

19. Sen S, Flynn MR, Du G, et al. Manganese accumulation in the olfactory bulbs and other brain regions of "asymptomatic" welders. Toxicol Sci 2011;121(1):161–7.

20. Casjens S, Pesch B, Robens S, et al. Associations between former exposure to manganese and olfaction in an elderly population: results from the Heinz Nixdorf Recall Study. Neurotoxicology 2017;58:58–65.

21. Guarneros M, Ortiz-Romo N, Alcaraz-Zubeldia M, et al. Nonoccupational environmental exposure to manganese is linked to deficits in peripheral and central olfactory function. Chem Senses 2013;38:783–91.

22. Triebig G, Triebig-Heller I, Bruckner T. Exposure study to examine chemosensory effects of ε-caprolactam in healthy men and women. Inhal Toxicol 2016;28(12): 561–71.

23. Bello G, Dumancas G. Association of 2,4-dichlorophenol urinary concentrations and olfactory dysfunction in a national sample of middle-aged and older U.S. adults. Int J Environ Health Res 2017;27(6):498–508.

24. Quandt SA, Walker FO, Talton JW, et al. Olfactory function in Latino farmworkers: subclinical neurological effects of pesticide exposure in a vulnerable population. J Occup Environ Med 2016;58(3):248–53.

25. Hisamitsu M, Okamoto Y, Chazono H, et al. The influence of environmental exposure to formaldehyde in nasal mucosa of medical students during cadaver dissection. Allergol Int 2011;60:373–9.

26. Altman KW, Desai SC, Moline J, et al. Odor identification ability and self-reported upper respiratory symptoms in workers post-9/11 World Trade Center site. Int Arch Occup Environ Health 2011;84:131–7.

27. McGee JK, Chen LC, Cohen MD, et al. Chemical analysis of World Trade Center fine particulate matter for use in toxicologic assessment. Environ Health Perspect 2003;111(7):972–80.
28. Aïdli SE, Kastalli S, Zaïem A, et al. Recurrent dysosmia induced by pyrazinamide. Fundam Clin Pharmacol 2009;23(5):539–41.
29. Riga M, Chelis L, Papazi T, et al. Hyposmia: an underestimated and frequent adverse effect of chemotherapy. Support Care Cancer 2015;23:3053–8.
30. Rolls ET. The cortical representation of taste and smell. In: Rouby C, Schaal B, Dubois D, et al, editors. Olfaction, taste, and cognition. New York: Cambridge University Press; 2002. p. 367.
31. Leyrer CM, Chan MD, Peiffer AM, et al. Taste and smell disturbances after brain irradiation: a dose volume histogram analysis of a prospective observational study. Pract Radiat Oncol 2014;4(2):130–5.
32. Koizumi T, Fukushima T, Tatai T, et al. Successful treatment of crizotinib-induced dysgeusia by switching to alectinib in ALK-positive non-small cell lung cancer. Lung Cancer 2015;88:112–3.
33. Sorokowski P, Karwowski M, Misiak M, et al. Sex differences in human olfaction: a meta-analysis. Front Psychol 2019;10(242):1–9.

Neurotoxicology Syndromes Associated with Drugs of Abuse

Rachel A. Caplan, MD[a,b,1], Jonah P. Zuflacht, MD[c,1], Jed A. Barash, MD, MHS[d], Corey R. Fehnel, MD, MPH[e,f],*

KEYWORDS

- Neurotoxicology • Opioids • Ethanol • Marijuana • Cocaine • Methamphetamine
- Psychostimulants • Hallucinogens

KEY POINTS

- The broad spectrum of signs and symptoms associated with opioid intoxication requires early recognition to provide proper treatment of patients presenting with this syndrome.
- Alcohol withdrawal can begin 2 days after cessation of chronic ethanol abuse and may lead to critical or even fatal illness.
- Habitual marijuana use is increasing and is associated with diminished lifetime achievement and motor vehicle accidents. Among adolescents, it has been associated with abnormal neural development and impairments of executive function, memory, and processing speed. Cannabinoids cross the placenta and are associated with low birth weight and executive dysfunction.
- Cocaine and other psychostimulants, which include amphetamine, methamphetamine, 3,4-methylenedioxymethamphetamine, cathinones, and khat, are peripheral sympathomimetics that inhibit catecholamine reuptake at nerve endings, leading to dramatic elevations in heart rate, blood pressure, and body temperature. Central nervous system effects are mediated through elevations in norepinephrine, dopamine, and serotonin leading to euphoria and increased alertness.
- Classic hallucinogens are serotonin agonists that result in both somatic and neuropsychiatric effects. In the acute setting, monitoring for autonomic instability may be warranted although the management is largely supportive. Anesthetics, inhalants, and other drugs of abuse can lead to nonspecific neurologic syndromes such as sympathetic hyperactivity, psychomotor agitation, and impaired awareness as well as more distinct complications such as decreased pain perception (phencyclidine, ketamine) and myelopathy (nitrous oxide).

[a] Department of Neurology, Massachusetts General Hospital, 55 Fruit Street WACC 721G, Boston, Massachusetts 02114, USA; [b] Department of Neurology, Brigham and Women's Hospital, 75 Francis Street, Boston MA 02115, USA; [c] Department of Neurology, Beth Israel Deaconess Medical Center, 330 Brookline Avenue, Kirstein 406D, Boston, MA 02215, USA; [d] Soldiers' Home, 91 Crest Avenue, Chelsea, MA 02150, USA; [e] Department of Neurology, Beth Israel Deaconess Medical Center, Harvard Medical School, 330 Brookline Avenue, Kirstein 471, Boston, MA 02215, USA; [f] Hinda and Arthur Marcus Institute for Aging Research, 1200 Centre Street, Boston, MA 02131, USA
[1] Co-first author.
* Corresponding author.
E-mail address: cfehnel@bidmc.harvard.edu

Neurol Clin 38 (2020) 983–996
https://doi.org/10.1016/j.ncl.2020.08.005
0733-8619/20/© 2020 Elsevier Inc. All rights reserved.

neurologic.theclinics.com

OPIOIDS
Epidemiology and Pharmacology

Oxycodone, fentanyl, and other related agents belong to a class of synthetic and semisynthetic prescription analgesics that have been at the center of an epidemic of misuse in the United States since the early 2000s. This public health crisis has been further complicated by rising rates of abuse of illegal opioids, including both heroin and illicitly manufactured fentanyl. In 2017, more than 47,000 Americans died as a result of an overdose on prescription and illicit opioids or about 130 people per day. That year, approximately 1.7 million US residents lived with a diagnosis of a substance use disorder associated with prescription opioids.[1]

Opioids promote analgesia primarily at mu opioid receptors with full agonist effects, although buprenorphine, a medication prescribed for opioid abuse, has partial agonist properties.[2] Mu receptors are distributed throughout the central and peripheral nervous system. Shorter- and longer-acting opioid preparations, including morphine (duration of effect, 3–6 hours) and transdermal fentanyl (duration of effect, 72 hours), are available.[3]

Acute and Chronic Complications

Opioid intoxication may have a varied presentation. From a neurologic perspective, opioids can cause euphoria, agitation, drowsiness, delirium, and miotic ("pinpoint") pupils.[4,5] In recent years, a sudden-onset amnestic syndrome in association with bilateral hippocampal damage on MR imaging has been reported in patients with a history of opioid abuse.[6,7] Other acute signs and symptoms from heroin use may include nausea, vomiting, constipation, xerostomia, pruritis, diaphoresis, and urinary retention.[8] Overdose may lead to respiratory depression and stupor. Treatment of overdose includes use of the opioid antagonist, naloxone, which can be administered repeatedly as needed by intranasal, parenteral, and pulmonary routes. For respiratory depression, ventilatory support is necessary and orotracheal intubation may also provide protection against a major complication of opioid overdose, aspiration.[9]

Signs and symptoms of opioid withdrawal are often described as flulike and may include myalgias and rhinorrhea; however, together with other features such as drug craving, pupillary dilation, diarrhea, and yawning, the picture may be more suggestive.[10] For heroin, withdrawal symptoms typically peak between 1 and 3 days but may last a week or longer. Although the syndrome is unpleasant, it is rarely fatal.[8] Treatment of withdrawal typically involves the administration of methadone or buprenorphine with tapering of dosing guided by stabilization of the patient's condition. Clonidine has also been used effectively as another option for autonomically mediated symptoms of withdrawal.[11]

Opioid abuse use is associated with longer-term complications. For example, infections with potentially enduring implications, including epidural abscess, have represented a growing complication of the opioid epidemic.[12] There is also evidence to suggest that opioid-dependent patients experience memory dysfunction across multiple domains in comparison to healthy counterparts.[13] Whether chronic opioid-associated memory deficits lie on a spectrum with the aforementioned acute opioid-associated amnestic syndrome is unknown and will require further study for clarification.

ALCOHOL (ETHANOL)
Epidemiology and Pharmacology

In 2015, more than 15 million American adults aged 18 years and older lived with an alcohol use disorder. Nearly two-thirds of these adults were men.[14] Moreover, excessive alcohol use—defined by underage, pregnant, binge, or heavy drinking—accounts for 88,000 deaths in the United States annually. Approximately 10% of deaths in working age adults are attributable to excessive alcohol consumption; in those who die, lifespan is shortened by an average of 30 years.[15]

Alcohol is primarily metabolized in the liver, where it is converted by alcohol dehydrogenase to acetaldehyde. With acute exposure, ethanol exerts inhibitory or enhancing effects at a variety of receptors in the brain, including N-methyl-D-aspartate (NMDA) and gamma-aminobutyric-acid (GABA)-ergic systems.[16] Factors that can influence the extent of acute intoxication include the volume and percentage of alcohol ingested, the interval over which it was ingested, and the size and tolerance of the person ingesting it.[17]

Acute and Chronic Complications

Alcohol generally has a depressant effect on the central nervous system, but presentation with intoxication is varied. At lower blood alcohol levels, ethanol is associated with changes in personality, impairments in judgment, and inattention. At moderate levels, dysarthria, ataxia, and nystagmus may become apparent. Finally, at higher levels, stupor, coma, or even death due to respiratory depression may occur. As such, use of other drugs, including those with sedative effects, should be considered with caution.[8] Appropriate ventilatory support, including intubation, may be initiated in cases of respiratory depression.[18] To prevent potential complications associated with alcohol abuse, including hypotension, hypoglycemia, electrolyte disturbances, and Wernicke-Korsakoff syndrome (see later section), patients are often treated with intravenous fluids that include dextrose, thiamine, and multivitamins.[8,17,18]

Patients in early withdrawal from excessive alcohol use (beginning 6 hours after stoppage or reduced intake) can present with a variety of signs and symptoms, including tremulousness and autonomic disturbances, both of which may last for 48 hours. Seizures may emerge during this window as well. Hallucinations reflect moderate withdrawal and can last 6 days. In contrast, delirium tremens—an encephalopathic state of late withdrawal that typically involves psychomotor agitation—may begin 2 days after cessation of chronic alcohol abuse and may persist for 2 weeks past the time of the last drink.[19] Before initiating treatment of withdrawal, it is critical to consider potential mimics or comorbid diagnoses, including meningitis and traumatic brain injury.[20] Symptom-driven treatment with benzodiazepines, as determined by a validated instrument (such as the Clinical Institute for Withdrawal Assessment Scale), is often the preferred strategy for withdrawal management.[21]

Ethanol abuse may be associated with acute or, more commonly, chronic myopathy.[22] Peripheral nerve damage in the form of a mixed sensorimotor polyneuropathy is another neuromuscular complication; patients typically report sensory changes and later, weakness, beginning in the distal lower extremities.[23] Whether alcohol-related neuropathy and dementia result from direct ethanol neurotoxicity or indirect effects mediated by other factors, such as nutritional deficiency, has been a source of debate.[24,25] A known complication of thiamine deficiency classically observed in patients with chronic alcoholism, Wernicke-Korsakoff syndrome, is characterized by ataxia, ophthalmoplegia, and a confusional state involving amnesia and confabulation.[26] Heavy alcohol use is also associated with an increased risk of ischemic and hemorrhagic stroke.[27] Lastly, Marchiafava-Bignami disease, a rare degenerative disorder of the corpus callosum, is a striking complication of chronic alcohol abuse with a poor outcome, often involving rapidly impaired consciousness and resulting in death within months of onset.[28]

MARIJUANA
Epidemiology and Pharmacology

Although alcohol and tobacco account for the greatest burden of disease, trends toward legalization of marijuana are expected to increase its use and drive a greater burden of marijuana-related disorders. Tetrahydrocannabinol (THC) will be the focus of this discussion as the compound offers the euphoric effects associated with recreational use. Conversely, cannabidiol has few psychotropic effects and has been associated with therapeutic properties of reduction in nausea, CB1 and CB2 receptor–modulated pain reduction, and potential antiinflammatory effects. The Food and Drug Administration recently approved cannabidiol for treatment of the Dravet epilepsy syndrome.[29]

Rates of marijuana use have steadily increased among select segments of the US population. The implications of these trends for the neurologic practitioner are 2-fold: (1) a likely increase in marijuana use–related neurologic disorders; and (2) a window of opportunity for improving the scientific understanding of both potential benefits and harms of marijuana use.

Evidence suggests a clear trend of increasing THC potency.[30] States with legalized recreational marijuana have experienced an increase in emergency department visits.[31] Although the effects of acute intoxication are generally transient, a proportion of individuals with known or unknown predisposition to psychiatric disorders may experience a *forme fruste* of psychosis associated with marijuana use. The neurologic and other health effects of habitual use of marijuana remains understudied. This remains particularly true for long-term health consequences, which are based on the older generation of less potent THC products.[32]

The wide distribution of cannabinoid receptors (CB1 throughout the central and peripheral nervous system) account for the myriad neurologic effects of the drug. Delta-9-THC is the main psychotropic compound derived from cannabis plants, which have endogenously produced analogues in anandamide and noladin, among others.[33] When smoked, effects occur within 10 to 20 minutes, with a rapid decline in serum concentration within 1 hour owing to rapid distribution to other tissues, accounting for the excretion of THC components detectable in toxicology screening for prolonged periods of time (59 hours in nonhabitual users).[34] Heavy users have detectable THC metabolites in urine for up to 2 months.[35]

Acute and Chronic Complications

Acute marijuana intoxication has the detrimental effects of impaired short-term memory, incoordination, and impaired judgment. Other effects include initial anxiety, followed by euphoria, disinhibition, and depersonalization with subjective perception of the slowing of time. Higher doses induce paranoia and psychosis. Systemic effects include scleral injection, tachycardia, hypertension, urinary retention, and decreased intraocular pressure.

Resting electroencephalogram recordings during intoxication may reveal slower alpha range frequencies whereas subtle changes in event-related potentials are seen with higher order cognitive tasks.[36] PET recordings reveal increased cerebral blood flow to the temporal lobes, including insular regions, parietal, and occipital cortex and the cerebellum.[37]

The mainstay of managing acute THC intoxication is time and reassurance. Severe symptoms are managed with benzodiazepines counteracting CB1-mediated blockade of GABA receptors. Although naloxone seems to block some effects of THC in animals, this has not carried over to humans.

Habitual users of marijuana are observed to experience emotional lability, anxiety, insomnia, hyperreflexia, diaphoresis, and salivation. The symptoms are not experienced by all and tend to resolve over 36 hours, whereas psychological need/dependence (craving) can persist much longer. Cardiovascular and neurovascular effects have drawn considerable attention in recent years, with reports of associated paroxysmal atrial fibrillation and transcranial Doppler evidence of increased cerebrovascular resistance.[38]

There is high-quality evidence suggesting that marijuana is addictive. Addiction is more strongly associated with use beginning in adolescence, where it has also been associated with abnormal brain development. Neurologic complications seem to be dose dependent. Marijuana is associated with diminished lifetime achievement, motor vehicle accidents, and chronic bronchitis. Among adolescents it has been associated with abnormal neural development and impairments of executive function, memory, and processing speed.[38] Cannabinoids readily cross the placenta and are associated with low birth weight and executive dysfunction. Lesser quality evidence supports its association with schizophrenia and depression or anxiety disorders.[39]

COCAINE, METHAMPHETAMINE, AND OTHER PSYCHOSTIMULANTS
Epidemiology and Pharmacology

Although cocaine emerged as an anesthetic in the late 1800s and, soon after, as a drug of abuse, the coca plant from which it is derived has been used by indigenous populations in South America for thousands of years.[40] The leaves of the coca plant have long been chewed by the Aymara people for social and medicinal purposes, including mitigation of altitude sickness in the Andes mountains. Cocaine has been isolated from mummified human remains in Northern Chile dating back 3000 years.[41] Cocaine, an alkaloid, was first isolated from the coca plant in around 1860 but did not generate much attention until Sigmund Freud praised it as a cure for mental illness in "Uber Coca" in 1884; that same year Karl Koller described it as an excellent local anesthetic.[42] Soon, it was being used widely in medicine, including for treatment of opium addiction; abuse became common, especially among medical professionals such as the pioneering surgeon and famous addict William Halsted.

Abuse of cocaine and other psychostimulants has remained prevalent and has even increased in the past several years. Cocaine and psychostimulants account for a high percentage of drug deaths and emergency room (ER) visits. In 2011, cocaine-related illness accounted for around 40% of 1.3 million drug-related ER visits reported in the 2011 Drug Abuse Warning Network report.[43] Out of more than 70,000 deaths from drug overdose in the United States in 2017, nearly 14,000 involved cocaine.[44] In addition, the opioid epidemic and the appearance of fentanyl-laced cocaine have driven a recent increase in the number of cocaine-related deaths; although nonopioid-related cocaine deaths decreased from 1.59 to 0.78 per 100,000 from 2006 to 2015, the rate of death from cocaine-related overdose involving heroin or synthetic opioids such as fentanyl has gone from 0.24 to 1.11 per 100,000 from 2010 to 2015.[45]

Cocaine and other psychostimulants, which include amphetamine, methamphetamine, 3,4-methylenedioxymethamphetamine (MDMA), cathinones, khat, and others, are peripheral sympathomimetics that inhibit catecholamine reuptake at nerve endings, raising the blood pressure, heart rate, and body temperature, sometimes to a life-threatening degree.[46] They also work in the brain, increasing the availability of norepinephrine, dopamine, and serotonin at the level of the synapse.[8] As a result, users experience a "rush," accompanied by euphoria, alertness, and increased confidence; agitation and hyperactivity also result. Psychostimulants, therefore, have a wide variety of effects on the nervous system.

Acute and Chronic Complications

Changes in behavior are one of the most well-known side effects of cocaine and stimulant abuse. Cocaine can cause paranoia, psychosis, and hallucinations. Discerning between acute intoxication and schizophrenia can be made more challenging by the large portion of people with mental illness who have comorbid substance abuse. Attempts to distinguish the 2 presentations have found that cocaine users have more unformed visual hallucinations (such as shadows and lights), whereas those with schizophrenia have more complex and bizarre delusions. Substance abusers are also more likely to have tactile hallucinations and complain of bugs crawling on the skin.[47] Cocaine use increases the frequency of hallucinations in people with schizophrenia.

Synthetic cathinones, the class of stimulants known as "bath salts," have become feared for producing psychosis as well as violent, even homicidal behavior; intoxicated patients frequently need to be physically restrained.[48] Whether chronic cocaine users suffer from cognitive impairment even after sustained abstinence is not certain; some studies do show long-term memory and attention deficits, whereas others indicate that these may become less severe after months of sobriety.[49]

Psychostimulant use, which can cause acute blood pressure elevation, vasospasm and a prothrombotic state, raises the risk of acute ischemic and hemorrhagic stroke. A case-control study in more than 2000 young adults, aged 15 to 49 years, found a 5.7-fold risk of ischemic stroke found in those who used cocaine in the preceding 24 hours.[50] Recent cocaine use has been associated with an increased risk of aneurysmal subarachnoid hemorrhage as well as higher rates of aneurysm rerurpture, delayed cerebral ischemia, and in-hospital mortality.[51] Methamphetamine is an increasingly recognized risk factor for intracerebral hemorrhage in the young, both with and without aneurysm or arteriovenous malformation rupture.[52] Chronic cocaine abuse is known to lead to accelerated atherosclerosis through repeated endothelial damage, raising stroke risk.[53] Beyond stroke, cocaine has been implicated in several cases of leukoencephalopathy, both in patients who had supposed toxic white matter damage resembling heroin-induced leukoencephalopathy, as well as in patients with likely demyelinating lesions thought to be an immune response to levamisole, a frequent cocaine adulterant.[54]

Seizure is another common manifestation of acute psychostimulant intoxication. Out of a group of 47 patients who presented to San Francisco General Hospital for seizure after recreational drug use, 32 had used cocaine and 11, amphetamine.[55] Nearly 10% of 474 patients presenting to a hospital in Minneapolis with cocaine intoxication experienced seizures, usually of generalized tonic-clonic semiology.[56] Status epilepticus has been seen; partial status may mimic psychosis from intoxication.

Acute rhabdomyolysis is known to result from cocaine abuse, as documented in a study of 39 patients presenting to the University of Miami Medical Center with an average creatine kinase (CK) greater than 12,000; six of these patients died due to complications including renal and liver failure as well as disseminated intravascular coagulation.[57] In the acute setting, users of stimulants are subject to developing a variety of movement disorders, including tremor, dyskinesias, and choreiform movements (in cocaine users, this is known as "crack dancing").[58] Chronic users of amphetamine and methamphetamine often exhibit "punding," purposeless, stereotyped, and repetitive motor behaviors such as compulsively sorting household objects.[59]

Acute management of stimulant intoxication involves treating tachycardia, hypertension, hyperthermia, and behavioral changes that result from sympathetic overactivation in the central nervous system. Benzodiazepines are a mainstay of therapy and address increases in heart rate and blood pressure as well as cocaine-associated chest pain and agitation.[60] Blood pressure should be lowered with antihypertensive medications. Although β-blockers are to be avoided in the setting of acute cocaine use due to a theoretic risk of coronary vasospasm from unopposed alpha-adrenergic activity, firm evidence on this risk is unclear,[61] and non–β-blocking vasodilators such as nitroglycerin or nitroprusside are preferred. Withdrawal from stimulants, which is characterized by anhedonia, lethargy, restlessness, cravings, and irritability, can be alleviated by β-blockers such as propranolol; GABA-ergic drugs are also being explored as a treatment of cocaine dependence.[62]

HALLUCINOGENS
Epidemiology and Pharmacology

Hallucinogens are "mind-altering" drugs that, in botanic forms, have been used by humans for millennia.[63,64] From Aristotle to the Aztecs, psychoactive plants, such as ayahuasca, psilocybe, and peyote, have had sacred roles in shamanistic practices and religious ceremonies.[8,65–68] Synthetic versions with similarly mystical properties, namely D-lysergic acid diethylamide (LSD), were first developed in the early 1940s by the Swiss pharmacologist Albert Hofmann.[69] Long banned by the federal government, LSD and other "classic" (ie, serotonergic) hallucinogens are now reemerging as both potent psychotherapeutic agents as well as novel research compounds.[70]

In 2010, more than 30 million people in the United States reported LSD, psilocybin, mescaline, or peyote ingestion at some point in their life.[71] According to the UN World Drug Report (2017), 16% of all new psychoactive drugs—defined as uncontrolled substances that have recently become available—fall under the category of classic hallucinogens.[72] LSD, by far the most potent, is also the most popular, with more than 10% of US adults in the most recent National Survey on Drug Use and Health endorsing lifetime use.[73,74]

Classic hallucinogens—with either a phenylalkylamine group such as amphetamine or an indolealkylamine ring like serotonin—act primarily by binding 5-HT$_2$ serotonin receptors.[8,75] Although activation of the 5-HT$_{2A}$ receptor, in particular, is necessary for the psychedelic effects, other serotonin, dopamine, and adrenergic receptors are also involved.[8,76,77] LSD reaches peak plasma concentrations within 1 to 2 hours of oral ingestion and has an elimination half-life of roughly 3 hours.[78] The pharmacodynamics are similar for psilocybin, N,N-dimethyltryptamine (the active psychoactive compound in ayahuasca), and mescaline (the active psychoactive compound in peyote), all of which produce peak physiologic effects within 1 to 4 hours.[79–82]

Acute and Chronic Complications

Within minutes of ingestion, users may develop signs of autonomic hyperactivity such as fever, tachycardia, mydriasis, and hypertension.[8,80] Serotonin syndrome, characterized by the triad of dysautonomia, altered mental status, and neuromuscular abnormalities (especially hyperreflexia), is possible in more severe cases.[83] The intended psychedelic effects typically begin later, although last longer, on the order of 6 to 12 hours.[8] They include perceptual distortions such as depersonalization, derealization, and hallucinations[84,85] as well as subjective experiences involving the transcendence of time and space, dissolution of the ego, and encounters with God.[86–88] The neuroanatomical basis of these bizarre effects is thought to result from opening of the so-called thalamic filter, allowing otherwise isolated brain regions to interact with one another.[89] Recent neuroimaging studies support this idea; LSD has been shown to increase blood flow to the visual cortex[86] and increase effective connectivity between the thalamus and posterior cingulate cortex.[90]

Management of acute hallucinogen intoxication is largely supportive because the somatic and neuropsychiatric effects are both self-limited and usually mild.[91] Verbal reassurance and a calm environment are often sufficient. Cardiac monitoring is useful in patients with autonomic instability. In more severe cases, such as those with persistent agitation, antipsychotics and benzodiazepines may be used.[92] Similar strategies have been used in the management of patients who have ingested new, synthetic hallucinogens such as 25C-NBOMe (also known as "Boom" or "Pandora").[93] Schizophrenia and other psychotic disorders can mimic acute hallucinogen intoxication.

Data on the long-term effects of hallucinogen use are limited. "Flashbacks," characterized by the spontaneous occurrence of hallucinogen-like symptoms, have been reported in anywhere from 15% to 77% of users.[8] Prolonged, recurrent symptoms reminiscent of acute hallucinogen intoxication, known as the hallucinogen-persisting perception disorder, are less common.[94] Although there are numerous case reports to the contrary, the long-term use of hallucinogenic drugs does not, in general, seem to be associated with lasting neuropsychological[95] or mental health[96] problems. Ayahuasca users, compared with control groups, perform similarly or better on most measures of psychiatric morbidity, well-being, and cognitive function.[97]

OTHER DRUGS OF ABUSE

Anesthetics, inhalants, and other drugs have also been associated with a variety of effects of the nervous system. MDMA, or ecstasy, used by around 1% of the US population in 2018,[98] is a synthetic drug structurally similar to amphetamine that also promotes hallucinations and feelings of intimacy with others. Similar to stimulants, it is a sympathomimetic, causing increases in body temperature and heart rate, and it can produce agitation, tremors, and seizure; abusers at prolonged "raves" can be subject to rhabdomyolysis.[8]

Phencyclidine (PCP, also called "angel dust") is a dissociative anesthetic with NMDA-blocking activity that was used widely in the 1970s but has since become less popular. Users experience euphoria and sensory distortion as well as agitation and psychosis, depending on the amount of drug used; a muted feeling of pain and body awareness heightens the risk of serious injury.[99] Physical examination may show nystagmus, miosis, or ataxia; at higher doses myoclonus, posturing, rhabdomyolysis, and vital sign instability may be seen.[8]

Ketamine, which became popular in 1980s rave culture, is another NMDA antagonizing dissociative anesthetic that has similar effects to PCP but is less toxic and shorter acting. The drug promotes feelings of expanded awareness and changes in perception that are seen in other psychedelics, and although death from overdose itself is very rare, users have suffered serious injury from accidents while intoxicated due to derealization and decreased pain perception.[100]

Nitrous oxide is an inhalant anesthetic that has become increasingly popular in the 2010s as a drug of abuse at clubs and music festivals, where it is inhaled from balloons. Infrequent use for a dissociative high has few side effects, but habitual users can develop myelopathy or even an acute demyelinating neuropathy as a result of functional B12 inactivation.[101]

Other inhaled drugs of abuse include household products such as solvents, gasoline, and glues, which due to their accessibility are often used by school-aged children and young teenagers; 58% of users in one survey had their first experience before starting high school. Acutely, inhalants are depressants and cause symptoms such as lethargy and ataxia, as well as systemic effects such as chemical airway burns and cardiac arrhythmias that can be fatal. Chronic users are subject to problems with cognition and coordination.[102]

CLINICS CARE POINTS

- Diagnosing the opioid-associated amnestic syndrome requires timely toxicologic screening and brain imaging; the window of detection for fentanyl and other opioids may last for several days, whereas that for the detection of characteristic hippocampal damage on MR imaging may last for approximately 1 week.
- Naltrexone is indicated for both opioid addiction and alcohol dependence.
- THC has psychological effects that are sought with recreational use. Cannabidiol has few psychological effects and has been associated with reductions in nausea, pain, and as a potential antiinflammatory.
- Cocaine and other psychostimulants account for roughly 40% of drug-related ER visits.
- Neurovascular complications of cocaine intoxication include ischemic stroke, aneurysmal subarachnoid hemorrhage, and intracerebral hemorrhage. Chronic cocaine use leads to accelerated atherosclerosis through repeated endothelial damage, chronically raising stroke risk.
- Acute management of cocaine and other psychostimulant intoxication involves treating tachycardia, hypertension, hyperthermia, and behavioral changes that result from sympathetic hyperactivity. Antihypertensive agents and benzodiazepines are both mainstays of therapy.
- Hallucinogens, in both organic and synthetic formulations, act primarily by binding 5-HT$_2$ serotonin receptors but also act on other serotonin, dopamine, and adrenergic receptors.
- Antipsychotics and benzodiazepines can be used in the acute setting to help address autonomic instability and mitigate neuropsychiatric symptoms associated with classic hallucinogens.

DISCLOSURE

The authors have no commercial or financial conflicts of interest nor funding to disclose.

REFERENCES

1. National Institute of Drug Abuse. Opioid overdose crisis. Available at: https://www.drugabuse.gov/drugs-abuse/opioids/opioid-overdose-crisis. Accessed October 4, 2019.

2. Pathan H, Williams J. Basic opioid pharmacology: an update. Br J Pain 2012; 6:11–6.

3. Argoff CE, Silvershein DI. A comparison of long- and short-acting opioids for the treatment of chronic noncancer pain: tailoring therapy to meet patient needs. Mayo Clin Proc 2009;84:610–2.

4. Vella-Brincat J, Macleod AD. Adverse effects of opioids on the central nervous systems of palliative care patients. J Pain Palliat Care Pharmacother 2007; 21(15–25).

5. Fareed A, Stout S, Casarella J, et al. Illicit opioid intoxication: diagnosis and treatment. Subst Abuse 2011;5:17–25.

6. Barash JA, Somerville N, DeMaria AJ. Cluster of an unusual amnestic syndrome - Massachusetts, 2012-2016. MMWR Morb Mortal Wkly Rep 2017;66(76):79.

7. Barash JA, Ganetsky M, Boyle KL. Acute amnestic syndrome with fentanyl overdose. N Engl J Med 2018;378:1157–8.

8. Brust JCM. Neurological aspects of substance abuse. 2nd edition. Philadelphia: Elsevier; 2004.

9. Boyer EW. Management of opioid analgesic overdose. N Engl J Med 2012;367: 146–55.

10. Kosten TR, Baxter LE. Effective management of opioid withdrawal symptoms: a gateway to opioid dependence treatment. Am J Addict 2019;28:55–62.

11. Schuckit MA. Treatment of opioid-use disorders. N Engl J Med 2016;375: 357–68.

12. Ronan MV, Herzig SJ. Hospitalizations related to opioid abuse/dependence and associated serious infections from 2002 to 2012. Health Aff (Millwood) 2016;35: 832–7.

13. Rapeli P, Fabritius C, Kalska H, et al. Memory function in opioid-dependent patients treated with methadone or buprenorphine along with benzodiazepine: longitudinal change in comparison to healthy individuals. Subst Abuse Treat Prev Policy 2009;4(6).

14. National Institute on Alcohol Abuse and Alcoholism. Alcohol Facts and Statistics. Available at: https://www.niaaa.nih.gov/alcohol-health/overview-alcohol-consumption/alcohol-facts-and-statistics. Accessed October 7, 2019.

15. Centers for Disease Control and Prevention. Excessive alcohol use: preventing a leading risk for death, disease, and injury at a glance. 2016. Available at: https://www.cdc.gov/chronicdisease/resources/publications/aag/alcohol.htm. Accessed October 7, 2019.

16. Most D, Ferguson L, Harris RA. Molecular basis of alcoholism. Handbook Clin Neurol 2014;125:89–111.

17. Vonghia L, Leggio L, Ferrulli A, et al. Acute alcohol intoxication. Eur J Intern Med 2008;19:561–7.

18. Yost DA. Acute care for alcohol intoxication: be prepared to consider clinical dilemmas. Postgrad Med 2002;112(14–26).

19. Jesse S, Brathen G, Ferrara M, et al. Alcohol withdrawal syndrome: mechanisms, manifestations, and management. Acta Neurol Scand 2017;135:4–16.

20. Mayo-Smith MF, Beecher LH, Fischer TL, et al. Management of alcohol withdrawal delirium. An evidence-based practice guideline. Arch Intern Med 2004;164:1405–12.

21. Sullivan JT, Sykora K, Schneiderman J, et al. Assessment of alcohol withdrawal: the revised clinical institute withdrawal assessment for alcohol scale (CIWA-Ar). Br J Addict 1989;84:1353–7.

22. Simon L, Jolley SE, Molina PE. Alcoholic myopathy: pathophysiologic mechanisms and clinical implications. Alcohol Res 2017;38:207–17.

23. Sadowski A, Houck RC. Alcoholic neuropathy 2019.

24. Chopra K, Tiwari V. Alcoholic neuropathy: possible mechanisms and future treatment possibilities. Br J Clin Pharmacol 2012;73:348–62.

25. Ridley NJ, Draper B, Withall A. Alcohol-related dementia: an update of the evidence. Alzheimers Res Ther 2013;5(3).

26. Arts NJ, Walvoort SJ, Kessels RP. Korsakoff's syndrome: a critical review. Neuropsychiatr Dis Treat 2017;13:2875–90.

27. Larsson SC, Wallin A, Wolk A, et al. Differing association of alcohol consumption with different stroke types: a systematic review and meta-analysis. BMC Med 2016;14:178.

28. Kohler CG, Ances BM, Coleman AR, et al. Marchiafava-Bignami disease: literature review and case report. Neuropsychiatry Neuropsychol Behav Neurol 2000; 13:67–76.

29. Abu-Sawwa R, Stehling C. Epidiolex (Cannabidiol) Primer: Frequently Asked Questions for Patients and Caregivers. J Pediatr Pharmacol Ther 2020;25(1): 75–7. https://doi.org/10.5863/1551-6776-25.1.75.

30. ElSohly MA, Mehmedic Z, Foster S, et al. Changes in Cannabis Potency Over the Last 2 Decades (1995-2014): Analysis of Current Data in the United States. Biol Psychiatry 2016;79(7):613–9.

31. Substance Abuse and Mental Health Services Administration, Drug Abuse Warning Network, 2010: National Estimates of Drug-Related Emergency Department Visits. HHS Publication No. (SMA) 12-4733, DAWN Series D-38. Rockville, MD: Substance Abuse and Mental Health Services Administration, 2012.

32. Volkow ND, Baler RD, Compton WM, et al. Adverse health effects of marijuana use. N Engl J Med 2014;379(23):2219–27.

33. Felder CC, Glass M. Cannabinoid receptors and their endogenous agonists. Annu Rev Pharmacol Toxicol 1998;38:179–200.

34. Busto U, Bendayan R, Sellers EM. Clinical pheramacokinetics of non-opiate abused drugs. Clin Pharmacokinet 1989;16(1):1–26.

35. Morgan JP. Marijuana metabolism in the context of urine testing for cannabinoid metabolites. J Psychoactive Drugs 1988;20:107.

36. D'Souza DC, Fridberg DJ, Skosnik PD, et al. Dose-related modulation of event-related potentials to novel and target stimuli by intravenous Δ^9-THC in humans. Neuropsychopharmacology 2012;37(7):1632–46.

37. O'leary DS, Block RI, Koeppel JA. Effects of smoking majirjuana on brain perfusion and cognition. Neuropsychopharmacology 2002;26:802.

38. Bolla KI, Brown K, Eldreth D. Dose-related neurocognitive effects of marijuana use. Neurology 2002;59:1337.

39. Zammit S, Allebeck P, Andreasson S. Self-reprted cannabis use as a risk factor for schizophrenia in Swedish conscripts of 1969; historical cohort study. BMJ 2002;325:1199.

40. Karch SB. Cocaine: History, Use, Abuse. J R Soc Med 1999;92(8):393–7.

41. Asser A, Pille T. Psychostimulants and Movement Disorders. Front Neurol 2015; 6:75.

42. Goerig M. Carl Koller, Cocaine, and Local Anesthesia. Reg Anesth Pain Med 2012;37(3):318–24.

43. Center for Behavioral Health Statistics and Quality. Selected tables of National estimates of drug-related emergency department visits 2011. Rockville (MD): Substance Abuse and Mental Health Services Administration; 2013.

44. Kariisa M. Drug Overdose Deaths Involving Cocaine and Psychostimulants with Abuse Potential — United States, 2003–2017. MMWR Morb Mortal Wkly Rep 2019;68(17):388–95.

45. Jones CM. Recent Increases in Cocaine-Related Overdose Deaths and the Role of Opioids. Am J Public Health 2017;107(3):430–2.

46. Schwartz BG, Rezkalla S, Kloner RA. Cardiovascular effects of cocaine. Circulation 2010;122(24):2558–69.

47. Mitchell J, Vierkant AD. Delusions and hallucinations of cocaine abusers and paranoid schizophrenics: a comparative study. J Psychol 1991;125(3):301–10.

48. Ross EA, Reisfield GM, Watson MC, et al. Psychoactive "bath salts" intoxication with methylenedioxypyrovalerone. Am J Med 2012;125(9):854–8.

49. Potvin S, Stavro K, Rizkallah E, et al. Cocaine and cognition: a systematic quantitative review. J Addict Med 2014;8(5):368–76.

50. Cheng YC, Ryan KA, Qadwai SA, et al. Cocaine Use and Risk of Ischemic Stroke in Young Adults. Stroke 2016;47(4):918–22.

51. Chang TR, Kowalski RG, Caserta F, et al. Impact of acute cocaine use on aneurysmal subarachnoid hemorrhage. Stroke 2013;44(7):1825–9.

52. Swor DE, Maas MB, Walia SS, et al. Clinical characteristics and outcomes of methamphetamine-associated intracerebral hemorrhage. Neurology 2019; 93(1):e1–7.

53. Bachi K, Mani V, Jeyachandran D, et al. Vascular disease in cocaine addiction. Atherosclerosis 2017;262:154–62.

54. Vosoughi R, Schmidt BJ. Multifocal leukoencephalopathy in cocaine users: a report of two cases and review of the literature. BMC Neurol 2015;15:208.

55. Alldredge BK, Lowenstein DH, Simon RP. Seizures associated with recreational drug abuse. Neurology 1989;39(8):1037–9.

56. Pascual-Leone A, Dhuna A, Altafullah I, et al. Cocaine-induced seizures. Neurology 1990;40(3 Pt 1):404–7.

57. Roth D. Acute rhabdomyolysis associated with cocaine intoxication. N Engl J Med 1989;320(10):667–8.

58. Asser A, Taba P. Psychostimulants and movement disorders. Front Neurol 2015; 6:75.

59. Fasano A, Barra A, Nicosia P, et al. Cocaine addiction: from habits to stereotypical-repetitive behaviors and punding. Drug Alcohol Depend 2008; 96(1–2):178–82.

60. Richards JR, Garber D, Laurin EG, et al. Treatment of cocaine cardiovascular toxicity: a systematic review. Clin Toxicol (Phila) 2016;54(5):345–64.

61. Hoffman RS. Cocaine and beta-blockers: should the controversy continue? Ann Emerg Med 2008;51(2):127–9.

62. Kampman KM. New Medications for the Treatment of Cocaine Dependence. Psychiatry 2005;2(12):44–8.

63. Bruhn JG, De Smet PAGM, El-Seedi HR, et al. Mescaline use for 5700 years. Lancet 2002;359(9320):1866.

64. Miller MJ, Albarracin-Jordan J, Moore C, et al. Chemical evidence for the use of multiple psychotropic plants in a 1,000-year-old ritual bundle from South America. Proc Natl Acad Sci U S A 2019;116(23):11207–12.

65. Dos Santos RG, Hallak JEC. Ayahuasca, an ancient substance with traditional and contemporary use in neuropsychiatry and neuroscience. Epilepsy Behav 2019;106300. https://doi.org/10.1016/j.yebeh.2019.04.053.

66. Elferink JGR. Some Little-Known Hallucinogenic Plants of the Aztecs. J Psychoactive Drugs 1988;20(4):427–35.

67. Metzner R. Teonanacatl: sacred mushroom of visions. El Verano, CA: Four Tree; 2004.

68. Shepard GHJ. Psychoactive botanicals in ritual, religion and shamanism. In: Elisabetsky E, Etkin N, editors. Ethnopharmacology. Oxford (United Kingdom): UNESCO/Eolss Publishers; 2005. p. 128–41.

69. Hoffman A. How LSD originated. J Psychedelic Drugs 1979;11:53.
70. Nichols DE. Psychedelics. Pharmacol Rev 2016;68(2):264–355.
71. Krebs TS, Johansen PO. Over 30 million psychedelic users in the United States. F1000Res 2013;2:98.
72. World drug report. Vienna, Austria; 2017.
73. Libanio Osorio Marta RF. Metabolism of lysergic acid diethylamide (LSD): an update. Drug Metab Rev 2019;51(3):378–87.
74. National Institutee of Drug Abuse. National Survey on Drug Use and Health: Trends in Prevalence of Various Drugs for Ages 12 or Older, Ages 12 to 17, Ages 18 to 25, and Ages 26 or Older; 2016 - 2018. 2019. Available at: https://www.drugabuse.gov/national-survey-drug-use-health. Accessed September 5, 2019.
75. Glennon RA. Arylalkylamine drugs of abuse: an overview of drug discrimination studies. Pharmacol Biochem Behav 1999;64(2):251–6.
76. Preller KH, Herdener M, Pokorny T, et al. The Fabric of Meaning and Subjective Effects in LSD-Induced States Depend on Serotonin 2A Receptor Activation. Curr Biol 2017;27(3):451–7.
77. Rickli A, Moning OD, Hoener MC, et al. Receptor interaction profiles of novel psychoactive tryptamines compared with classic hallucinogens. Eur Neuropsychopharmacol 2016;26(8):1327–37.
78. Dolder PC, Schmid Y, Steuer AE, et al. Pharmacokinetics and Pharmacodynamics of Lysergic Acid Diethylamide in Healthy Subjects. Clin Pharmacokinet 2017;56(10):1219–30.
79. Carbonaro TM, Johnson MW, Hurwitz E, et al. Double-blind comparison of the two hallucinogens psilocybin and dextromethorphan: similarities and differences in subjective experiences. Psychopharmacology (Berl) 2018;235(2):521–34.
80. Liechti ME. Modern Clinical Research on LSD. Neuropsychopharmacology 2017;42(11):2114–27.
81. Dos Santos RG, Valle M, Bouso JC, et al. Autonomic, neuroendocrine, and immunological effects of ayahuasca: a comparative study with d-amphetamine. J Clin Psychopharmacol 2011;31(6):717–26.
82. Kovacic P, Somanathan R. Novel, unifying mechanism for mescaline in the central nervous system: electrochemistry, catechol redox metabolite, receptor, cell signaling and structure activity relationships. Oxid Med Cell Longev 2009;2(4):181–90.
83. Volpi-Abadie J, Kaye AM, Kaye AD. Serotonin syndrome. Ochsner J 2013;13(4):533–40.
84. Dolder PC, Schmid Y, Muller F, et al. LSD Acutely Impairs Fear Recognition and Enhances Emotional Empathy and Sociality. Neuropsychopharmacology 2016;41(11):2638–46.
85. Griffiths RR, Johnson MW, Richards WA, et al. Psilocybin occasioned mystical-type experiences: immediate and persisting dose-related effects. Psychopharmacology (Berl) 2011;218(4):649–65.
86. Carhart-Harris RL, Muthukumaraswamy S, Roseman L, et al. Neural correlates of the LSD experience revealed by multimodal neuroimaging. Proc Natl Acad Sci U S A 2016;113(17):4853–8.
87. Letheby C, Gerrans P. Self unbound: ego dissolution in psychedelic experience. Neurosci Conscious 2017;2017(1):nix016.
88. Griffiths RR, Hurwitz ES, Davis AK, et al. Survey of subjective "God encounter experiences": Comparisons among naturally occurring experiences and those

occasioned by the classic psychedelics psilocybin, LSD, ayahuasca, or DMT. PLoS One 2019;14(4):e0214377.

89. Geyer MA, Vollenweider FX. Serotonin research: contributions to understanding psychoses. Trends Pharmacol Sci 2008;29(9):445–53.

90. Preller KH, Razi A, Zeidman P, et al. Effective connectivity changes in LSD-induced altered states of consciousness in humans. Proc Natl Acad Sci U S A 2019;116(7):2743–8.

91. Taylor RL. Management of "Bad Trips" in an Evolving Drug Scene. JAMA 1970; 213(3):422.

92. Solursh LP. Use of Diazepam in Hallucinogenic Drug Crises. JAMA 1968; 205(9):644.

93. Zygowiec J, Solomon S, Jaworski A, et al. 25C-NBOMe Ingestion. Clin Pract Cases Emerg Med 2017;1(4):295–7.

94. Orsolini L, Papanti GD, De Berardis D, et al. The "Endless Trip" among the NPS Users: Psychopathology and Psychopharmacology in the Hallucinogen-Persisting Perception Disorder. A Systematic Review. Front Psychiatry 2017;8: 240–55.

95. Halpern JH, Pope HGJ. Do hallucinogens cause residual neuropsychological toxicity? Drug Alcohol Depend 1999;53(3):247–56.

96. Johansen PØ, Krebs TS. Psychedelics not linked to mental health problems or suicidal behavior: a population study. J Psychopharmacol 2015;29(3):270–9.

97. Barbosa PC, Mizumoto S, Bogenschutz MP, et al. Health status of ayahuasca users. Drug Test Anal 2012;4(7–8):601–9.

98. Abuse NIoD. MDMA (Ecstasy/Molly). 2019. Available at: http://www.drugabuse. gov/drugs-abuse/mdma-ecstasymolly. Accessed October 15, 2019.

99. Bey T, Patel A. Phencyclidine Intoxication and Adverse Effects: A Clinical and Pharmacological Review of an Illicit Drug. Cal J Emerg Med 2007;8(1):9–14.

100. Kalsi SS, Wood DM, Dargan PI. The epidemiology and patterns of acute and chronic toxicity associated with recreational ketamine use. Emerg Health Threats J 2011;4:7107.

101. Thompson AG, Leite MI, Lunn MP, et al. Whippits, nitrous oxide and the dangers of legal highs. Pract Neurol 2015;15(3):207–9.

102. Howard MO. Inhalant Use and Inhalant Use Disorders in the United States. Addict Sci Clin Pract 2011;6(1):18–31.

UNITED STATES POSTAL SERVICE ®

Statement of Ownership, Management, and Circulation
(All Periodicals Publications Except Requester Publications)

1. Publication Title	2. Publication Number	3. Filing Date
NEUROLOGIC CLINICS	000 – 712	9/18/2020

4. Issue Frequency	5. Number of Issues Published Annually	6. Annual Subscription Price
FEB, MAY, AUG, NOV	4	$326.00

7. Complete Mailing Address of Known Office of Publication (Not printer) (Street, city, county, state, and ZIP+4®)

ELSEVIER INC.
230 Park Avenue, Suite 800
New York, NY 10169

Contact Person: Malathi Samayan
Telephone (Include area code): 91-44-4299-4507

8. Complete Mailing Address of Headquarters or General Business Office of Publisher (Not printer)

ELSEVIER INC.
230 Park Avenue, Suite 800
New York, NY 10169

9. Full Names and Complete Mailing Addresses of Publisher, Editor, and Managing Editor (Do not leave blank)

Publisher (Name and complete mailing address)
Dolores Meloni, ELSEVIER INC.
1600 JOHN F KENNEDY BLVD. SUITE 1800
PHILADELPHIA, PA 19103-2899

Editor (Name and complete mailing address)
STACY EASTMAN, ELSEVIER INC.
1600 JOHN F KENNEDY BLVD. SUITE 1800
PHILADELPHIA, PA 19103-2899

Managing Editor (Name and complete mailing address)
PATRICK MANLEY, ELSEVIER INC.
1600 JOHN F KENNEDY BLVD. SUITE 1800
PHILADELPHIA, PA 19103-2899

10. Owner (Do not leave blank. If the publication is owned by a corporation, give the name and address of the corporation immediately followed by the names and addresses of all stockholders owning or holding 1 percent or more of the total amount of stock. If not owned by a corporation, give the names and addresses of the individual owners. If owned by a partnership or other unincorporated firm, give its name and address as well as those of each individual owner. If the publication is published by a nonprofit organization, give its name and address.)

Full Name	Complete Mailing Address
WHOLLY OWNED SUBSIDIARY OF REED/ELSEVIER, US HOLDINGS	1600 JOHN F KENNEDY BLVD. SUITE 1800 PHILADELPHIA, PA 19103-2899

11. Known Bondholders, Mortgagees, and Other Security Holders Owning or Holding 1 Percent or More of Total Amount of Bonds, Mortgages, or Other Securities. If none, check box. ▶ ☐ None

Full Name	Complete Mailing Address
N/A	

12. Tax Status (For completion by nonprofit organizations authorized to mail at nonprofit rates) (Check one)
The purpose, function, and nonprofit status of this organization and the exempt status for federal income tax purposes:
☒ Has Not Changed During Preceding 12 Months
☐ Has Changed During Preceding 12 Months (Publisher must submit explanation of change with this statement)

PS Form 3526, July 2014 [Page 1 of 4 (see instructions page 4)] PSN: 7530-01-000-9931   PRIVACY NOTICE: See our privacy policy on www.usps.com.

---

13. Publication Title	14. Issue Date for Circulation Data Below
NEUROLOGIC CLINICS	MAY 2020

15. Extent and Nature of Circulation			Average No. Copies Each Issue During Preceding 12 Months	No. Copies of Single Issue Published Nearest to Filing Date
a. Total Number of Copies (Net press run)			237	218
b. Paid Circulation (By Mail and Outside the Mail)	(1)	Mailed Outside-County Paid Subscriptions Stated on PS Form 3541 (Include paid distribution above nominal rate, advertiser's proof copies, and exchange copies)	119	111
	(2)	Mailed In-County Paid Subscriptions Stated on PS Form 3541 (Include paid distribution above nominal rate, advertiser's proof copies, and exchange copies)	0	0
	(3)	Paid Distribution Outside the Mails Including Sales Through Dealers and Carriers, Street Vendors, Counter Sales, and Other Paid Distribution Outside USPS®	74	65
	(4)	Paid Distribution by Other Classes of Mail Through the USPS (e.g. First-Class Mail®)	0	0
c. Total Paid Distribution (Sum of 15b (1), (2), (3), and (4))		▶	193	176
d. Free or Nominal Rate Distribution (By Mail and Outside the Mail)	(1)	Free or Nominal Rate Outside-County Copies Included on PS Form 3541	26	24
	(2)	Free or Nominal Rate In-County Copies Included on PS Form 3541	0	0
	(3)	Free or Nominal Rate Copies Mailed at Other Classes Through the USPS (e.g. First-Class Mail)	0	0
	(4)	Free or Nominal Rate Distribution Outside the Mail (Carriers or other means)	0	0
e. Total Free or Nominal Rate Distribution (Sum of 15d (1), (2), (3) and (4))		▶	26	24
f. Total Distribution (Sum of 15c and 15e)		▶	219	200
g. Copies not Distributed (See Instructions to Publishers #4 (page 43))		▶	18	18
h. Total (Sum of 15f and g)		▶	237	218
i. Percent Paid (15c divided by 15f times 100)		▶	88.12%	88%

* If you are claiming electronic copies, go to line 16 on page 3. If you are not claiming electronic copies, skip to line 17 on page 3.

16. Electronic Copy Circulation		Average No. Copies Each Issue During Preceding 12 Months	No. Copies of Single Issue Published Nearest to Filing Date
a. Paid Electronic Copies	▶		
b. Total Paid Print Copies (Line 15c) + Paid Electronic Copies (Line 16a)	▶		
c. Total Print Distribution (Line 15f) + Paid Electronic Copies (Line 16a)	▶		
d. Percent Paid (Both Print & Electronic Copies) (16b divided by 16c × 100)	▶		

☒ I certify that 50% of all my distributed copies (electronic and print) are paid above a nominal price.

17. Publication of Statement of Ownership
☒ If the publication is a general publication, publication of this statement is required. Will be printed ☐ Publication not required.
in the NOVEMBER 2020 issue of this publication.

18. Signature and Title of Editor, Publisher, Business Manager, or Owner

Malathi Samayan - Distribution Controller   *Malathi Samayan*   Date: 9/18/2020

I certify that all information furnished on this form is true and complete. I understand that anyone who furnishes false or misleading information on this form or who omits material or information requested on the form may be subject to criminal sanctions (including fines and imprisonment) and/or civil sanctions (including civil penalties).

PS Form 3526, July 2014 (Page 3 of 4)   PRIVACY NOTICE: See our privacy policy on www.usps.com.

Moving?

Make sure your subscription moves with you!

To notify us of your new address, find your **Clinics Account Number** (located on your mailing label above your name), and contact customer service at:

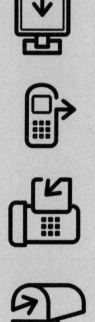

Email: journalscustomerservice-usa@elsevier.com

800-654-2452 (subscribers in the U.S. & Canada)
314-447-8871 (subscribers outside of the U.S. & Canada)

Fax number: 314-447-8029

Elsevier Health Sciences Division
Subscription Customer Service
3251 Riverport Lane
Maryland Heights, MO 63043

*To ensure uninterrupted delivery of your subscription, please notify us at least 4 weeks in advance of move.